CLINICAL APPLICATION
OF LEUKOCYTE DEPLETION

Clinical Application of Leukocyte Depletion

*Proceedings of the 3rd Hokkaido Symposium
on Transfusion Medicine*

EDITED BY S. SEKIGUCHI

Director, Hokkaido Red Cross Blood Centre
Sapporo, Japan

OXFORD

BLACKWELL SCIENTIFIC PUBLICATIONS

LONDON EDINBURGH BOSTON
MELBOURNE PARIS BERLIN VIENNA

© 1993 by
Blackwell Scientific Publications
Editorial Offices:
Osney Mead, Oxford OX2 0EL
25 John Street, London WC1N 2BL
23 Ainslie Place, Edinburgh EH3 6AJ
238 Main Street, Cambridge
  Massachusetts 02142, USA
54 University Street, Carlton
  Victoria 3053, Australia

Other Editorial Offices:
Librairie Arnette SA
2, rue Casimir-Delavigne
75006 Paris
France

Blackwell Wissenschafts-Verlag GmbH
Meinekestrasse 4
D-1000 Berlin 15
Germany

Blackwell MZV
Feldgasse 13
A-1238 Wien
Austria

First published 1993

Set by Semantic Graphics, Singapore
Printed and bound in Great Britain
at the University Press, Cambridge

DISTRIBUTORS

Marston Book Services Ltd
PO Box 87
Oxford OX2 0DT
(*Orders*: Tel: 0865 791155
      Fax: 0865 791927
      Telex: 837515)

USA
Blackwell Scientific Publications, Inc.
238 Main Street
Cambridge, MA 02142
(*Orders*: Tel: 800 759–6102
      617 876–7000)

Canada
Times Mirror Professional Publishing, Ltd
130 Flaska Drive
Markham, Ontario L6G 1B8
(*Orders*: Tel: 800 268–4178
      416 470–6739)

Australia
Blackwell Scientific Publications Pty Ltd
54 University Street
Carlton, Victoria 3053
(*Orders*: Tel: 03 347–5552)

A catalogue record for this title
is available from the British Library

ISBN 0–632–03716–4

Library of Congress
Cataloging in Publication Data

Hokkaido Symposium on Transfusion Medicine
  (3rd: 1991)
  Clinical application of leukocyte depletion:
  proceedings of the 3rd Hokkaido Symposium
  on Transfusion Medicine /
  edited by S. Sekiguchi.
       p.   cm.
    Includes bibliographical references and
     index.
    ISBN 0–632–03716–4
    1. Leucocyte-poor blood products—
    Therapeutic use—Congresses.
  I. Sekiguchi, Sadayoshi, 1933–
  II.Title.
    [DNLM: 1. Blood Transfusion
    —methods—congresses.
  2. Hemofiltration—congresses.
  3. Leukocytes—congresses.
  WH 200 H721L 1992]
  RM171.4.H65 1992
  615′.39—dc20

Contents

Preface

Preparing, providing, and transfusing leukocyte-poor blood and blood components is one of the most important issues in the field of transfusion medicine at present. There are many side-effects of blood transfusion such as nonhemolytic febrile reaction, viral infection, alloimmunization, and graft-versus-host reaction. Prevention of such blood-transfusion-associated complications by irradiation and/or removal of immunocompetent leukocytes has been studied for the last decade. Knowledge of the mechanism of the complications, in addition to the fact that the leukocytes in the blood products cause these complications, has been accumulated, and the technology of removing leukocytes, mainly leukocyte-removal filters, has developed rapidly in the past few years. The mechanism of alloimmunization in the blood transfusion may be explained by the present knowledge of immunology, but it is still unclear how the transfused donor's leukocytes stimulate the recipient's immune system. A number of clinical studies have proved that the transfusion of leukocyte-depleted blood products reduces the occurrence of alloimmunization. Careful studies, including multicenter studies performed in Japan, are reported in this book.

The question of how many leukocytes should be removed to prevent these side-effects is of significant importance. Among the possible methods used to remove or reduce the leukocytes in blood products, leukocyte-removal filters have been shown to be the most efficient. The efficiency of filters, both for red-cell and platelet concentrates, has been improved rapidly. However, the mechanism of leukocyte depletion by filters is still not fully understood, and it is necessary to clarify this to develop high-performance filters. As the efficiency of filters increases, the number of residual leukocytes is reduced. It is necessary to establish a method to count the residual leukocytes in filtered blood products. The method should be easy to operate, reliable, and sensitive. The occurrence of side-effects depends not only on the number of leukocytes transfused to the patients, but also the population of leukocytes. The type of residual leukocytes in the filtered blood products should be known. Ultraviolet B irradiation is known to abolish the stimulatory effect of leukocytes in mixed lymphocyte reactions. Ultraviolet irradiation is one method that can be used instead of, or in addition to, the leukocyte depletion by filters, though the mechanism of inactivation of leukocytes by ultraviolet is still not clear. Leukocyte depletion of blood products should also reduce the risk of leukocyte-transmitted viral infection. The possibility of reducing viral infection by filters is also reported. The cost effectiveness of leukocyte-removal filters is another aspect to consider. All of the above topics are discussed herein.

This symposium was held on July 5 and 6, 1991, in Sapporo, as the 3rd Hokkaido Symposium on Transfusion Medicine. The discussions after the oral presentations were tape recorded and the transcript is included here. I would like to thank all the authors who contributed to the proceedings. I also wish to thank the staff of the Research Department of Hokkaido Red Cross Blood Center and Blackwell Scientific Publications Ltd for getting the proceedings through the process of publication.

Sadayoshi Sekiguchi, MD

Part 1
Production Aspects

1 · Collection of leukocyte-depleted platelets using the CS-3000 Plus separator and TNX-6 chamber

H.M. Cullis

Business Development, Baxter Healthcare Corporation, Fenwal Division, 1425 Lake Cook Road, Deerfield, IL 60015, USA

Abstract

Since the CS-3000 was first offered for sale in 1979, platelet collections using the PLT chamber and procedure number 1 have produced platelet concentrates that generally averaged 5×10^7 white blood cells and 4.2×10^{11} platelets. This year, Fenwal offered the TNX-6 upgrade to the CS-3000, which produces platelet collections with similar numbers of platelets but with only 2×10^6 to 6×10^6 white blood cells.

This increase in purity was achieved by altering the shape of the centrifuge chamber and by altering the computer program which controls the plasma pump speed. There was no change to the disposable plastic tubing kit or to the operation of the machine.

The development of platelet separation techniques provided some insight into how to avoid the formation of a white blood cell layer on top of packed red blood cells in a centrifugal field. Counts of contaminating white blood cells obtained from hemapheresis departments have confirmed the propriety of these changes.

The collection process will be described and the data obtained from hemapheresis centers will be presented.

Introduction

The CS-3000 Plus with TNX-6 collection protocol was developed to perform hemapheresis for platelets while collecting few leukocytes. The objective was to limit the total numbers of leukocytes to the range between 2×10^6 and 6×10^6 in an average platelet collection. (The name of the separator chamber, TNX-6, stands for 10 to the sixth.) The development objective has been achieved; hemaphersis centers are currently using the procedure to collect platelets with very few leukocytes.

When the number of leukocytes in a platelet concentrate is in the range of 10^6, it is difficult to count them. To illustrate this problem, 200 ml of whole blood contains about 10^9 leukocytes, and two drops of whole blood contain about 10^6 leukocytes. Consider how difficult it is to dilute two drops of blood to 200 ml and then to count the number of leukocytes. Consider also that there are about 400 000 platelets for each leukocyte. As you will see, many institutions are not willing to devote the time necessary to do such counts.

It is appropriate to ask, why is it desirable to exclude leukocytes from platelet collections? After all, the donors lose more leukocytes in a normal blood donation than in a platelet donation. Besides, filters can remove leukocytes from the platelets at the time of transfusion. To answer these points, I will list some reasons why clinicians and researchers in the USA try to avoid the collection, storage, and transfusion of leukocytes with platelets:

1 *Immunization* — Leukocytes in transfused platelets may cause undesirable immune responses in the recipient.

2 *Unintentional engraftment* — Leukocytes may engraft in the donor.

3 *Transmission of intracellular pathogens* — Leukocytes may carry viruses, such as cytomegalovirus and human immunodeficiency virus.

4 *Stored leukocytes produce soluble leukokines*, for example, endogenous pyrogen factor, which cannot be filtered and are undesirable to transfuse. Soluble products of leukocyte metabolism and products of leukocyte activation present problems both for the stored platelets and for the recipient. Even if platelet concentrates are filtered to remove intact leukocytes prior to transfusion, there is concern that during storage the leukocytes may produce and release leukokines. These leukokines may be pyrogenic, and may cause platelets to aggregate. The leukocytes may be disrupted in the filtering process and the soluble proteins may be infused.

5 *Leukocytes will metabolize nutrients intended for banked platelets* — If large numbers of leukocytes are stored with platelets, the leukocytes, having higher metabolic activity, will compete with platelets for nutrients. The products of metabolism may produce carbon dioxide which may alter the pH, or may produce adenosine diphosphate which could stimulate the platelets to aggregate.

It would obviously be better if platelet transfusions contained few or no leukocytes. There are advantages in not collecting them in the first place: this is both possible and practical.

The scope of this chapter does not include clinical matters. Other authors will discuss in detail the problems which may occur when leukocytes are stored and transfused with platelets.

Perhaps the title of this chapter should be "How to avoid collecting leukocytes when collecting platelets." I will discuss the following subjects as they relate to collection of platelets by hemapheresis for transfusion:

1 How platelets are collected and concentrated in general.
2 How platelet collection using the CS-3000 is different.
3 Why leukocytes accompany platelets.
4 Which leukocytes are collected with platelets.
5 How leukocytes are avoided with the TNX-6.
6 What operating parameters affect the collection of platelets and leukocytes.

Finally, I will present data on TNX-6 yields from a number of institutions collecting platelets in the USA.

Materials and methods

How platelets are collected and concentrated

In general, platelets are separated from bags of whole blood using centrifugation. The first or primary separation process centrifugally causes the sedimentation of erythrocytes beneath the plasma and platelets, which are lighter and are therefore displaced to the centrifugal "top" of the bag. The platelet-rich plasma is then removed, and a second centrifugation process is employed to concentrate platelets from the plasma.

The primary separation

All formed elements of blood are heavier or more dense than plasma (Fig. 1.1). If placed in a strong centrifugal field for a long time, all cells and platelets will sediment to the bottom of the plasma. But if the centrifugal field is weak or if the time is short, only the cells that sediment the fastest will go to the bottom of the plasma; the cells that sediment more slowly will remain suspended in the plasma. Erythrocytes have a density of 1.092 and they will sediment 60 times faster than platelets, whose density is only 1.055. It is this physical difference which permits the primary separation of red cells from platelet-rich plasma.

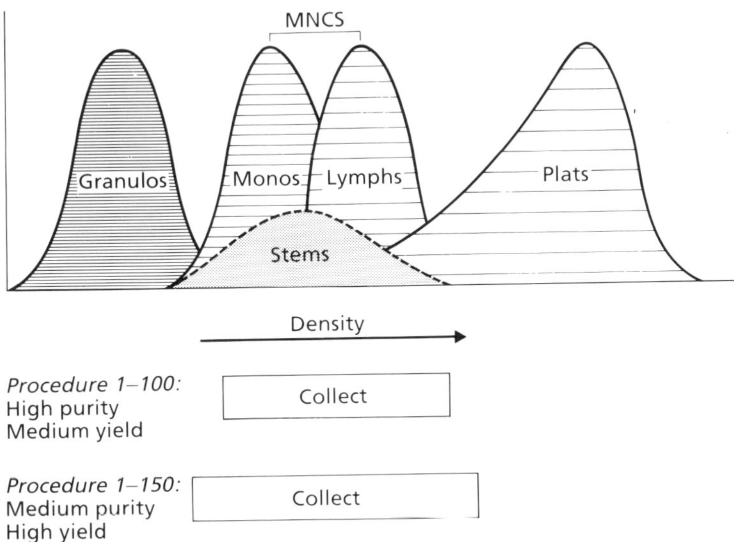

Fig. 1.1 Densities of cells. Granulos, granulocytes; Monos, monocytes; Lymphs, lymphocytes; Plats, platelets; Stems, stem cells. (Source: Yang J.)

When blood is centrifuged to make platelet-rich plasma, the application of **g** (gravitational) force for an appropriate length of time will cause the red cells to sediment to a concentration of 65–80%. As illustrated in Figure 1.2, erythrocytes are sedimented quickly, but most of the platelets sediment more slowly and they tend to remain with the plasma. None the less, there is some sedimentation of platelets, and the major portion of the platelets will reside near the erythrocyte layer. It is necessary to remove all the platelet-rich plasma in order to collect platelets efficiently.

From Figure 1.2 it can be seen that erythrocytes sediment quickly to a concentration of about 71%, but that greater packing requires proportionately more time. One reason for this is that at a concentration of 71% the space between red cells is less than the width of one red cell. Sialic acid on the surface of the red cells provides a negative charge, which tends to repel individual red cells when they approach each other. Platelets, which, like the erythrocytes, are negatively charged, are similarly repelled by the red cells. The platelets are therefore repelled into the plasma portion of the centrifuged mass. The process is self-controlling, and will exclude platelet-rich plasma from the cell mass if sufficient **g** forces, enough time to sediment, and prompt removal of platelet-rich plasma are achieved. If excessive centrifugal force is exerted, or if the platelet-rich plasma is not removed promptly, the platelets will tend to sediment into the top of the red cells, where the red cell concentration is always less than 65%.

Once the primary centrifugation is done, the platelet-rich plasma is removed in preparation for the secondary concentration of platelets. The platelet-rich plasma is centrifuged separately to pack the platelets into a small volume, so that excess plasma can be removed. The result is a platelet concentrate which can be transfused to supplement coagulation processes without creating fluid overload in the patient.

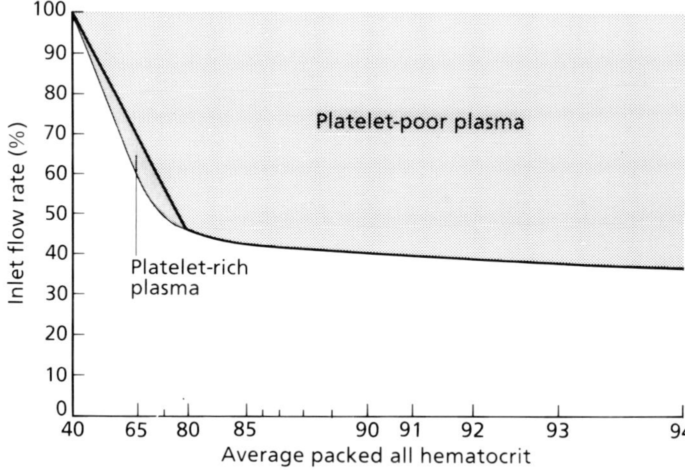

Fig. 1.2 Platelet separation chart showing platelet-rich plasma above red cells at 70% hematocrit. (Source: Brown R.)

How the CS-3000 collects platelets

The CS-3000 is the closed-system sealless centrifuge system for platelet hemapheresis, first sold in 1979. This system collects platelets directly from a donor instead of from bags of whole blood. It uses the same process described above, except that the primary and secondary centrifugation processes are conducted simultaneously. All of the collection is under computer control (Fig. 1.3).

In the CS-3000 centrifuge, a primary separation process is conducted in the separation chamber to separate platelet-rich plasma from erythrocytes and leuko-cytes. The platelet-rich plasma is pumped to a secondary collection chamber where platelets are concentrated, while the platelet-poor plasma is returned to the donor. (The plasma may also be collected if desired, either for addition to the platelet concentrate or for other uses.) The process is continuous, and all stages are controlled by a computer.

In the primary separation process, whole blood from the donor is continuously pumped into a separation chamber in the centrifuge. All of the platelet-rich plasma which is displaced above the red cells is pumped from the sedimented red cells as soon as it is formed. The degree of red cell packing is controlled by whole blood flow rate, and by centrifugal force. The platelet-rich plasma is continuously pumped through an optical density monitor on its way to the collection/concentration chamber.

The optical density of the removed platelet-rich plasma is continuously monitored by a filter photometer set at 540 nm. This photometer is particularly sensitive to the optical density contributed by erythrocytes, but it is also sensitive to reasonable concentrations of leukocytes. If erythrocytes or leukocytes exceed a given concentration in the optical path, the optical density increases, and the computer takes action

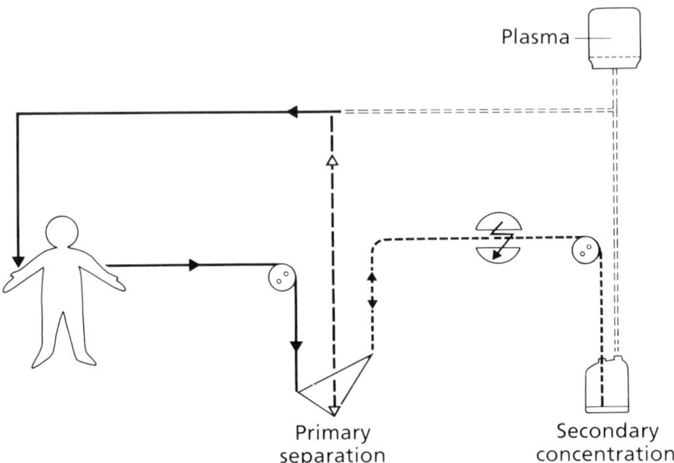

Fig. 1.3 CS-3000 flow diagram.

to prevent collection of these cells. Usually the action taken is to reverse the flow of plasma temporarily, and thus to return the cellular mixture to the separation chamber. It should be noted that the plasma pump direction does not affect the flow of blood from the donor or back to the donor. The donor blood flow is controlled exclusively by the whole blood pump, which does not reverse. The plasma pump controls only a loop of plasma flow within the tubing kit. It cannot pull blood from the donor or return blood to the donor.

The platelet-rich plasma is continuously transferred to the secondary collection chamber in the centrifuge. In this collection chamber the platelets are sedimented away from the plasma. This concentrates the platelets into a small volume of plasma appropriate for transfusion, and permits the plasma to be continuously returned to the donor, if this is desired. Alternately, the clear plasma may be collected independently of the platelet concentrate.

A computer controls the CS-3000. In the collection of platelet concentrate, the computer controls the direction and rate of the plasma pump. The computer program increases or decreases the rate of the plasma pump to remove all the platelet-rich plasma as soon as it has formed above the erythrocytes.

The optical detector determines when red cells are in the tubing, and this signals the computer to reverse the pump to put the red cells back into the red cell chamber. Then, based on computer calculation, the flow rate is set to achieve periodic depletions of the platelet-rich plasma.

This is, in overall outline, the same process as the general one described earlier. How then does the CS-3000 avoid collecting leukocytes?

Why leukocytes accompany platelets

The first question is, where are the leukocytes? When red cells are centrifugally packed to 70–75% concentrations, a considerable fraction of the lymphocytes, having densities less than 1.075, will accumulate at the surface of the erythrocytes, as shown in Figure 1.4, which illustrates the behavior of blood cells as blood is centrifuged. At the left axis, blood has just started to be centrifuged. The separation is shown as time progresses to the right. Lymphocytes will be found at the surface of the erythrocyte layer at a given point in time during centrifugation. This is about the time when the most platelets are available. It is these lymphocytes which can become contaminates of platelet concentrates. Most platelets will accumulate at the surface of the erythrocytes when the hematocrit of the erythrocytes is about 70%. But there are also lymphocytes just below the platelets. The leukocytes are less dense than erythrocytes, ranging from 1.065 to 1.085. They therefore sediment slightly more slowly than erythrocytes when they are both in physiologic concentration. When the red cells have first reached this concentration, there is very little separation of leukocytes from erythrocytes. This permits easy detection of leukocytes, because they are mixed with erythrocytes.

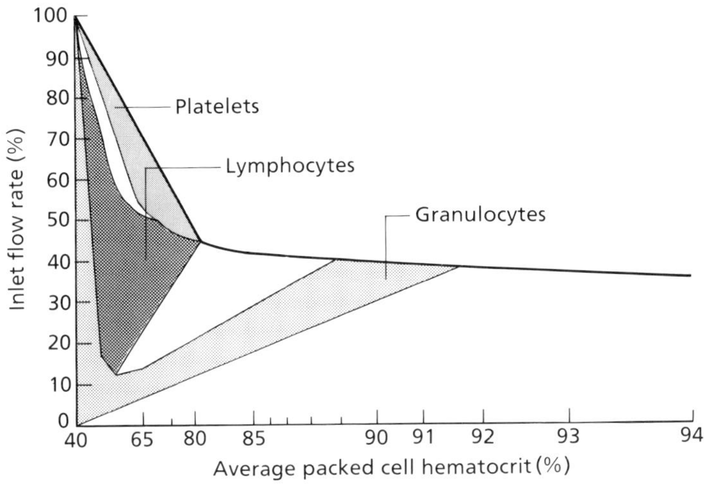

Fig. 1.4 Sedimentation of all blood components showing lymphocytes separating. (Source: Brown R.)

Which leukocytes are collected with platelets?

At this point, the density of the erythrocyte mass is not sufficiently high to cause leukocytes to float. These lymphocytes have similar sedimentation characteristics to erythrocytes. As plasma is pumped from the chamber, these lymphocytes, mixed with erythrocytes, are also removed and are pumped past the optical detector. These cells can be optically detected and are prevented from being transferred to the secondary platelet concentration. It is these small lymphocytes, similar in size and density to reticulocytes, which the TNX-6 procedure must avoid collecting. The few cells which are collected are virtually 100% lymphocytes and more than 70% of these have markers for T cells.

How the TNX-6 avoids collecting leukocytes

The TNX-6 process includes two major changes which permit the collection of platelets with very few leukocytes: (i) a new chamber shape for the primary separation process; and (ii) a revised computer routine for detecting the onset of erythrocytes and leukocytes.

How does TNX-6 chamber contribute to the process? It concentrates all erythrocytes and lymphocytes in the same manner that is used for leukocyte collection, employing a chamber nearly identical to that used in granulocyte hemapheresis. First, look at the Granulo chamber (Fig. 1.5). The Granulo chamber is designed to collect and concentrate leukocytes. There is a funnel-shaped area leading to the leukocyte exit port at the top center. Next, for comparison, look at the TNX-6 chamber (Fig. 1.6):

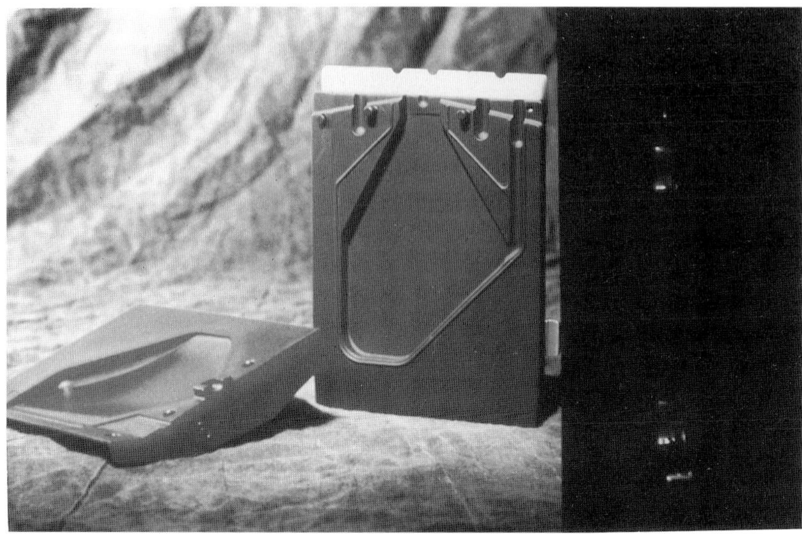

Fig. 1.5 The Granulo chamber.

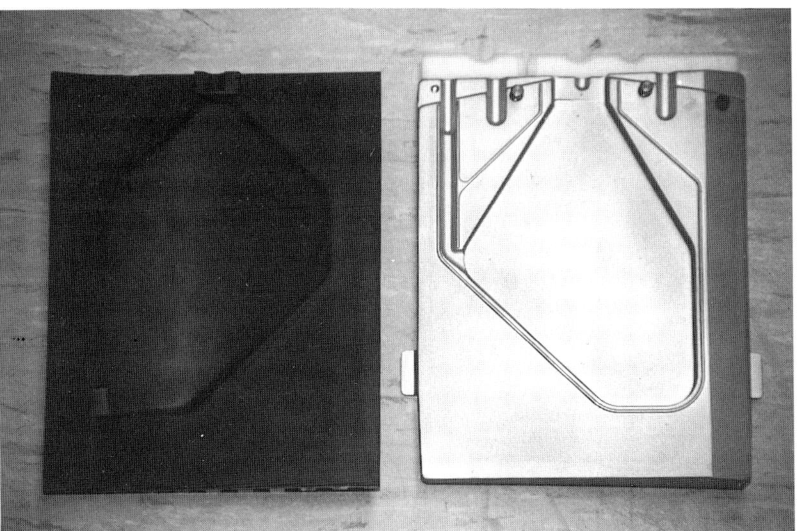

Fig. 1.6 The TNX-6 insert.

The TNX-6 chamber shown here is almost the same as the leukocyte or Granulo chamber in Figure 1.5, except that the area has been made more shallow by filling in part of this cavity.

The side-view of the TNX-6 chamber shown in Fig. 1.7 shows the filled-in portion, in contrast to the Granulo chamber.

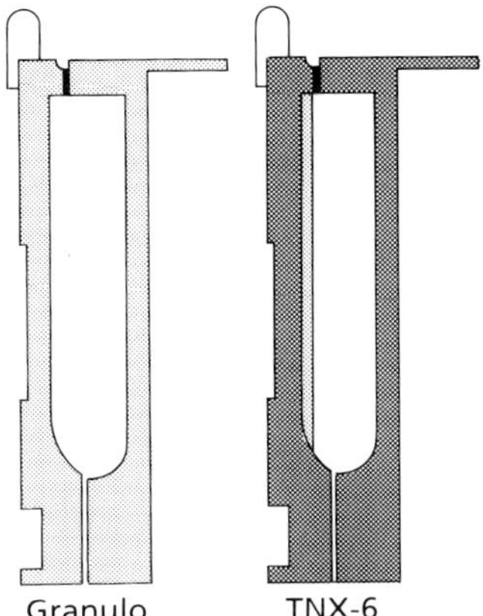

Fig. 1.7 Side-view of the Granulo chamber and the TNX-6.

The TNX-6 chamber concentrates cells so that many are presented to the optical detector at one time. When this happens, the optical detector can take decisive action to reverse the plasma flow to avoid collection of leukocytes. If the pump could not reverse, there would be occasions when large numbers of leukocytes would be collected with the platelets. In addition, the chamber is designed to accumulate platelets and preserve them just above the surface of the erythrocytes.

Figure 1.8 illustrates the process of accumulating platelets. The computer program causes the plasma removal rate to be increased for each 400–500 ml of plasma processed, so as to remove all the platelet-rich plasma to the secondary concentration chamber.

The TNX-6 chamber replaces the PLT chamber which has been used since 1979. The TNX-6 chamber is adapted from the Granulo chamber with only a few changes.

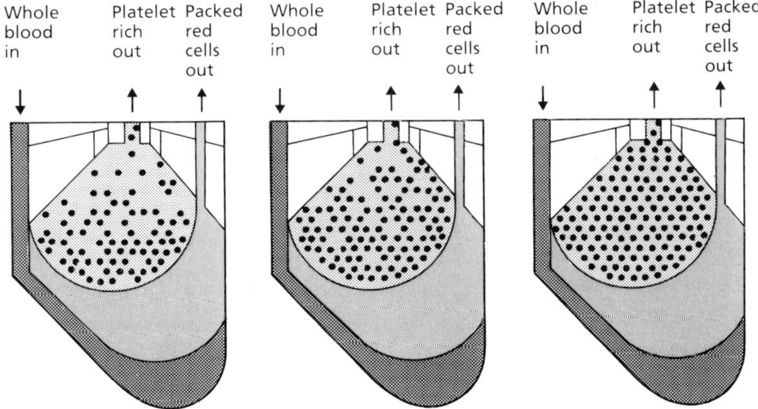

Fig. 1.8 TNX-6 chamber filling. (Source: Yang J.)

The changes are important; the TNX-6 cannot be used to collect leukocytes. Unlike the Granulo chamber, in the TNX-6 chamber the plasma removal port is placed at the extreme centrifugal top of the chamber in such a way that no reservoir of plasma can accumulate above the port. With no plasma reservoir and with its funnel shape, the TNX-6 concentrates light white blood cells and erythrocytes so that they are abruptly presented to the optical detector at a single moment, just as the last of the plasma is depleted.

An improvement was made to the optical detector computer program. The computer constantly monitors the optical density of the platelet-rich plasma. In the past, a fixed threshold was selected, at which the plasma pump would reverse and return cells to the collection chamber. Because the optical density of plasma will vary among different donors, it was necessary to select an optical threshold which was assured of being above that of the most dense plasma. Accordingly, the threshold was set so high that some leukocytes and some erythrocytes would be collected with the platelets.

Two machines were operated side by side to illustrate the difference between the old program and the new program (Fig. 1.9). One was equipped with the old computer program and the original PLT chamber; the other with the CS-3000 Plus and the TNX-6 chamber.

A nurse operating the machines can see the difference: with the older system, the plasma line takes on a visibly red appearance well before the optical detector senses the presence of red cells. At the conclusion of this collection, the platelet product

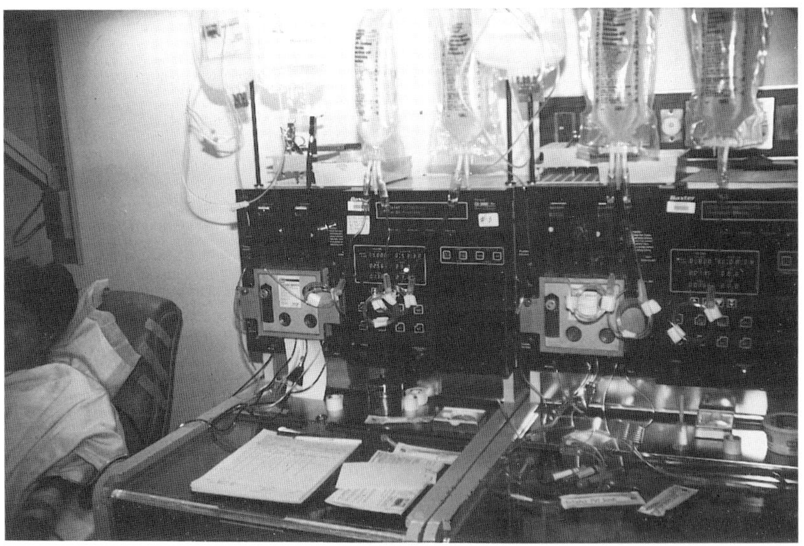

Fig. 1.9 Two CS-3000 Plus machines side by side.

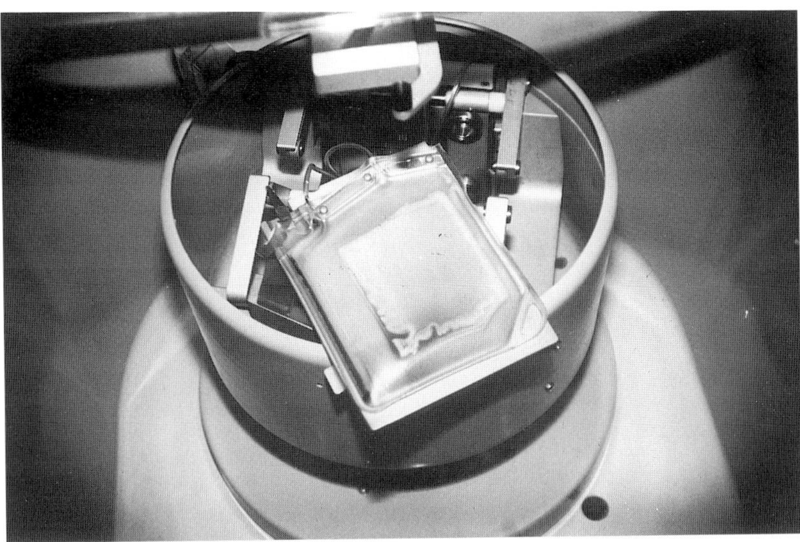

Fig. 1.10 Platelet product with red cells.

would usually contain about 0.5 ml of erythrocytes and many leukocytes. Figure 1.10 shows what such a product looked like.

In contrast, with the CS-3000 Plus and the TNX-6 chamber, the optical detector senses the presence of cells much sooner. The computer monitors the optical density of the individual donor's plasma, and selects a threshold just slightly above the plasma density. This permits an optical threshold to be selected which is precisely related to the optical density of the plasma of any given donor. It also permits much more accurate discrimination between platelet-rich plasma and blood cells.

Figure 1.11 shows the appearance of the platelet-rich plasma line with the CS-3000 Plus and the TNX-6 chamber. This picture, taken just before triggering the optical detector, shows no visible trace of red cells in the line.

At the conclusion of this hemapheresis, the collected product looks like the collection bag shown in Figure 1.12.

Selection of operating parameters

Sometimes it is desirable to alter the parameters of collection to suit the donor or the recipient. The collection can be made at flow rates from 30 to 60 ml/min, and at centrifuge speeds ranging from 1400 to 1600 rpm. Optical thresholds may range from 6 to 24. The flow rate, centrifuge speed, and optical threshold are selected by the operator from the menu on the control panel of the CS-3000.

The speed of the centrifuge may be reduced with negligible loss in platelet yield. In the past, it was necessary to centrifuge whole blood at 372 **g** (1600 rpm) in order to

 Chapter 1

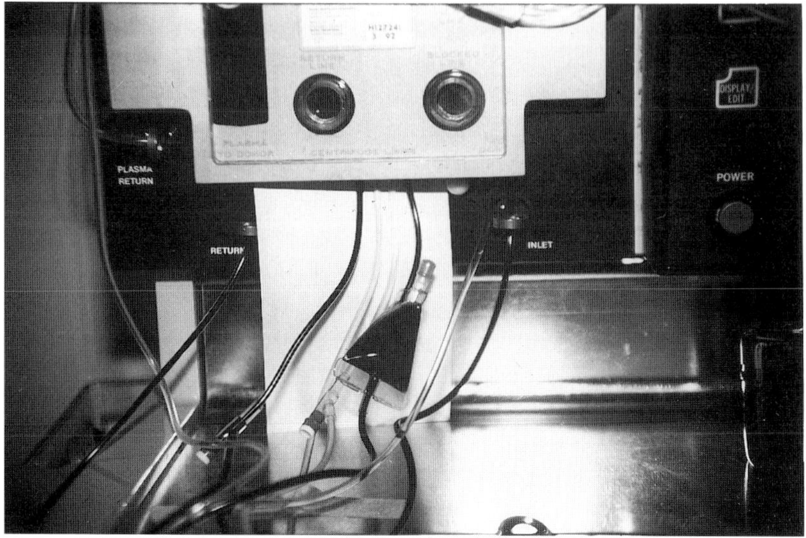

Fig. 1.11 Clear tubing lines with TNX-6.

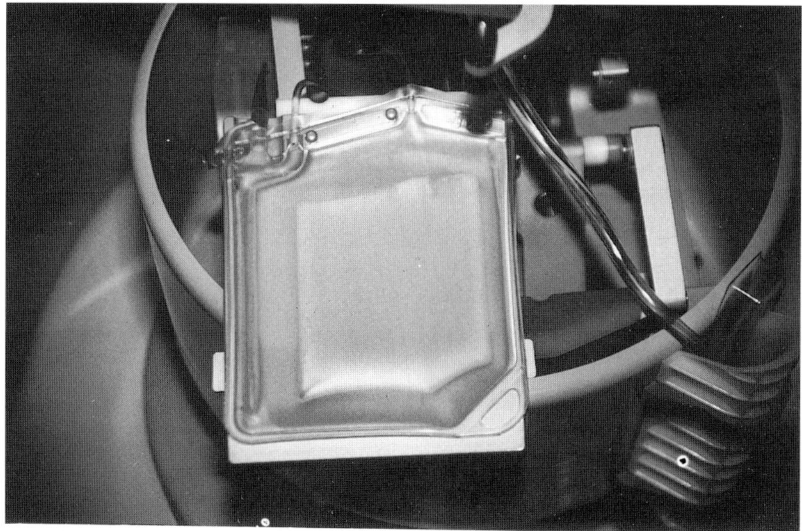

Fig. 1.12 Clean TNX-6 collection bag.

insure that leukocytes would be separated with the erythrocytes. The TNX-6 chamber concentrates lymphocytes so they may be detected at lower centrifuge speeds. When whole blood is being drawn, the centrifuge speed may be reduced from 1600 rpm (at 60 ml/min draw rate) to 1400 rpm (at 40 ml/min) without increased leukocyte

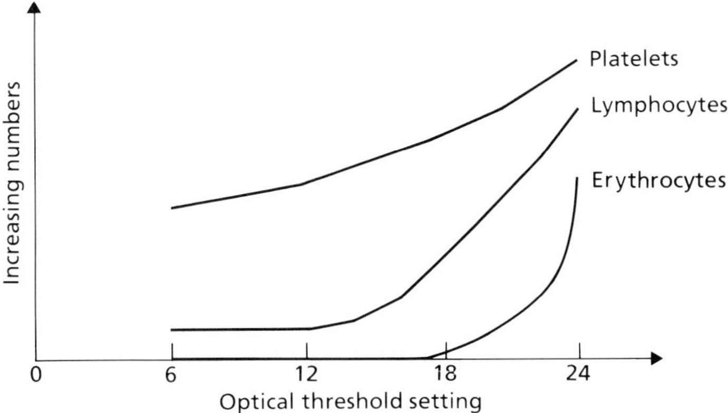

Fig. 1.13 Optical settings with the TNX-6.

collection. The lower sedimenting force permits easier, faster resuspension of the platelets.

The selection of an optical threshold may be based on particular donor or recipient needs. If it is desirable to collect more platelets from a given donor and if the number of leukocytes is not critical, the optical threshold may be increased; the number of platelets collected will be increased as a result of the higher setting (Fig. 1.13). For example, if the optical interface setting is increased from 6 to 12, the number of platelets and white blood cells collected will increase by about 10%. If a setting of 18 is selected, the platelet yield will increase by an additional 10%, but the trade-off is that lymphocyte collection will also be increased. Settings above 24 will not only result in increased platelet and leukocyte numbers, but will include measurable numbers of erythrocytes in the product.

Results

Data on platelet yields

Between January and April 1991, data from several hemapheresis centers in the USA were sent to the Fenwal home office for analysis and comparison. The names of the centers are abbreviated to initials, to maintain confidentiality. The first line in Table 1.1 shows all the data that we gathered in 1990; that information is not included in the averages for 1991.

The prehemapheresis counts are included as a measure of platelet counting ability and an indication of any bias that may exist in the data. In these centers, there does not appear to be any bias.

Only four institutions did routine leukocyte counts on the platelet collection, and among those four SP did not use hemacytometer counts. Perhaps this indicates the

Table 1.1 TNX-6 platelet yields from institutions in the USA

Institution	n	plt pre	s.d.	plt e11	s.d.	wbc e6	s.d.	vol proc	plt/l e11
1990									
Total	214			4.2	5.9	4.9	2.1	5000	
1991									
SO	39	263	46	3.6	0.7			3800	0.95
WM	31	262	49	3.8	1.1			4000	0.95
SB	63	274	46	3.9	0.9			4000	0.98
SP	13	260	58	4.1	1.2	7.8	0.9	4000	1.03
TA	47	269	58	4.0	0.7			4200	0.93
OB	4	258	40	4.2	0.1			4500	0.93
TH	34	277	50	5.0	1.2	1.4	1.1	4500	1.11
OC	20	244	27	4.3	0.6			4500	0.95
ON	29	247	47	4.1	1.0	5.4	7.6	5000	0.82
LS	18	238	38	4.8	0.9	2.1	2.0	5000	0.96
SD	18	243	61	4.3	1.2			5000	0.86
CH	15	247	53	4.5	1.2			5000	0.90
WT	60	279	39	5.7	1.5			6000	0.95
Total	391			(n = 13)		n = 4			
Average		258		4.3		4.2			0.95
Standard deviation		14		0.56		2.9			0.07

difficulty of counting cells when the concentration is in the range of $1/\mu l$. In any event, it appears that leukocyte levels in the 10^5–10^6 range are quite predictable and reliable.

Perhaps the most important point drawn from these data is that almost all the institutions using this method were able reliably to produce 0.95 times 10^{11} platelets per liter of blood processed. This reliability has permitted the CS-3000 Plus to predict the platelet yield with an internal program accessible through the control panel menu.

Conclusions

1   The TNX-6 platelet collection program permits the hemapheresis of large numbers of platelets with far fewer leukocytes than other methods; contamination by leukocytes will be limited to 10^5–10^6 per platelet collection.

2   Platelet yields with the TNX-6 are consistently about 0.95×10^{11} per liter of whole blood processed.

3   The CS-3000 Plus permits the operator to select operating parameters either to maximize platelet yield or to minimize leukocyte levels.

Discussion

WHYTE: For the purpose of diminishing lymphocytes for the alloimmunization purpose of decreasing them, it is probably important that the antigen-presenting cell, the dendritic cell, is also removed and that the reduction in lymphocyte count is only a marker for that reduction. The dendritic cell looks like a small lymphocyte. Where does its density fall, and do you know if you have any diminishment of alloimmunization with this method? It is better than, for example, filtration.

CULLIS: Well, that's a very tough question. The density of the dendritic cell is 1.062, which would indicate that these are likely to be the dendritic antigen-presenting cells that we would like to collect at other times. Effectiveness, or should we say, effectiveness in failing to stimulate antigen production by the recipient is not available yet, so I could not tell you about that.

SNIECINSKI: At the COHMC with the CS-3000 Plus and TNX chamber [for collection of platelet concentrates] we studied a different optical threshold varying from 6 to 13. Your graph shows that until a threshold of 13 or 14 the number of leukocytes actually does not increase significantly. But we had a very different experience when collecting platelets at the optical threshold setting of 13. In fact the number of white cells that were collected in those components were equal to the number of white cells collected by 2997 single-stage, which would be at the level of 10^9 white cells per platelet concentrate. Can you comment on that?

CULLIS: I did not know of those numbers. It must be unique to your center. In the data I received from our survey of 13 centers, I did not see those high numbers, so I would have to look into that. I really couldn't comment at this time. [If true, all lymphocytes would have been collected (Ed.).]

AKASHI (Osaka Red Cross Blood Center): For most voluntary blood donors in Japan, offering two arms on hemapheresis is less comfortable than offering one arm. Do you have any program to develop a machine needing only one arm?

CULLIS: Yes, we do. The program is currently pending before the Food and Drug Administration in the United States and there is a special tubing kit with a single needle and the one-arm procedure, that draws and returns in much the same way as a discontinuous flow technique. It does have the penalty of being longer in processing time because the one needle is shared and part of the time is drawing, part return.

2·Comparison of a "top and bottom" system with a conventional quadruple-bag system for blood-component preparation and storage

S. Nakajo, S. Chiba, T.A. Takahashi, and S. Sekiguchi

Hokkaido Red Cross Blood Center, Yamanote 2-2, Nishi-ku, Sapporo 063, Japan

Abstract

A "top and bottom" bag is a blood collection bag that has one outlet at the top and two outlets at the bottom. After high-speed centrifugation, whole blood (400 ml) is separated automatically into components by semiautomated component extractors such as the Separator and the Optipress. The red cells and the plasma are expelled simultaneously into different component bags and the buffy coat remains in the blood collection bag.

We investigated the composition of blood components prepared by the top and bottom system and compared it to that of blood prepared by the conventional quadruple-bag system. The residual leukocytes in the buffy coat-poor red cell concentrate (BPRCC) prepared by the top and bottom system were significantly lower than those prepared by the conventional system. The BPRCC prepared by the Optipress and the Separator contained $5.8 \pm 3.3 \times 10^8$ and $4.7 \pm 2.7 \times 10^8$ leukocytes/bag, respectively (mean $\pm$ s.d., $n = 10$). The average number of residual lymphocytes was less than 5.39×10^6 cells/bag and 5.31×10^6 cells/bag in the BPRCC prepared by the Optipress and the Separator, respectively.

In contrast, the BPRCC prepared by the conventional quadruple-bag system contained more than 5×10^7 lymphocytes/bag. A sufficient number of platelets could be collected from the buffy coat prepared by the top and bottom system. Furthermore, the characteristics of red cells in the BPRCC prepared by the top and bottom system during storage were well maintained compared to those prepared by the conventional system.

Thus, we conclude that the top and bottom system can be used to prepare BPRCC from whole blood with high efficiency, especially as concerns the removal rate of lymphocytes. The BPRCC prepared by the top and bottom system should contribute to a decrease in febrile reactions caused by contaminating leukocytes as well as other side-effects of blood transfusion.

Introduction

It is known that transfusion reactions such as febrile reactions, alloimmunization virus infection and graft-versus-host disease (GvHD) are caused by the administration of blood components containing contaminating leukocytes [1,2]. Various leukocyte removal-filters have been developed recently to reduce or deplete these leukocytes effectively from blood components. We routinely prepare leukocyte-poor red cells from concentrated red cells (CRCs) using a Sepacell R-500NN filter (Asahi Medical, Tokyo, Japan) following requests from hospitals [3]. However, this filtration procedure cannot be adopted for the routine preparation of blood components in blood centers because of cost-effectiveness and the restricted expiration date. In addition to filtration procedures, several techniques were developed to deplete leukocytes from whole blood, one of which is the removal of the buffy coat after centrifugation [4–6]. In this method, plasma is separated from whole blood after centrifugation, then the buffy coat is removed, after which additive solution is used to prepare BPRCC that decreases the number of leukocytes, extends the expiration date up to 42 days, and gives more plasma for fractionation. Moreover, it is possible to prepare platelet concentrate (PC) from buffy coat [5,6].

At present, there are two types of bag systems — the conventional quadruple-bag system, which consists of a collection bag and three satellite bags for red cells; and the top and bottom bag system, which has outlets at the top and bottom of the collection bag.

In both systems, the preparation procedure needs to be automated to obtain high-quality blood components and for labor efficiency. Automatic systems for blood-component preparation have been developed and are used in some European countries.

We investigated the composition of blood components prepared by the top and bottom system and the conventional bag system, and the handling of various semiautomated component extractors, in particular comparing BPRCC from the top and bottom system with that of the conventional bag system.

Materials and methods

Bag systems and semiautomated component extractors

Figures 2.1 and 2.2 and Table 2.1 show the bag systems and semiautomated component extractors used in this investigation.

The top and bottom bag consists of a collection bag that has upper and lower outlets (Fig. 2.3a). After centrifugation, plasma is expelled through the upper outlet, red cells pass through the bottom outlet to a satellite bag which contains an additive solution, and buffy coat remains in the collection bag [7–9]. In contrast, the conventional bag has only one outlet at the top and consists of a collection bag and three satellite bags, one for an additive solution (Fig. 2.3b). At first, plasma is separated, then buffy coat is transferred to one satellite bag and returned to the additive solution in the collection bag.

We also examined manually prepared blood components for comparison.

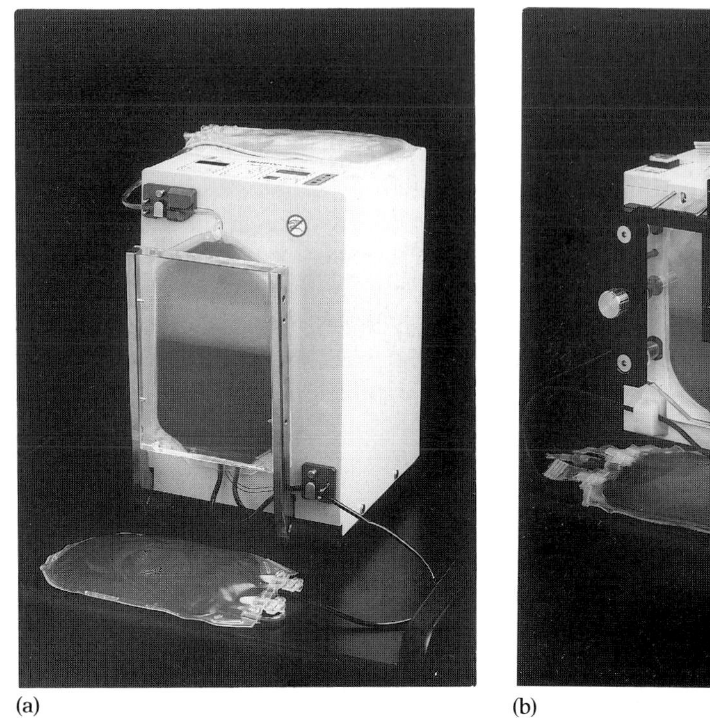

(a)   (b)

Fig. 2.1 Semiautomated component extractors (top and bottom bag system). (a) Separator; (b) Optipress.

Table 2.2 summarizes the characteristics of each semiautomated component extractor.

Table 2.1 Details of the bag systems and semiautomated component extractors used in the investigation

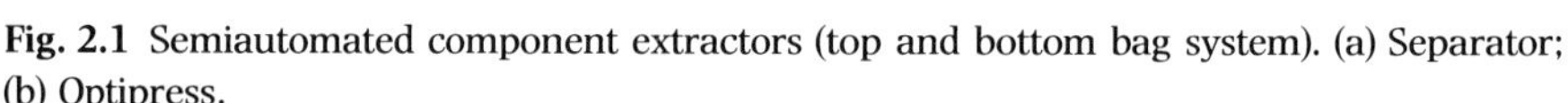

Bag system	Bag (manufacturer)	Semiautomated component extractor (manufacturer)
Top and bottom	Biopack U (Biotrans, Dreieich, Germany)	Separator (Biotrans, Dreieich, Germany)
	Optipac (Baxter, Deerfield, USA)	Optipress (Baxter, Deerfield, USA)
Conventional	Quadruple bag (Kawasumi, Japan)	Compomat (NPBI, Emmer-compascuume, The Netherlands)
		Terumo AC-211 (Terumo, Japan)

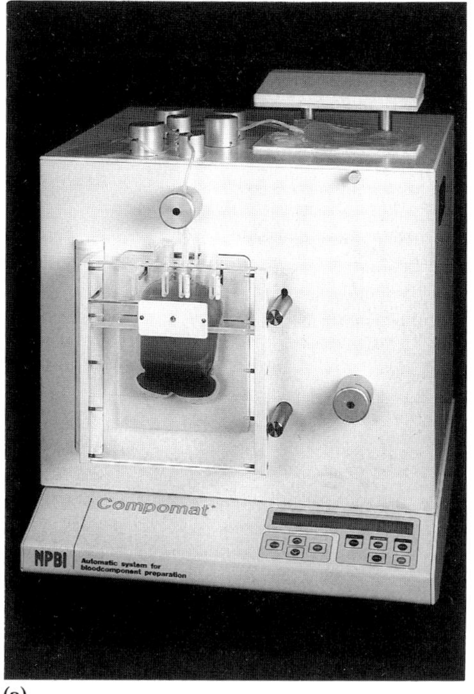
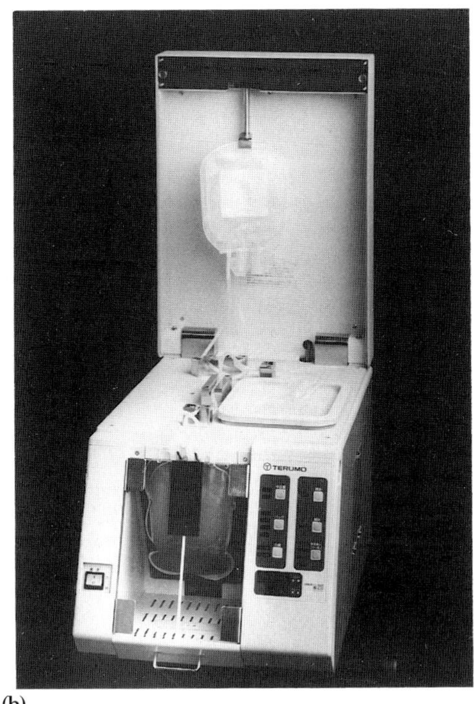

(a) (b)

Fig. 2.2 Semiautomated component extractors (conventional bag system). (a) Compomat; (b) Terumo.

Preparation of blood

We collected 400 ml of whole blood in a PVC bag containing 56 ml of citrate phosphate dextrose (CPD). The blood was transferred to a conventional quadruple-bag

Table 2.2 Characteristics of the semiautomated component extractor

	Top and Bottom		Conventional	
	Separator	Optipress	Compomat	Terumo
Method of pressure				
Type of pressure plates	Lower press	Parallel press	Parallel press Slide shutter	Upper press
Motive power	Motor	Air cylinder	Air cylinder	Motor
Measure of BC weight	Thickness of bag	Thickness of bag	Slide shutter position	Weight
	Digital control	Manual control	Volume × time	

BC, buffy coat.

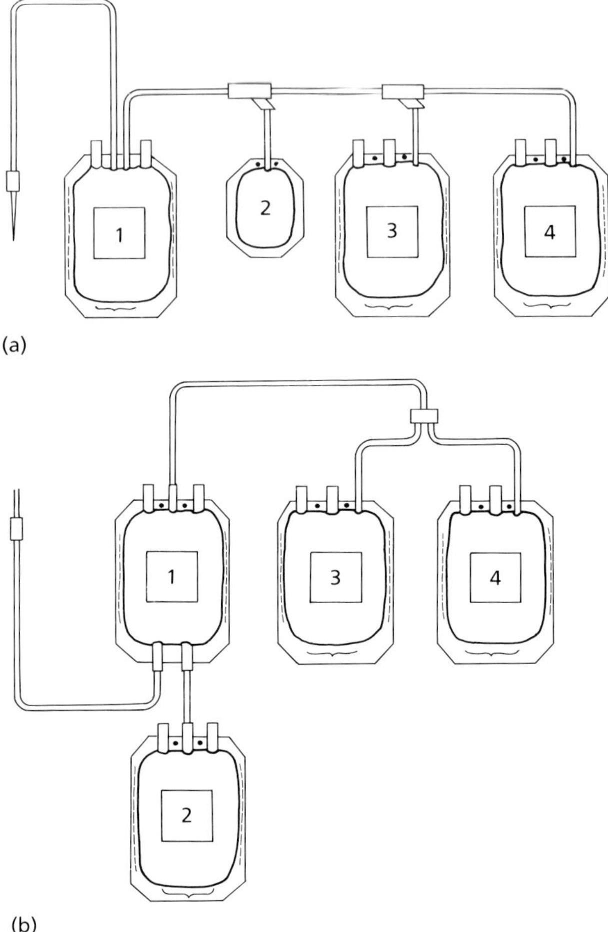

(a)

(b)

Fig. 2.3 Bag systems. (a) Conventional bag system: 1 collection bag; 2 buffy coat; 3 platelets; 4 plasma. (b) Top and bottom bag system: 1 collection bag; 2 red cells; 3 platelets; 4 plasma.

system or a top and bottom bag using a sterile connection device (SCD-312, Haemonetics, USA) and separated into components within 4 h of collection.

We used mannitol adenine phosphate solution as the additive solution [10].

Preparation of components

Buffy coat method

In both systems, the whole blood was centrifuged at 4540 g for 6 min at 22°C, after which separation of red cells and plasma was carried out by each semiautomated

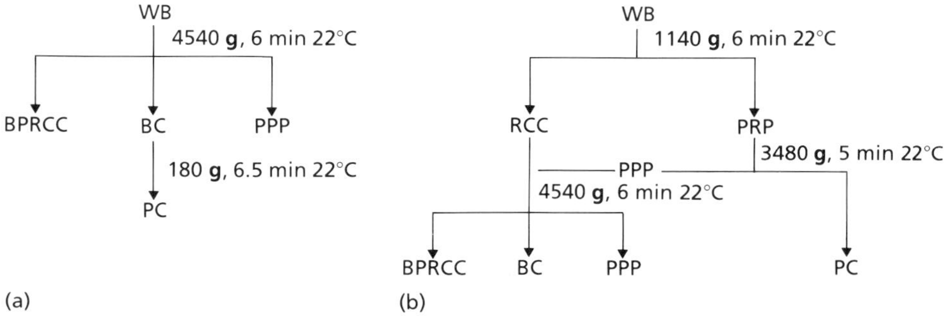

Fig. 2.4 Preparation of blood components. (a) Buffy coat method; (b) platelet-rich plasma method. BC, buffy coat; BPRCC, buffy coat-poor red cell concentrate; PC, platelet concentrate; PPP, platelet-poor plasma; PRP, platelet-rich plasma; RCC, red cell concentrate; WB, whole blood.

component extractor (Fig. 2.4a). The volume of the buffy coat was adjusted to 70 ml in the Separator, the Optipress and the Terumo machines, but it was adjusted to 80 ml in the Compomat because of mechanical conditions. For preparation of PC, the buffy coat was then centrifuged at 180 g for 6.5 min at 22°C, 40 ml of the supernatant was transferred into the satellite bag and platelets were concentrated in plasma.

In the case of PC preparation in the Separator, the buffy coat remaining in the collection bag was transferred into another satellite bag. PC was prepared as described above.

We also manually prepared BPRCC from whole blood and PC from buffy coat. After centrifugation as described above, plasma was expelled at the interface between red cells and plasma, about 32 g of leukocyte-rich upper layer was harvested as buffy coat and 42 g of plasma was added to the buffy coat.

Platelet-rich plasma

After centrifugation at 1140 g for 6 min at 22°C, platelet-rich plasma (PRP) was isolated in one of the two satellite bags (Fig. 2.4b). The connecting tube was stopped by using a clamp without a seal, and all four bags were placed in the centrifuge a second time (3480 g, 5 min, 22°C) to precipitate the platelets. After centrifugation, platelets were resuspended in 40 ml of platelet-poor plasma (PPP) and the remaining PPP was returned to the red cells. After the whole blood with a reduced amount of platelets was centrifuged (2500 g, 10 min, 22°C), separation of cells and plasma was performed using the Optipress.

Cell counting

The numbers of red cells, leukocytes, and platelets and the hematocrit value were counted by using a Coulter Counter S Plus IV (Coulter Electronics, USA). The subpopulations of leukocytes in BPRCC were determined by the cytospin method [11].

Biochemical functions of red cells

Adenosine triphosphate (ATP) and 2,3-diphosphoglycerate (2,3-DPG) were assayed with an ATP kit (BMY, Tokyo, Japan) and 2,3-DPG kit (BMY, Tokyo, Japan), respectively. The plasma-free hemoglobin level was determined by the *O*-tridin method. The plasma glucose concentration was determined enzymatically. Osmotic fragility was measured by the coil planet centrifuge method [12]. Red cell morphology was judged by light microscopy [13].

Sedimentation profile of leukocytes after hard spinning

After the whole blood collected in a Biopack U was centrifuged (4540 **g**, 6 min, 22°C) 20 ml aliquots of red cells from the bottom outlet and plasma from the top outlet were fractionated and the numbers of leukocytes counted.

We estimated the sedimentation profiles of leukocytes based on the percentage of leukocytes contained in each fraction compared to total leukocytes.

Operation time

We measured the time it took to prepare BPRCC automatically using each semi-automated component extractor. We divided the procedure into three steps as follows: (i) pretreatment — taking the bag out of the centrifuge cup to hanging the bag; (ii) separation time — from pushing the start button to the end of preparation; (iii) posttreatment — the time from taking off the bag to sealing the tube.

Results

Sedimentation profile of leukocytes after hard spinning

To remove the buffy coat effectively, the leukocytes should be concentrated at the interface of red cells and plasma. We estimated the sedimentation profile of leukocytes after centrifugation.

Figure 2.5 shows that when the blood was centrifuged at 4540 **g** for 6 min, approximately 80% of the leukocytes were concentrated in 20 ml of buffy coat layer.

Thus we determined that centrifugation should be done at 4540 **g** for 6 min.

Characteristics of BPRCC

Table 2.3 presents the results of cell counts in BPRCC prepared in each bag system. Leukocyte removal in the top and bottom system was good compared with the conventional bag system. A significantly higher removal rate was obtained with the Optipress (87.2 ± 5.8%, mean ± s.d., $n = 10$) compared to the other machines.

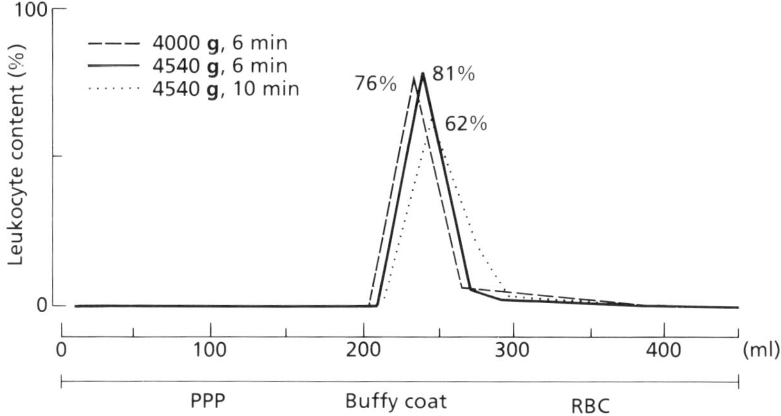

Fig. 2.5 Sedimentation profiles of leukocytes. PPP, platelet-poor plasma; RBC, red blood cells.

The number of residual lymphocytes was confirmed by the cytospin method. It was less than 5.3×10^6 per bag in the top and bottom system. Most of the residual leukocytes were granulocytes.

We measured biochemical functions of red cells prepared by the buffy coat method (Table 2.4), but found no significant difference between the two systems.

Properties of PC

The properties of PC prepared in this test are illustrated in Table 2.5. PC preparation was performed by the buffy coat method using the Separator or by the PRP method using the Optipress.

In both systems, the number of platelets in PC met the standard (4×10^{10}/bag), but the volume of PC did not meet the criteria (40 ml) in four of five cases with the Separator and 15 of 20 cases with the Compomat.

Yield of plasma

The yield of plasma was $74.1 \pm 2.0\%$ ($n = 10$) with the Separator, $84.3 \pm 1.1\%$ ($n = 7$) with the Optipress, $75.5 \pm 2.2\%$ ($n = 10$) with the Compomat, $71.7 \pm 3.3\%$ ($n = 10$) with the Terumo, and $81.5 \pm 8.0\%$ ($n = 10$) by the manual method.

Operation time

Figure 2.6 shows the time it took to prepare 1 unit of BPRCC. This indicates that the separation time of the conventional bag system was shorter than that of the top and bottom system.

Table 2.3 Properties of buffy coat-poor red cell concentrates (mean ± s.d.)

	Top and bottom			Conventional		
	Separator	Optipress (BC method)	Optipress (PRP method)	Compomat	Terumo	Manual
n	10	10	7	10	10	10
Volume (ml)	272.5 ± 13.9	248.8 ± 10.2	259.3 ± 8.0	252.7 ± 7.2	285.0 ± 19.9	250.0 ± 25.9
Hematocrit (%)	56.4 ± 1.9	55.0 ± 0.7	56.3 ± 1.7	58.2 ± 1.3	61.3 ± 1.5	61.1 ± 4.5
Leukocyte						
Cells/bag ($\times 10^8$)	5.8 ± 3.3	4.7 ± 2.7	3.1 ± 2.0	7.7 ± 3.1	14.2 ± 6.2	9.2 ± 2.9
Removal rate (%)	78.4 ± 10.4	83.9 ± 6.6	88.9 ± 3.7	72.0 ± 6.6	56.8 ± 11.3	65.7 ± 4.6
Lymphocyte						
Cells/bag ($\times 10^7$)	0.5 > *	0.5 > *	0.4 > *	6.2 ± 2.7	19.6 ± 11.2	10.1 ± 0.4
Removal rate (%)	99.3 <	99.6 <	99.8 <	93.9 ± 2.3	79.5 ± 13.3	89.3 ± 2.3
Red cell						
Cells/bag ($\times 10^{11}$)	16.3 ± 1.8	14.7 ± 0.1	15.4 ± 1.2	15.5 ± 0.8	16.5 ± 0.1	16.0 ± 1.3
Recovery rate (%)	85.6 ± 1.8	77.2 ± 1.6	78.2 ± 0.8	83.9 ± 1.2	91.6 ± 2.2	86.2 ± 2.2
Platelet						
Cells/bag ($\times 10^9$)	0.5 ± 0.2	0.6 ± 0.4	0.4 ± 0.1	6.7 ± 2.6	17.2 ± 7.1	24.8 ± 10.9
Removal rate (%)	99.5 ± 0.1	99.4 ± 0.3	99.7 ± 0.1	94.1 ± 2.3	81.1 ± 12.2	73.6 ± 13.1

* Cytospin method.
BC, buffy coat; PRP, platelet-rich plasma.

Table 2.4 Characteristics of buffy coat-poor red cell concentrates (mean ± s.d.)

Days of storage	0	7	14	21	28	35	42
Adenosine triphosphate	2.40 ± 0.15	2.23 ± 0.22	1.88 ± 0.16	1.24 ± 0.06	1.09 ± 0.11	1.09 ± 0.11	0.98 ± 0.14
(µmol/g Hb)	2.99 ± 0.50	2.47 ± 0.39	2.44 ± 0.32	1.21 ± 0.15	1.18 ± 0.21	1.10 ± 0.17	0.87 ± 0.25
2,3-Diphosphoglycerate	8.2 ± 1.5	1.0 ± 0.5	0.1 ± 0.1	0.1 ± 0.0	0.1 ± 0.0		
(µmol/g Hb)	9.7 ± 0.7	1.3 ± 0.4	0.2 ± 0.1	0.1 ± 0.0	0.1 ± 0.0		
Supernatant Hb	20 ± 2	30 ± 2	36 ± 7	48 ± 10	59 ± 14	68 ± 7	102 ± 30
(mg/dl)	27 ± 4	33 ± 2	31 ± 5	39 ± 2	52 ± 6	64 ± 5	84 ± 11
Glucose	523 ± 3	462 ± 8	427 ± 11	387 ± 9	366 ± 6	329 ± 8	306 ± 6
(mg/dl)	504 ± 3	470 ± 8	427 ± 11	358 ± 9	352 ± 6	320 ± 8	294 ± 6
Osmotic fragility	93 ± 2	95 ± 1	95 ± 2	95 ± 2	92 ± 3	90 ± 4	92 ± 3
(HMP mosmol/kg)	98 ± 3	98 ± 3	98 ± 1	97 ± 1	98 ± 4	98 ± 1	97 ± 1
Morphology score	99.7 ± 0.2	95.1 ± 1.7	89.8 ± 4.0	88.6 ± 4.5	90.1 ± 2.6	80.3 ± 3.1	78.2 ± 1.3
	98.2 ± 3.4	90.8 ± 6.9	88.2 ± 9.0	84.2 ± 9.0	80.3 ± 9.4	75.9 ± 10.0	74.4 ± 7.8

Upper figures, Separator ($n = 5$); lower figures, Terumo ($n = 4$).
Hb, hemoglobin; HMP, hemolysis maximum point.

Table 2.5 Properties of platelet concentrates (mean ± s.d.)

	Top and bottom		Conventional		
	Separator (n = 5)	Optipress (PRP method; n = 5)	Compomat (n = 15)	Terumo (n = 10)	Manual (n = 5)
Volume (ml)	36.1 ± 2.0	42.9 ± 3.0	46.1 ± 4.6	41.9 ± 3.9	33.6 ± 6.2
Platelets ($\times 10^{10}$)	7.9 ± 1.2	7.2 ± 1.8	6.1 ± 1.3	5.5 ± 2.3	4.5 ± 1.4
Leukocytes ($\times 10^{7}$)	6.3 ± 7.4	4.8 ± 3.1	2.5 ± 3.8	1.4 ± 1.6	2.9 ± 2.5

PRP, platelet-rich plasma.

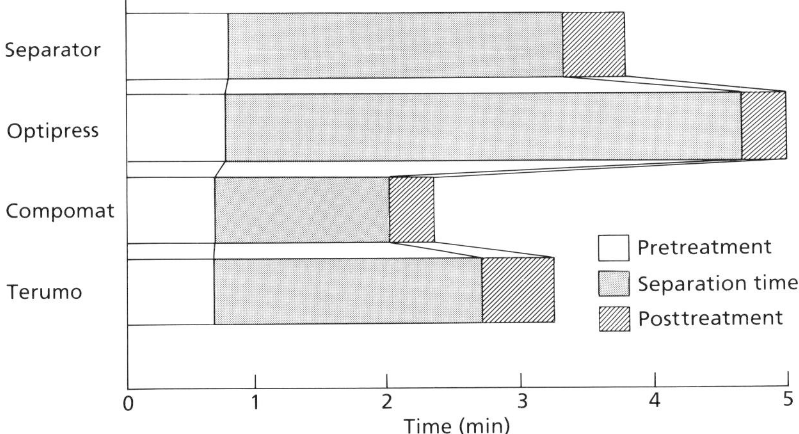

Fig. 2.6 Operation time for the buffy coat-poor red cell concentrate.

Summary

The febrile reactions occurring most frequently as a result of transfusions can be prevented in most cases by the removal of 1 log (90%) of leukocytes in the blood components [2]. A simple method for leukocyte depletion is to centrifuge the blood and subsequently remove the buffy coat.

We examined the preparation of BPRCC in the top and bottom system, and compared it with the conventional bag system. With the top and bottom system it was possible to prepare BPRCC that contained fewer leukocytes than in the conventional bag system (Table 2.3).

When the Compomat was compared with the Separator, the volume of the buffy coat in the Compomat was 10 ml greater than in the Separator and, furthermore, the buffy coat layer was fully removed by using the slide-shutter. Nevertheless, leukocyte removal in the Compomat was lower than in the Separator. This was because it was difficult to remove leukocytes smoothly and effectively by top-out expulsion, and the remaining leukocytes in the tube were returned to the collection bag when additive solution was added to the buffy coat. In contrast to the conventional bag system, the buffy coat remained in the collection bag in the top and bottom system. In particular, there was extensive removal of lymphocytes in BPRCC prepared by the top and bottom system. Lymphocytes tend to concentrate at the interface between red cells and plasma after centrifugation, since the specific gravity of lymphocytes is higher than that of other cells. The number of residual lymphocytes in BPRCC was reduced to the level of 10^6 or less per bag. Moreover, filtration of BPRCC might help prevent alloimmunization [1].

With regard to PC preparation, in both systems the number of platelets met the standard, but in some cases the volume was below the standard. The hematocrit of the buffy coat increased to about 30% and the centrifugation adopted in this test was probably not optimal.

When using the Optipress, PC was prepared by the PRP method. A high hematocrit level (54%) made it difficult to prepare PC from the buffy coat.

PC is prepared from pooled buffy coats in Europe [14]. However, the preparation of pooled PC is not approved in Japanese blood centers. This pooling procedure is so reasonable that we believe it should be used in Japan as well.

The operating time needed to prepare 1 unit of BPRCC automatically using the conventional bag system tended to be shorter than that with the top and bottom system. Since red cells passing through the bottom outlet have high viscosity, red cell flow seems to be slower, and it takes a little longer. However, if much blood is separated using several semiautomated component extractors, the operation time will differ in this situation. Further investigations are needed to evaluate the operation of semiautomated component extractors.

References

1 Sekiguchi S, Takahashi TA. Leukocyte-depleted blood products and their clinical usefulness. In: Brozović B, ed. *The Role of Leukocyte Depletion in Blood Transfusion Practice.* Oxford: Blackwell Scientific Publications, 1989:26–34.

2 Synder EL. Clinical use of white cell-poor blood components. *Transfusion* 1989;29:568–571.

3 Segawa K, Hasegawa H, Hosoda M, Takahashi TA, Sekiguchi S. A new leukocyte removal filter-Imugard E for red cell concentrates. Comparison of the efficacy with Sepacell R-500N. *Jpn J Transfus Med* 1990;36:497–503.

4 Prins HK, de Brunjin JCGH, Henrichs HPJ, Loos JA. Prevention of microaggregate formation by removal of 'buffy-coats'. *Vox Sang* 1980;39:48–51.

5 Loos H. Automation in blood component preparation. In: Murawski K, ed. *Transfusion Medicine — Recent Technological Advances.* New York: Alan R Liss, 1986:333–341.

6 Uda M, Ohkuma S, Ishii A, Nishizaki T. Preparation of blood components with a saline-adenine-glucose-phosphate-maltose quadruple-pack system. *Transfusion* 1985;25:325–329.

7 Högman CF, Erikson L, Hedlund K, Wallvik J. The bottom and top system: a new technique for blood component preparation and storage. *Vox Sang* 1988;55:211–217.

8 Kretschmer V, Khan-Blouki K, Biermann E, Söhngen D, Eckle R. Improvement of blood

component quality — automatic separation of blood components in a new bag system. *Infusionstherapie* 1988;15:232–239.

9 Pitersz RNI, Dekker WJA, Reesink HW. Comparison of a conventional quadruple-bag system with a 'top-and-bottom' system for blood processing. *Vox Sang* 1990;59:205–208.

10 Shimizu T, Furuta M, Kouketsu K *et al*. *In vitro* evaluations of 4 red cell additive solutions studies in 7 blood centers. *Jpn J Transfus Med* 1989;35:640–646.

11 Takahashi TA, Hosoda M, Sekiguchi S. Cytospin method for the determination of residual leukocytes in leukocyte-depleted platelet concentrates. *Jpn J Transfus Med* 1989;35:497–503.

12 Takahashi TA, Yamamoto S, Hasegawa H *et al*. A new type of blood component collector: plasma separation by gravity without any electrical devices. *Jpn J Transfus Med* 1989;35:73–79.

13 Usry RT, Moor GL, Manalo FW. Morphology of stored, rejuvenated human erythrocytes. *Vox Sang* 1975;28:176–183.

14 Eriksson L, Högman CF. Platelet concentrates in an additive solution prepared from pooled buffy coats. 1. *In vitro* studies. *Vox Sang* 1990;59:140–145.

Discussion

YUASA (Juntendo University): We at medical institutions expect a supply of buffy coat-depleted red cell concentrates in future. You mentioned a good removal of leukocytes with your method; the top and bottom system. What do you think of the effect of filtration on the residual number of leukocytes together with your centrifugation method? Do you have any idea of the number of residual leukocytes if you combine the centrifugation method and the leukocyte removal filter?

NAKAJO: We have not yet examined this point, but I suppose the residual leukocytes will decrease in number. The efficiency of filtration seems to be improved.

MIYAHARA: When we applied filtration method after buffy coat depletion, the number of residual leukocytes decreased to less than 1×10^6 in red cell concentrates. We have not examined this method to platelet concentrates, but I expect a lower number. I suppose the range in 1×10^5 might be possible.

SEKIGUCHI: The best way to remove the leukocytes from the conventional blood products is to use the filtration method just after the depletion of buffy coat. In our results, an extra 1 log reduction was obtained.

3 · Preparation of leukocyte-poor blood components by the nonbutton platelet concentrate method using quadruple- and quintuple-bag systems

M. Miyahara*

Japanese Red Cross Okayama Blood Center, 3-36 Izumi-cho, Okayama 700, Japan

Abstract

To prepare leukocyte-poor blood components in a closed system, we devised a nonbutton platelet concentrate (NBPC) method using a quadruple-bag system. By this method, leukocyte-poor PCs composed of 1.9×10^7 of residual leukocytes (leukocyte removal efficiency 98.3%) and red cell concentrates with 8.5×10^8 of residual leukocytes (efficiency 66.5%) were prepared. The efficiency of leukocyte removal from red cells was improved by combining it with filtration. The quintuple-bag system with a small Imugard filter made it possible to obtain leukocyte-depleted red cells with a mean 1.4×10^7 leukocytes/bag (efficiency 99.1%) in a closed system. Moreover, better results were obtained when filtration through a Sepacell filter was carried out on the red cells prepared by an NBPC method, though the procedure was performed in an open system. The mean residual leukocytes obtained were 8.2×10^5/bag (efficiency 99.97%). These data indicate that the NBPC method is useful in the preparation of leukocyte-poor blood components capable of preventing or reducing human leukocyte antigen (HLA) alloimmunization in a closed system.

Introduction

One of the problems of blood components such as red cell concentrates (RCCs) and PCs prepared by the conventional method is that they contain a large number of leukocytes. Repeated transfusions of these components commonly induce the appearance of leukocyte antibodies due to HLA alloimmunization. These antibodies may cause nonhemolytic febrile transfusion reaction [1–3] and refractoriness to platelet transfusion [4–6]. Although several leukocyte-poor red cells (LPRCs) prepared by centrifugation or filtration methods are now available from blood centers, these products are prepared in an open system and they are not necessarily efficient enough at leukocyte removal to prevent these adverse reactions.

* Née M. Uda.

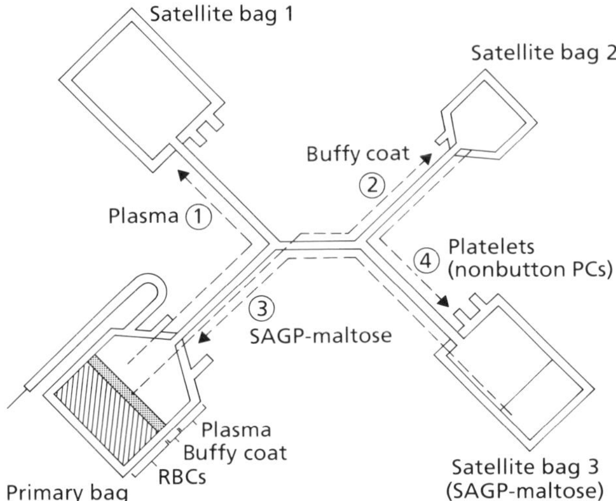

Fig. 3.1 A quadruple-bag system for the nonbutton platelet concentrate (PC) method. RBCs, red blood cells; SAGP, saline adenine glucose phosphate; 1–4, numerical order of transference of blood components from one bag to another.

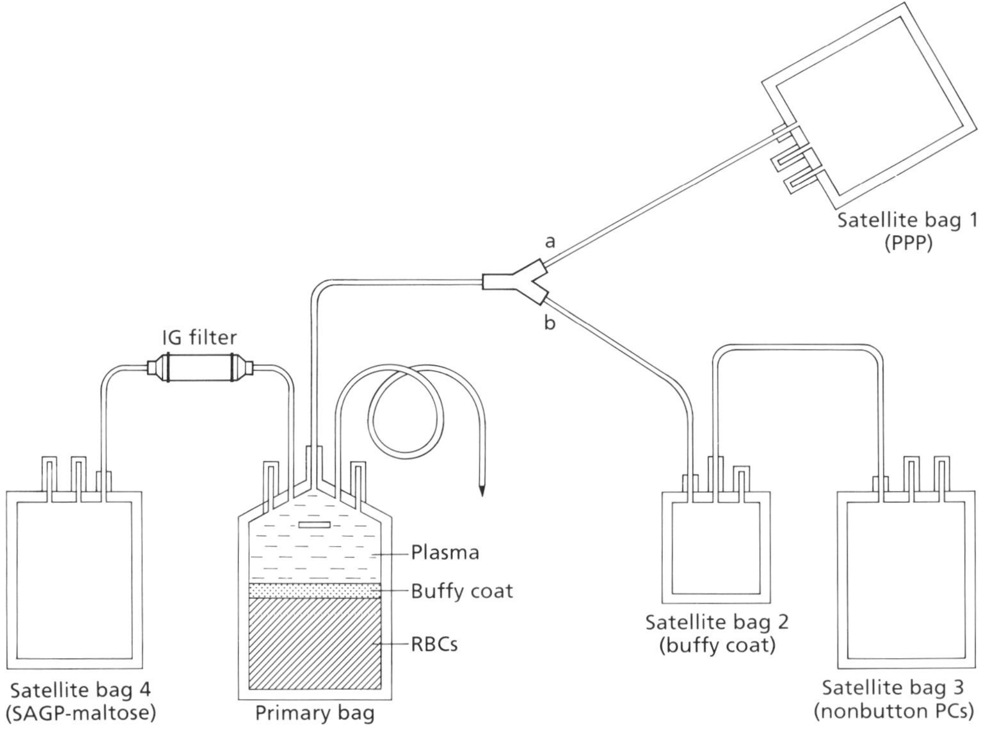

Fig. 3.2 A quintuple-bag system with a small Imugard (IG) filter for the nonbutton platelet concentrate (PC) method. PPP, platelet-poor plasma; RBCs, red blood cells; SAGP, saline adenine glucose phosphate.

In order to prepare LPRCs in a closed system, the author has attempted to use an NBPC method incorporating a quadruple-bag system (Fig. 3.1) [7,8], which had previously been devised as a gentler method for preparing PCs without forming a platelet button. The NBPC method involves two steps in centrifugation. In the first step, platelets are concentrated in a buffy coat layer by high-speed centrifugation, and then separated from red blood cells. In the second step, contaminating leukocytes and red blood cells in the buffy coat are precipitated by low-speed centrifugation, leaving the lighter platelets in the supernatant plasma as the NBPCs. A number of leukocytes should be removed from both RCCs and PCs during these processes. A major feature of the method is that buffy coat removal and isolation of platelets from red cells can be processed simultaneously.

Moreover, a quintuple-bag system with a small Imugard (IG) filter was devised to improve the efficacy of the NBPC method (Fig. 3.2). In addition, filtration using Sepacell, a newly developed second-generation filter, was performed on the LPRCs prepared by the NBPC method.

This chapter gives details of these techniques and how efficient they are in removing leukocytes from blood components. Attempts to operate the NBPC method automatically using an automatic plasma extractor (Fig. 3.3) are also discussed.

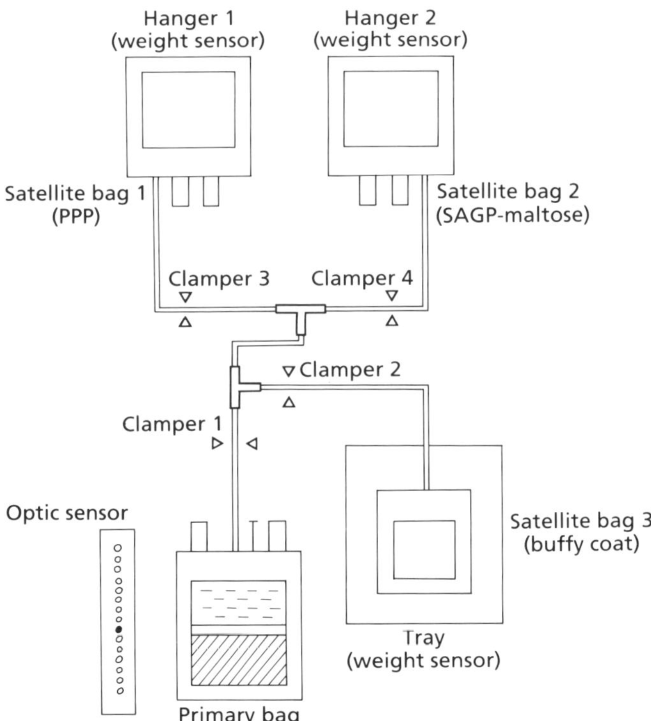

Fig. 3.3 A quadruple-bag system for the nonbutton platelet concentrate method using an automatic plasma extractor. PPP, platelet-poor plasma; SAGP, saline adenine glucose phosphate.

Materials and methods

Preparation of leukocyte-poor blood components

Nonbutton platelet concentrate method using a quadruple-bag system

Blood (400 ml) was collected in the primary bag of a quadruple-bag system (Fig. 3.1) manufactured by Kawasumi Kagakukogyo (Tokyo, Japan) according to my specifications: the primary bag contains 60 ml of acid citrate dextrose (ACD) solution and the third satellite bag contains 140 ml of saline adenine glucose phosphate (SAGP)-maltose solution [8]. In the first step, the whole blood was centrifuged at 3500 g for 6 min, and approximately 100 ml of the supernatant plasma was transferred into the first satellite bag. After the buffy coat was transferred to the second satellite bag with approximately 70 ml of residual plasma, the SAGP-maltose solution in the third satellite bag was added to the primary bag to prepare buffy coat-poor red cells with a hematocrit of approximately 60%. In the second step, the contaminating leukocytes and red blood cells in the second satellite bag were sedimented by centrifugation at 180 g for 3 min. The platelets remaining in the supernatant plasma were transferred to the empty third satellite bag to obtain NBPCs.

Nonbutton platelet concentrate method using an automatic plasma extractor

The procedure is basically the same as for the manual method, described above. An automatic plasma extractor, model ACS-210 (Terumo, Tokyo, Japan), has an optic sensor to detect the interface of buffy coat and plasma and three weight sensors to detect the volume of satellite bags (Fig. 3.3). The extractor was operated under the following conditions: the optic sensor was adjusted to position 8, the volume of buffy coat to be collected was adjusted to 30 ml, and the volume of plasma including buffy coat to be transferred to the second satellite bag was 70 ml.

*Nonbutton platelet concentrate method using a quintuple-bag system
with a small Imugard filter*

Blood (400 ml) was collected in the primary bag of a quintuple-bag system (Fig. 3.2) manufactured by Terumo (Tokyo, Japan) according to my specifications: the primary bag contains 60 ml of ACD solution, the fourth satellite bag contains 140 ml of SAGP-maltose solution [8], and a small column contains 6–7 g of Imugard filter. In the first step, the whole blood was centrifuged at 3500 g for 6 min. Approximately 100 ml of the supernatant plasma was transferred into the first satellite bag, and then the buffy coat was transferred to the second satellite bag with approximately 70 ml of residual plasma. After the connecting tubes were sealed at positions a and b, the satellite bags 1 and 2 were separated from the primary bag. In the second step, the contaminating leukocytes and red blood cells in the second satellite bag were sedimented by centrifugation at 180 g for 5 min. The platelets remaining in the supernatant plasma were transferred to the empty third satellite bag to obtain the NBPCs. In the final step, the SAGP-maltose solution in the fourth satellite bag was added to the primary bag through the filter column to resuspend red blood cells. After the primary bag was hung, the red cell suspensions were filtered through a small column containing Imugard filter to prepare leukocyte-depleted red cells at both room temperature and 4–6°C. The length of the connecting tubes from the primary bag to the fourth satellite bag had previously been adjusted to 60 cm.

Filtration through Sepacell R-500NN and Imugard 400Y filters

The LPRCs prepared by the NBPC method using a quadruple-bag system or RCCs were filtered through Sepacell R-500NN (Asahi Medical, Tokyo, Japan) or Imugard 400Y (Terumo, Tokyo, Japan) at room temperature according to their procedures.

Blood cell counts

Red blood cells, platelets, and leukocytes of more than 300/μl were counted by an electronic counter, model E-5000 (Sysmex, Kobe, Japan).

Leukocyte counts

Method for harvesting the leukocytes

The data on residual leukocytes in blood components listed in Tables 3.1–3.3 were determined by the method of Vakkila and Myllyla [9]. Red cells (10–15 ml) were hemolyzed with about 150 ml of 0.83% NH_4Cl in 0.01 mol/l $KHCO_3$ (pH 7.4) at 4°C for about 5 min. The remaining leukocytes were centrifuged at 700 **g** for 10 min, and then washed with cold phosphate buffered saline followed with RPMI-1640 medium (GIBCO Lab., NY) containing 5% fetal calf serum. After the leukocyte pellets were carefully resuspended with RPMI-1640 medium, they were transferred to the graduated tube. The leukocytes were centrifuged again at 550 g for 10 min, and then resuspended in RPMI-1640 medium so that the total volume was adjusted to 1 ml. The harvested leukocytes were stained with Türk reagent and counted in a Burker chamber.

Propidium iodide method

The data on residual leukocytes in blood components listed in Table 3.4 were determined by the modification method of Kao and Scornick [10]. The mixture of 200 μl of sample and 800 μl of propidium iodide solution containing 0.005 w/v%

Table 3.1 Properties of platelet concentrates prepared by the nonbutton platelet concentrate (NBPC) method and the conventional platelet-rich plasma (PRP) method

	PRP method ($n = 22$)	NBPC method ($n = 20$)
Volume (ml)	44 ± 5	41 ± 8
Platelet yield		
($\times 10^4/\mu l$)	156 ± 37	155 ± 33
($\times 10^{10}$/bag)	6.48 ± 1.40	6.92 ± 1.46
(%)	68.4 ± 10.6	69.5 ± 9.4
Red cell contamination		
($\times 10^2/\mu l$)	8.2 ± 6.0	0.39 ± 0.28
($\times 10^8$/bag)	3.38 ± 2.52	0.18 ± 0.14
(%)	0.016 ± 0.012	0.0009 ± 0.0007
Leukocyte contamination		
($\times 10^2/\mu l$)	2.4 ± 1.7	0.43 ± 0.69
($\times 10^7$/bag)	9.8 ± 7.0	1.9 ± 1.4
(%)	4.2 ± 3.1	0.71 ± 1.01

Table 3.2 Results of the nonbutton platelet concentrate method using an automatic plasma extractor ($n = 11$)

Product	Volume (ml)	Platelet yield (%)	Leukocyte contamination (%)	Ratio (%) of granulocytes: lymphocytes in residual WBC
Red cell concentrates	234 ± 13	7.7 ± 3.3	38.9 ± 10.8	$10:90$
Platelet-poor plasma	157 ± 2	1.9 ± 2.2	0.2 ± 0.1	NT
Platelet concentrates	42 ± 4	62.9 ± 5.8	1.7 ± 0.9	NT
Buffy coat	33 ± 7	27.6 ± 5.8	61.2 ± 10.1	$46:54$

WBC, white blood cells; NT, not tested.

Table 3.3 Leukocyte removal of red cell concentrates by the nonbutton platelet concentrate method using a quintuple-bag system with a small Imugard (IG) filter ($n = 5$)

Filters	Cotton weight (g)	Filtration temperature (°C)	Filtration time (min)	Leukocytes removal (%)	Residual leukocytes ($\times 10^7$/bag)	Ratio (%) of lymphocytes: granulocytes in residual WBC
IG-S6	6	RT	70	95.5 ± 2.4	9.54 ± 4.68	$17:83$
IG-S6	6	4–6	180	97.0 ± 2.3	5.05 ± 3.06	$35:65$
IG-S7	7	RT	120	97.8 ± 1.5	3.96 ± 1.48	$30:70$
IG-S7	7	4–6	280	99.1 ± 0.7	1.41 ± 0.57	$67:33$

RT, room temperature; WBC, white blood cells.

Table 3.4 Leukocyte removal from red cell concentrates by various combinations of the nonbutton platelet concentrate (NBPC) method and filtrations (*n* = 5)

Method	Filtration temperature (°C)	Residual leukocytes ($\times 10^6$/bag)	Leukocyte removal (%)	System (open or closed)
IG-400Y*	RT	175.0 ± 120.8	93.8 ± 4.2	Open
NBPC + IG-400Y†	RT	15.60 ± 9.10	99.1 ± 0.2	Open
NBPC + IG-S7‡	4–6	14.10 ± 5.70	99.1 ± 0.7	Closed
Sepacell§	RT	4.73 ± 3.29	99.82 ± 0.14	Open
NBPC + Sepacell**	RT	0.82 ± 0.70	99.97 ± 0.03	Open

* Prepared by filtration through Imugard 400Y.
† Prepared by a combination of the NBPC method and filtration using Imugard 400Y.
‡ Prepared by the NBPC method using a quintuple-bag system with a small Imugard filter (IG-S7).
§ Prepared by filtration through Sepacell R-500NN.
** Prepared by a combination of the NBPC method and filtration using Sepacell R-500NN.
RT, room temperature.

propidium iodide and 0.03 v/v% Nonidet P-40 were mixed well and then incubated at room temperature for 15 min. After the solution was centrifuged at 800 **g** for 5 min, 800 µl of the supernatant was discarded. The stained leukocytes were resuspended with the remaining solution (200 µl), and then 5 µl of the suspension was spotted and smeared on a slide glass for immunofluorescence study. The smear was covered with a cover glass and all leukocytes in the well were counted with the fluorescence microscope, model BH-2 (Olympus, Tokyo, Japan).

Determination of the ratio of granulocytes/lymphocytes

Measurement of size distribution

The ratio of granulocytes to lymphocytes shown in Table 3.5 was determined by measuring leukocyte size distribution using an electronic cell counter, model E-5000 (Sysmex, Kobe, Japan).

Table 3.5 Leukocyte removal from red cell concentrates by the nonbutton platelet concentrate method using a quadruple-bag system (*n* = 15)

	Residual leukocytes ($\times 10^8$/bag)	Efficacy (%) of leukocyte removal
Total leukocytes	8.46 ± 2.94	66.5 ± 3.2
Lymphocytes	0.61 ± 0.32	92.8 ± 3.2
Granulocytes	7.24 ± 2.82	53.3 ± 16.3

Peroxidase staining method

The ratio of granulocytes to lymphocytes shown in Table 3.3 was determined by the peroxidase method using a peroxidase staining kit containing 2,7-diaminofluorene as a substrate (Muto Pure Chemicals, Tokyo, Japan).

Results

The properties of PCs prepared by the NBPC method using a quadruple-bag system (Fig. 3.1) and the conventional platelet-rich plasma method are shown in Table 3.1. There was no significant difference in the platelet yield between them, but the numbers of leukocytes and red blood cells remaining in the PCs prepared by the NBPC

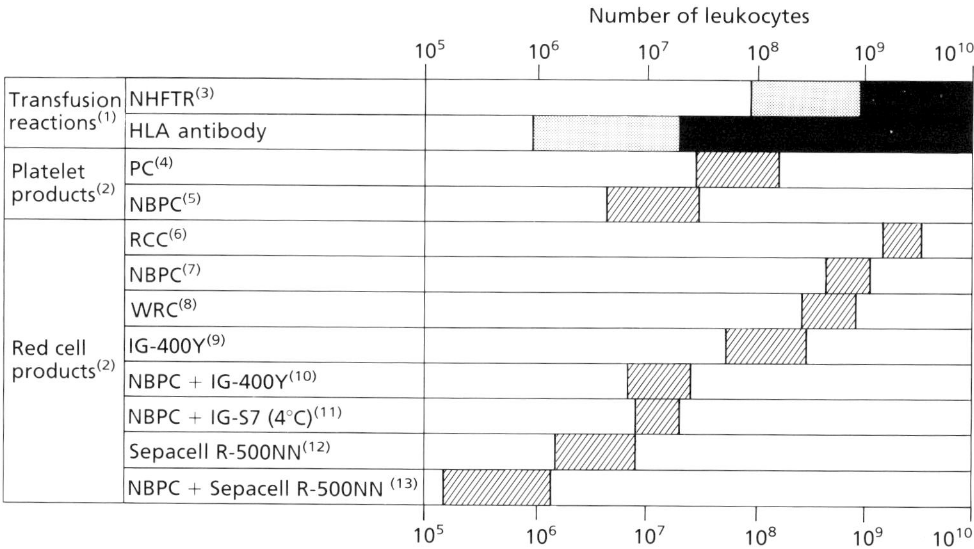

Fig. 3.4 The number of leukocytes remaining in various leukocyte-poor blood components and how effective they were in preventing transfusion reactions. [1]■ Observed; □ rarely observed; □ not observed. [2]▨ The number of leukocytes remaining in blood components. [3]NHFTR, nonhemolytic febrile transfusion reactions. [4]PC, platelet concentrates prepared by the conventional method. [5]Leukocyte-poor platelet concentrates prepared by the nonbutton platelet concentrate (NBPC) method. [6]Red cell concentrates (RCC) prepared by the conventional method. [7]Leukocyte-poor red cell concentrates prepared by the NBPC method. [8]Washed red cells (WRC) prepared by the conventional method. [9]Leukocyte-poor red cells prepared by filtration with the Imugard 400Y (IG-400Y) filter. [10]Leukocyte-depleted red cells prepared by a combination of the NBPC method and filtration using the Imugard 400Y filter. [11]Leukocyte-depleted red cells prepared by the NBPC method using a quintuple-bag system with a small Imugard filter (IG-S7). [12]Leukocyte-depleted red cells prepared by filtration using a Sepacell R-500NN filter. [13]Leukocyte-depleted red cells prepared by a combination of the NBPC method and filtration using the Sepacell R-500NN filter.

method were much lower than those in the PCs prepared by the conventional method. The volume of PCs was inclined to vary more widely in the NBPC method than in the conventional method. Approximately 66% of leukocytes were also removed from RCCs by the NBPC method, as shown in Table 3.5. Most of the residual leukocytes were granulocytes, suggesting that the method removes lymphocytes preferentially.

Table 3.2 shows the results of the distributions of platelets and leukocytes in various blood components prepared by the NBPC method using an automatic plasma extractor (Fig. 3.3). The mean numbers of remaining leukocytes in RCCs and PCs were similar to those of the components prepared by the manual NBPC method. However, the reproducibility of the volume of PCs was slightly improved by the automatic NBPC method.

Table 3.3 shows the results of preparation of leukocyte-depleted red blood cells by the NBPC method using a quintuple-bag system (Fig. 3.2) with a small Imugard filter containing 6–7 g of cotton wool. More than 95% of leukocyte removal efficiency was obtained in all conditions, even though the small filter column was used. The efficiency was better than that of LPRCs prepared by the conventional method using the Imugard 400Y filter (Table 3.4). Moreover, lowering the temperature of the procedure caused a marked increase in leukocyte removal from RCCs, though it required a longer filtration time (Table 3.3). As a result, the remaining leukocytes decreased to the level of approximately 1.4×10^7 when the IG-S7 filter was used at 4–6°C.

Furthermore, a simple combination of the NBPC method and filtration using a Sepacell filter gave leukocyte-depleted red cells containing the fewest leukocytes. That is, the RCCs prepared by the technique contained a mean 8.2×10^5 of residual leukocytes/bag, as shown in Table 3.4. However, the residual leukocytes increased to the level of 4.7×10^6 when only filtration using Sepacell was carried out.

These data are summarized in Figure 3.4.

Summary

There is much debate on how many leukocytes should be removed from blood components for preventing transfusion reactions due to leukocytes. Early studies have suggested that if blood products contain less than 1×10^9 of leukocytes per transfusion, the risk of febrile reactions could be reduced [11,12]. However, it has been found that the incidence of HLA alloimmunization depends not only on the absolute numbers of leukocytes at a single transfusion but also on frequency and intervals of transfusions [6,13]. In addition, various inherited and acquired factors in individuals affect their immune response to leukocytes. Therefore, it is difficult to indicate the exact number of leukocytes to be removed, but it is now generally admitted that HLA alloimmunization can be avoided by transfusing leukocyte-depleted blood components containing fewer than $0.5–1.5 \times 10^7$ leukocytes per transfused unit (Fig. 3.4) [6,9,14].

The author has shown in this paper that PCs and RCCs prepared by the NBPC method contained on average 1.8×10^7 and 8.5×10^8 leukocytes per unit, respectively. These products are probably effective for reducing febrile transfusion reactions, but are not necessarily efficient enough at leukocyte removal to prevent HLA alloimmunization. It seemed difficult to remove granulocytes effectively by only centrifugation, because granulocytes were not so easily located as lymphocytes in a buffy coat by high-speed centrifugation.

It was found that effective leukocyte removal from RCCs was achieved by combining the NBPC method (buffy coat removal) and filtration. For instance, the use of a quintuple-bag system with a small Imugard filter made it possible to prepare leukocyte-depleted red cells with a mean contamination of 1.4×10^7 leukocytes per unit in a closed system. Moreover, better results of leukocyte removal were obtained when filtration through Sepacell filter was carried out on the LPRCs previously prepared by the NBPC method, though the procedure was performed in an open system. The mean number of contaminating leukocytes of the product was 8.2×10^5 per unit — almost equal to one-sixth that (4.7×10^6) of red cells prepared by filtration alone. These products should be effective in avoiding HLA immunization. Consequently, this technique is considered effective in preparing LPRCs, because centrifugation (by the NBPC method) removes lymphocytes preferentially, as described above and filtration eliminates granulocytes more effectively than lymphocytes [15].

The number of contaminating leukocytes in various leukocyte-poor blood components and their efficacy are summarized in Figure 3.4. The author considers that these products can be used in the following ways: (i) the LPRCs, with approximately 8×10^8 of residual leukocytes prepared by the NBPC method, are used for general transfusions or as starting material for filtration; (ii) leukocyte-depleted PCs with 1×10^7 of residual leukocytes prepared by the NBPC method and leukocyte-depleted red cells prepared by the use of a quintuple-bag system are used for reducing HLA alloimmunization; and (iii) leukocyte-depleted red cells prepared by combining buffy coat removal (the NBPC method) and filtration through Sepacell filter are for preventing HLA immunization, especially in massive blood transfusions.

The major advantage of the NBPC method is that leukocyte-poor blood components, including RCCs and PCs, can be prepared in a closed system. Thus, the system enables the expiry period of these products to be prolonged, with the result that these products can be widely adopted in transfusion. In addition, this technique has many other merits: (i) damage to platelets is minimized by not forming a platelet button during their isolation; (ii) the preservative can be added to the red cells after their isolation, allowing adjustment of the preservative and hematocrit of RCCs; and (iii) about 25% more plasma than usual can be harvested.

In spite of these advantages, some difficulties remain to be solved before the NBPC method can be applied routinely: it is a complicated procedure and its reproducibility is somewhat low. It was found that these problems could be improved by the use of an automatic plasma extractor such as Terumo ACS-210. The apparatus has an optic sensor to detect the interface of buffy coat and plasma layers in the primary bag, as well as weight sensors to control the collecting volume to the satellite bags, as shown in Figure 3.3. The conditions of these sensors are changeable. Thus, the extractor made it possible to obtain an easy operation and good reproducibility.

In conclusion, the NBPC method, especially the technique using a quintuple-bag system with a small Imugard filter, is considered to be useful to prepare leukocyte-depleted blood components containing less than approximately 1×10^7 leukocytes per unit in a closed system.

References

1 Dauset J. Leukoagglutinins. IV. Leukoagglutinins and blood transfusion. *Vox Sang* 1954;4:190–198.
2 Brittingham TE. Immunologic studies on leukocytes. *Vox Sang* 1957;2:242–248.
3 Brittingham TE, Chaplin HJ Jr. Febrile transfusion reactions caused by sensitivity to donor leukocytes and platelets. *JAMA* 1957;165:819–825.
4 Herzig RH, Herzig GP, Bull MI *et al.* Correction of poor platelet transfusion responses with leukocyte-poor HLA matched platelet concentrates. *Blood* 1975;46:743–750.
5 Eernisse JG, Brand A. Prevention of platelet refractoriness due to HLA antibodies by administration of leukocyte-poor blood components. *Expl Hematol* 1981;9:77–83.
6 Fisher M, Chapman JR, Ting A, Morris TJ. Alloimmunization to HLA antigens following transfusion with leukocyte-poor and purified platelet suspensions. *Vox Sang* 1985;49:331–335.
7 Uda M, Okada H, Ishii A, Nishizaki T. Non-button PC method: a gentler procedure for preparing platelet concentrates. *Jpn J Transfus Med* 1985;31:385–390.
8 Uda M, Ohkuma S, Ishii A, Nishizaki T. Preparation of blood components with saline-adenine-glucose-phosphate-maltose quadruple-pack system. *Transfusion* 1985;25:325–329.
9 Vakkila J, Myllyla G. Amount and type of leukocytes in leukocyte-free red cell and platelet concentrates. *Vox Sang* 1987;53:76–82.
10 Kao KJ, Scornik JC. Accurate quantitation of the low number of white cells in white cell-depleted blood components. *Transfusion* 1989;29:774–777.
11 Brittingham TE, Chaplin H Jr. The antigenicity of normal and leukemic human leukocytes. *Blood* 1961;17:139–165.
12 Perkins HA, Pane R, Ferguson J, Wood M. Nonhemolytic febrile transfusion reactions. Quantitative effects of blood components with emphasis on isoantigenic incompatibility of leukocytes. *Vox Sang* 1966;11:578–600.
13 Murakami S, Sato K, Orii T. The incidence of antileukocyte antibodies in blood transfusion. *Immunohaematology* 1980;2:1–7.
14 Sirchia G, Parravicini A, Rubulla P, Greppi N, Scalamogna M, Morelati F. Effectiveness of red blood cells filtered through cotton wool to prevent antileukocyte antibody production in multitransfused patients. *Vox Sang* 1982;42:190–197.
15 Kikugawa K, Minoshima K. Filter columns for preparation of leukocyte-poor blood for transfusion. *Vox Sang.* 1978;34:281–290.

Discussion

Iᴛᴏ (Kyoto University Medical School): It is said that fewer leukocytes are observed in blood products after the second filtration. Dr Meryman made the same comment in his presentation. I suppose, the reason for this is probably that the competition among leukocytes exists in the first filtration but it may not be so in the second filtration. Can we reduce the number of residual leukocytes to almost zero by repeated filtrations or do any of the subsets still remain in the blood products? Is it required to use different kinds of filters?

MIYAHARA: Do you mean repeated filtration with the same filter?

ITO: Dr Meryman used the same Pall filter. Is it better to combine the different kind of filters to get more efficient removal?

MIYAHARA: I cannot comment on this with certainty, however, I suppose about 1 log reduction will be possible. I cannot say which is more effective, double filtrations or the combination of centrifugation and single filtration, but I think the removal of buffy coat would be applied to all blood products with a removal efficiency of 60–70%. The leukocyte-depleted products will be easily produced from this buffy coat-removed product. The combination of different kinds of removal methods will be better than a double filtration method. One example is the combination of centrifugation, while lymphocytes are removed preferentially, and filtration, while granulocytes are depleted. Alternatively, double filtration with different type of filters might be interesting.

SEKIGUCHI: It is unknown whether double filtration with the same filter that can remove by 3 log in a single filtration can achieve 6 log reduction. The mechanism of leukocyte depletion has not been clarified yet. If we could make it clear, we would propose various combinations of several methods such as double filters and others.

MIYAHARA: As you know, microaggregate filters are often used at the bedside. Dr Wenz reported how to improve leukocyte removal efficiency of microaggregate filters. He had tried centrifugation under low temperature just before filtration, because the formation of microaggregates is essential for removing leukocytes by microaggregate filters. But I think the leukocyte removal is still too low to avoid HLA alloimmunization. The Pall filter that you mentioned is not for microaggregates but for leukocyte depletion, isn't it?

TAKAHASHI: It seems to me that it is the uniform concept that leukocyte depletion should be performed at blood centers. I think we should perform leukocyte depletion and quality control of blood products at blood centers and deliver them to the clinical side. I'm sure this is the method used all over the world.

4 · Properties of the Factor VIII/von Willebrand factor complex in stored banked blood

A. Farrugia, S. Douglas, G. Whyte, R. Harrap, G. Raines,*
S. Sykes,* H. Aumann,† A. Street,† and A. Oates‡

*Red Cross Blood Bank, Victoria, Departments of *Clinical Chemistry and †Haematology, Alfred Hospital,
and ‡Commonwealth Serum Laboratories, Victoria, Australia*

Abstract

We have studied the storage properties of Factor VIII/von Willebrand factor (vWF) in banked blood (Fig. 4.1), using a range of biologic and immunologic assays. Von Willebrand activity, as assessed by collagen-binding and ristocetin cofactor assays, started to decay in blood units stored at 4°C at 5 days postcollection. This loss in activity was accompanied by a loss of high molecular weight multimers of vWF in SDS agarose electrophoresis and two-dimensional crossed immunoelectrophoresis. However, storage of blood filtered with a high-efficiency leukocyte-removal filter, Sepacell R-500CS, resulted in significantly improved stability of both vWF and Factor VIII activity ($P < 0.05$) for 10 days post-blood collection. Multimeric structure of vWF was also improved in filtered blood. Measurements performed at both 4 and 22°C indicated a preferential loss of all activities at banked blood temperatures; however, loss was decreased at 22°C and parallel biologic and immunologic assays suggested a combination of physical loss and proteolytic degradation. White cell removal resulted in a decreased loss at both temperatures for Factor VIII, but only improved vWF preservation at 4°C.

We conclude that part of the storage lesion of Factor VIII/vWF in banked blood is due to physical removal/degradation from interactions with white cells. This effect may contribute to the hemostatic aberrations observed upon transfusion of large volumes of banked blood.

Discussion

BROZOVIĆ: It's a very interesting, fascinating presentation. Do you intend to apply the same technique on platelet concentrates which are stored at 22°C, where we know there is an interaction between vWF platelets and endothelium?

WHYTE: Yes. It will be very interesting, particularly the present findings of macroaggregates, those fluffy clouds of platelets which appear in stored platelets, because they are a problem to which I don't have an answer at the moment.

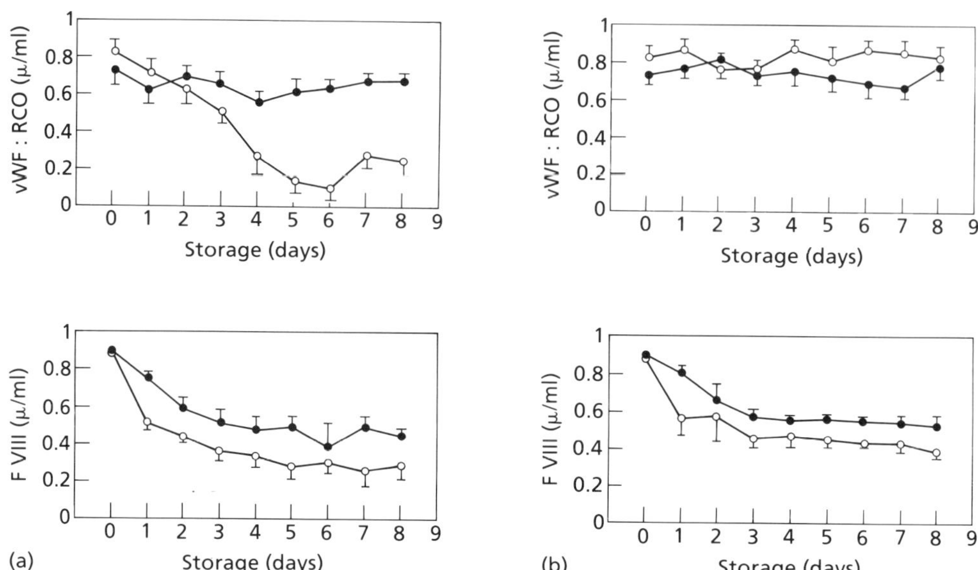

Fig. 4.1 Factor VIII (F VIII) and von Willebrand factor (vWF) in stored blood at (a) 4°C and (b) 22°C. Mean ± s.d. of 6 u. ● filtered; ○ unfiltered. RCO, ristocetin cofactor.

SNIECINSKI: Very, very interesting data. These fluffy macroaggregates may explain the failure of filters in certain cases during filtration of the platelet components when the filters become clotted and it is impossible to filter platelet concentrates. The reason for that has not been known, so that may be another explanation of that phenomenon.

WHYTE: Yes, it may be a totally temperature-dependent, but perhaps a very early, degradation effect of vWF.

Part 2
Laboratory Aspects

5 · Multicenter studies on leukocyte depletion by filtration of red cell and platelet concentrates: methodology and controls

M. Masse and the Produits Sanguins Labiles (PSL)
Working Group

Centre Régional de Transfusion Sanguine, 1 Boulevard A. Fleming, 25020 Besançon, France

Abstract

The ever-improving performances of the filtration procedure make it possible to obtain blood products with a residual leukocyte content of between 10^5 and 10^6. Such improvements make it necessary to use identical protocols together with standardized counting methods. In order to assess precisely filtration results, the French working group Produits Sanguins Labiles PSL, composed of 21 transfusion teams, has carried out two large-scale studies on filtration of 1400 red blood cell (RBC) suspensions, equally divided into RBCs and buffycoat (BC)-free RBCs, and on filtration of over 700 platelet concentrates (PCs), collected with different cell separators (first- and second-generation), prepared with the platelet-rich plasma (PRP) or BC pool method. All postfiltration white cell counts were performed with a Nageotte hemacytometer (volume of chamber: 50 µl; limit of sensitivity: 0.2 white blood cells (WBCs/µl). This method has been validated and its precision (below 25%) determined by a technical consensus. In order to increase 10- to 20-fold the sensitivity of this technique, a modified method, including a concentration step of sample, before counting, is validated in reference ranges, varying from 0.01 to 12 WBCs/µl, with a good correlation coefficient (from 0.929 to 0.996).

Results show significant differences among the studied filters (six for RBCs and five for platelets). Eighty percent of filtered BC-free RBC units contained less than 1×10^6 WBCs/µl, compared to only 40% of filtered standard RBC. Before filtration, two groups of platelet suspensions are distinguished: with a high (Group I) or low level (Group II) of contaminating WBC. Here again, filtration results are significantly better with the second group: more than 95% on the filtered platelet suspension, in this group, contained less than 1×10^6 residual WBCs, compared to only 60% in Group I.

Introduction

Since the 1950s, it has been clearly established that removing the BC from blood units could prevent and suppress posttransfusion nonhemolytic febrile reactions [1]. Significant work has continued to demonstrate the beneficial effect of leukocyte-depleted blood components [2]. It is generally admitted that refractoriness to platelets, human leukocyte antigen (HLA) alloimmunization or transmission of viruses such as cytomegalovirus (CMV) or human T lymphotropic virus I (HTLV-I) can be reduced or avoided by transfusing leukocyte-depleted RBCs or platelets, in other words containing less than 1×10^6 nucleated cells per transfused unit [3–6].

Efficient removal of these contaminating leukocytes is obtained by filtration. It is currently unequivocally recognized that filtration is the simplest and most efficient method for preparing leukocyte-depleted red cells and platelets [7]. Numerous publications have focused on comparing commercially available filters [8,9]. Constant progress has been made with regard to filtering materials, which has led to a more than 3 log depletion. The ever-improving performances of the filtration procedures [10,11] make it possible to obtain blood products (red cells and platelets) with a residual leukocyte content comprised between 10^5 and 10^6, and, in the near future, less than 10^5. Such improvements make it necessary to observe some criteria to appreciate the efficiency of filtration [12,13]. A review of different publications shows extremely variable results with the commercial filters now available [14–18]. These differences can partly be accounted for by the heterogeneity of the blood products to be filtered [19], and also by the absence of standardized protocols and validated counting methods, able to detect very low concentrations, of nearly 1 WBC/µl.

In order to evaluate accurately the current performance of filtration and to assess filtration results, the French working group PSL, incorporating 21 transfusion centers and quality control laboratories, has carried out two large-scale studies for over 1 year. The first study includes some 1400 RBC suspension filtrations, equally divided into standard RBCs and BC-free RBCs. The other study was performed on over 700 platelet suspension filtrations, prepared with different apheresis machines, random PCs and BC pools. The success and therefore the interest of this national study rest for a large part on the large number of controls (over 3000) performed with a single and simple counting method, using the Nageotte chamber (Marienfeld KG, Bad Mergentheim, Germany). This counting method has been validated and its precision determined by a technical consensus.

Materials and methods

Filtration of red blood cells

Blood was drawn from healthy donors into triple or quadruple bags from different manufacturers. The mean volume of whole blood drawn was 431 ± 76 ml, and the mean original hemoglobin mass, prior to any manipulation, was 60 ± 10 g. Two types of blood suspensions were prepared after hard or soft-spin centrifugation: standard blood concentrates (or RBC concentrates) and leukocyte-depleted blood concentrates (or BC-poor RBC concentrates). BC removal was performed manually or automatically using three pieces of equipment: Optipress (Baxter Healthcare,

Deerfield, IL, USA), Compomat (NBPI, Amstelveen, The Netherlands), and EX-30 (Terumo France, St Quentin en Yvelines, France). The BC was removed 0–15 days postcollection.

About 1400 filtrations were carried out and analyzed, using six commercially available filters with homogeneous filter lots. Each filter was tested in at least three different blood transfusion centers. A common protocol was respected throughout the study. RBC concentrates and BC-poor RBC concentrates were filtered by gravity (difference in height: 120 cm) immediately after removal from storage at 4 °C and a single unit was filtered through each filter. Filtration temperature never exceeded 10 °C. For each filter, filtration procedures were performed as prescribed by the manufacturer. The following filters were chosen on the basis of their availability at the time of the study: Erypur and Optima g-2 (Organon Teknika, Boxtel, Holland), IgE (Terumo, Tokyo, Japan), Leukotrap (Cutter Biological, West Haven, NY, USA), Pall RC-50 (Pall Biomedical, Glen Cove, NY, USA), and Sepacell R-500N (Asahi Medical, Tokyo, Japan). The Leukotrap filter (filter A) is a closed kit (it is an on-line filter) and it includes the filter and harvesting bags. The filter is primed with the additive solution contained in one of the bags, prior to red cell filtration. The Erypur filter (filter B) is used with an automated system (Prestomat, Organon Teknika) which incorporates a priming and a rinsing stage. The filters C (IgE), G (Optima g-2), and E (R-500N) were rinsed, after filtration, with 50 ml of saline. The filters D (RC-50) and F (R-500N) were used directly without priming or rinsing.

The samples needed for the different controls were collected immediately after each filtration, either on 20 cm tubing or by sterile transfer into a bag, after multistripping homogenization. We took into account prefiltration and postfiltration values of volume, hemoglobin, and WBC content of each RBC unit. The volume of RBC suspensions was calculated by dividing net weight by a factor of 1.05. Pre- and postfiltration RBC concentration and prefiltration WBC counts were determined using different automated counters.

Filtration of platelet suspensions

Four groups of PCs were prepared:

1 Group I (PC): pooled PCs obtained following the conventional PRP method. The pools are made from 7–12 donors.

2 Group II (BC-PC): pooled BC PCs obtained with the BC method. Two different methods were used to prepare platelets from diluted BC: from single or from pooled BC with a conventional quadruple bag or a "top and bottom" bag. With regard to the importance of leukocyte depletion by filtration, the pooled method was more effective. The pools are made up from BC of six to seven donors.

3 Group III (APC1): this group concerns apheresis platelet concentrates, obtained with first-generation equipment: CS-3000 (Baxter Healthcare, Deerfield, IL, USA), IBM-2997 (Cobe, Lakewood, CO, USA), V-50 (Haemonetics, Braintree, MA, USA).

4 Group IV (APC2): a new generation of equipment Cobe Spectra (Cobe, Lakewood, CO, USA) provided us with a new generation of platelet concentrates.

Two groups of apheresis platelets were defined according to the initial level of contaminating WBCs:

1 APC1: high WBC contamination (5×10^8).
2 APC2: low WBC contamination ($<10 \times 10^6$).

The different PCs were filtered by gravity at room temperature. For each filter, procedures were performed as prescribed by the manufacturers. About 740 filtrations were carried out using five commercially available filters: Pall PL-100, Pall PL-50, Sepacell PL-10, Sepacell PL-5, and Terumo IG-500 (past-generation filter). The filtrations were distributed as follows: IG-500: Groups I and II; PL-100: Groups I and III; PL-50: Groups II and IV; PL-5N: Groups II and IV; PL-10N: groups I–IV.

Several parameters were measured or calculated before each filtration. We took into account volume, platelet, and WBC content as well as time of filtration. The volume of platelet suspensions was calculated by dividing net weight by 1.03. The number of residual leukocytes was determined by manual counting using the Nageotte chamber.

Postfiltration WBC counting method

The number of residual leukocytes was determined by manual counting using a Nageotte hemocytometer. The counting chamber has a volume of 50 µl and the theoretical limit of sensitivity is 0.2 WBC/µl. This simple, inexpensive method uses 50 µl of filtered RBC solution or filtered platelet suspension, diluted 1 : 10 in Plaxan lysis solution (Fiers, Kortrijk, Belgium). The sample is allowed to settle for 20 min and optical reading is performed by microscope (20-fold magnification). Each Nageotte hemocytometer is made up of two identical chambers (2×20 µl). The second chamber is counted when no leukocyte is found in the first one. Optical reading is made easier by the use of a metal-based Nageotte chamber. The maximum counting time per hemacytometer is 20 min. The method is adapted to the detection of low leukocyte concentrations ranging from 10^5 to 10^6 WBCs per filtered unit.

Reliability

In order to determine the accuracy of this method, nine samples with concentrations varying from 0.5 to 40 leukocytes per µl were counted simultaneously in one laboratory by seven technicians, following the same protocol and using identical equipment. The samples were prepared by serially diluting an RBC concentrate, whose BC had been previously removed and thus partially WBC-depleted. The actual WBC concentration of these samples was estimated from the mean of seven countings. The coefficient of variation (CV) was calculated for each concentration.

Validation

With a view to testing our counting method, we prepared four theoretic ranges of increasing leukocyte concentration by adding known volumes of fresh suspensions of mononuclear cells, to pure RBC or platelet suspensions (obtained after three successive filtrations). Each range included 30 samples of different concentration, covering a wide range: (a) 0.2–12; (b) 0.02–0.4; (c) 0.02–0.5; and (d) 0.02–0.8 WBCs/µl. Each tested range corresponds to a different preparation of sample: (a) RBC suspension diluted 10-fold, as previously described; (b) pure RBC sample; (c) RBC suspension concentrated two-fold; and (d) pure platelet suspension. For (b), (c), and (d) samples, a large volume (15 ml) of lysis solution (either Plaxan, for RBC solution, or acetic acid 3%, for platelet suspension), is added to 1 ml (b, d), or 2 ml (c) of pure sample. After allowing to rest for 6 min and centrifuging at 1600 g for 6 min, the supernatant is discarded and the final volume of the suspension is adjusted at 1 ml precisely.

Results

Prefiltration

Red blood cell suspensions

A total of 1435 products, grouped into RBC concentrates (n = 745) and BC-poor RBC concentrates (n = 690), were assayed before filtration. For RBC concentrates, mean volume was 288 ± 49 ml, total hemoglobin content 58 ± 11 g, hematocrit 62 ± 7%, and there was a mean value of 22.6 ± 10.1 × 10^8 WBCs/unit. For BC-poor RBC concentrates, mean volume was 247 ± 41 ml; total hemoglobin mass 54 ± 9 g; hematocrit 66 ± 8%; and there was a mean value of 8.4 ± 5.5 × 10^8 WBCs/unit. It must be noted that, despite the great disparity in methods (manual or automated), BC removal led to an approximate 65% WBC depletion, along with a mean hemoglobin loss of 4 g, i.e. 93% RBC recovery. Thus, the total hemoglobin mass of the BC-poor RBC group is significantly lower than that of the non-BC-depleted group ($P < 10^{-4}$).

Platelet suspensions

The heterogeneity of platelet suspensions, especially concerning the initial level of contaminating leukocytes is illustrated in Table 5.1. There is an important difference before filtration between the number of WBCs in Groups I and II on the one hand, and Groups III and IV on the other hand. This is why two "families" of platelet suspensions are distinguished: one family (PC and APC1) with high levels of WBCs and the other one (BC-PC and APC2) with low levels of WBCs.

Table 5.1 Prefiltration results of platelet suspensions

Platelet suspension	No. tested	Volume (ml)	Platelets 10^{11}	Leukocytes 10^6	No. donors/ unit
PC	253	454 ± 79	5.7 ± 1.3	411 ± 226	9
APC1	182	318 ± 93	5.3 ± 1.9	340 ± 412	1
BC-PC	195	276 ± 43	4 ± 0.7	66 ± 102	6
APC2	107	420 ± 77	5.2 ± 1.0	5.2 ± 7.9	1

APC1, apheresis platelet concentrates group 1; APC2, apheresis platelet concentrate group 2; BC-PC, buffy coat platelet concentrate; PC, platelet concentrate.

Hemoglobin loss

The amount of hemoglobin lost during filtration (expressed in g) constitutes the greatest limiting factor; it depends on certain features of the filter (fiber quality, volume of filter housing), and on the filtration procedure (priming, saline rinsing, air rinsing, no rinsing). Table 5.2 shows the postfiltration total hemoglobin according to filter type and red cell suspension, varying from 54 to 39 g. This table shows that the hemoglobin loss due to filtration differs greatly from filter to filter: it varies from 5.7 g for the Leukotrap filter to 17.3 for the R-500N filter. Leukotrap, IgE, and RC-50 filters induce a relatively low loss (<7 g); Erypur and R500 filters (with rinsing) induce intermediary losses ranging from 7.1 to 9.2 g. Finally, Optima g-2 and Sepacell filters (without rinsing) result in considerable losses, ranging from 14 g (24%) to 17 g (30%). The mean difference in hemoglobin content (about 4 g), observed prior to filtration between the two groups, is still found postfiltration. This shows that hemoglobin loss, due to filtration only, is identical for the two groups of RBC concentrates. No significant difference was observed ($P > 0.05$).

Table 5.2 Total hemoglobin (Hb) and hemoglobin loss, according to filter type and red blood cell (RBC) suspension (mean ± s.d.)

Filters	Group I RBC concentrates			Group II BC-poor RBC		
	n	Total Hb (g)	Hb loss (%)	n	Total Hb (g)	Hb loss (%)
Leukotrap	8	54 ± 6	5.7 ± 2.2	54	47 ± 7	6.4 ± 2.2
Erypur	88	53 ± 9	8.0 ± 4.4	72	43 ± 7	7.1 ± 5.1
IgE	104	53 ± 9	6.4 ± 3.4	76	51 ± 7	5.8 ± 2.9
RC-50	148	50 ± 11	6.6 ± 4.0	110	48 ± 9	6.9 ± 1.9
R-500	121	47 ± 11	9.2 ± 6.7	88	41 ± 9	8.7 ± 3.3
R-500 no rinsing	65	50 ± 8	16.5 ± 2.1	63	42 ± 6	17.3 ± 2.5
Optima g-2	113	43 ± 9	13.9 ± 3.9	172	39 ± 9	14.0 ± 4.4

BC, buffy coat.

Platelet recovery

The amount of platelets lost during filtration (expressed as a percentage or in number of platelets) constitutes the limiting factor. It depends on the volume of filter housing and on the filtration procedure, but also on the presence of microaggregates. This undesirable phenomenon must be avoided before starting the filtration. These observations make it necessary to give a prudent interpretation of results. According to platelet suspensions, platelet recovery is 90–91% with PL50, 89–91% with Ig500, 88–91% with PL-100, 86–88% with PL-10N, and 85–87% with PL-5N.

Leukocyte-depletion

Red cell filtration

In terms of leukocyte-depletion, the comparative efficiencies of the six filters, Erypur, Optima g-2, IgE, R-500N, Leukotrap, and RC-50, are illustrated in Table 5.3. In our study, the efficiency of the IgE filter is much lower than that of other filters: the median of residual leukocytes obtained after filtering RBC concentrates through IgE is 40×10^6, whereas it ranged from 0.4 to 4.1×10^6 with the other filters. Similarly, BC-poor RBC concentrates filtered with the IgE filter have a median of 7×10^6 residual leukocytes versus only 0.1–0.9×10^6 with the other filters. In addition to residual WBC median postfiltration, this table shows the distribution (expressed as a percentage) of the results around the 5×10^6 limit. Considerable differences can be observed, arising from filter type and type of RBC suspension filtered (RBC concentrates versus BC-poor RBC concentrates). With the exception of the IgE filter, whose performance

Table 5.3 Residual white blood cells (WBCs; median $\times 10^6$) according to filter and red blood cell (RBC) suspension

Filters	n	Group I RBC concentrates Median $\times 10^6$	% values $<5 \pm 10^6$	n	Group II BC-poor RBC Median $\times 10^6$	% values $<5 \times 10^6$
Leukotrap	9	4.1	70	54	0.9	91
Erypur	94	2.7	61	78	0.4	99
IgE	112	40	12	79	7	46
RC-50	148	1.7	74	110	0.3	99
R-500N	225	1.5	87	166	0.5	100
Optima g-2	114	0.4	89	173	0.1	100
Cumulative (except IgE)	590	1.5	80	581	0.3	99

BC, buffy coat.

Table 5.4 Residual white blood cells (WBCs; median $\times 10^6$) according to filter and platelet suspension

Filters	Median $\times 10^6$		Median $\times 10^6$	
	PC	APC1	BC-PC	APC2
Ig-500	1.9		<0.04	
PL-100	1.5	1.6		
PL-50			<0.11	<0.17
PL-10N	1.1	1.1	<0.04	<0.12
PL-5N			<0.04	<0.06
All filters:				
Median $\times 10^6$	1.5	1.2	<0.05	<0.11
% $< 5 \times 10^6$	90	82	100	100
% $< 1 \times 10^6$	34	42	95	99
% $< 5 \times 10^5$	2	3	69	50

is markedly inferior, the median of residual WBCs is 1.5×10^6 for RBC concentrates ($n = 590$) and 0.34×10^6 for BC-poor RBC concentrates ($n = 581$). The results are significantly different ($P < 10^8$: Wilcoxon test). Furthermore, 20% of the same filtered RBC concentrates contain more than 5×10^6 WBCs, versus only 1% of the filtered BC-poor RBC concentrates. These two observations confirm the beneficial effect of BC removal on reducing the final content of contaminating leukocytes.

Platelet suspension filtration

In Table 5.4, comparative efficiencies of the five filters do not show significant differences within each group of platelet suspensions. The median of residual WBCs ranges from 1.1 to 1.9×10^6 for the BC and APC1 groups. For the other groups (BC-PC and APC2 groups) a significant difference (more than 1 log) was observed, since the median of residual WBCs varied from 0.04 to 0.17×10^6. Furthermore, this median value was over-estimated. Indeed, we noted that the sensitivity limit of our counting method proved insufficient, since in more than 50% of the counts we found fewer than 0.2 WBC/µl (or no leukocytes detectable on the Nageotte chamber).

White blood cell counting method

Reliability

For this study we adopted the Nageotte chamber and tried to determine the accuracy of this counting method. Figure 5.1 shows the CV obtained from nine samples with leukocyte concentrations varying from 0.5 to 42.9 WBCs/µl, and tested by seven

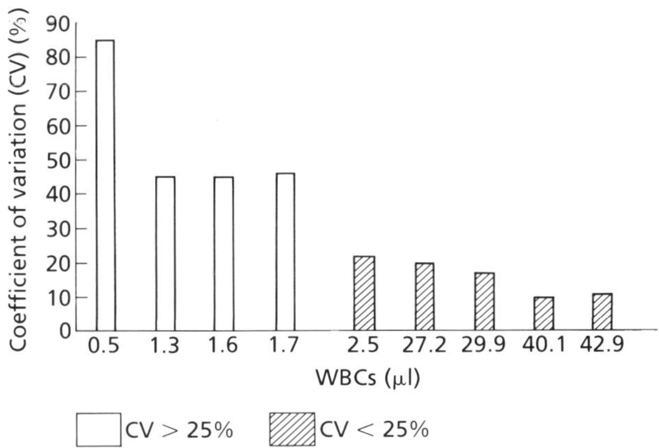

Fig. 5.1 Reliability of white blood cell (WBC) counting method, expressed as a coefficient of variation (CV).

different technicians. The higher the concentration, the lower the CV. If a maximal CV of 25% is admitted, this chart affirms that in our study, only the results obtained with concentrations higher than 2.5 WBCs/μl (0.7×10^6 WBCs per filtered unit) can be considered reliable. This implies that even very experienced operators need to be extremely careful when counting samples with very low leukocyte concentrations (<1 WBC/μl). Like any counting method, the method we adopted for this study has a limit of detection. Here it would be a theoretic limit of 1 WBC counted, i.e. 0.2 WBCs/μl. It is obvious that this theoretic limit, based on the detection of one single cell, cannot yield accurate results. The interlaboratory controls carried out for this study provide an approach to determining the limit of the Nageotte chamber. Indeed, we observed during the study that in spite of a standardized procedure and extremely rigorous sampling, the reliability limit was 2.5 WBCs/μl with a CV of 25%.

Validation

We undertook to test a modification of our counting method, by introducing a concentration step of RBC or platelet samples, to detect leukocyte concentrations as low as 0.01 WBC/μl in RBC suspension and 0.02 WBC/μl in platelet suspension.

We chose to correlate our method with known ranges of WBC concentration (mononuclear cells), varying from 0.01 to 12 WBCs/μl, and to evaluate its accuracy. The results of the validation of the counting method are summarized in Figure 5.2. This figure shows the validated methods using the Nageotte chamber. Method (a) corresponds to the Nageotte method previously described and used for the PSL investigations. Methods (b) and (c) are especially used for RBC suspensions. Method (d) was used for platelet suspensions.

This validation was carried out on four groups of about 30 samples. In this figure,

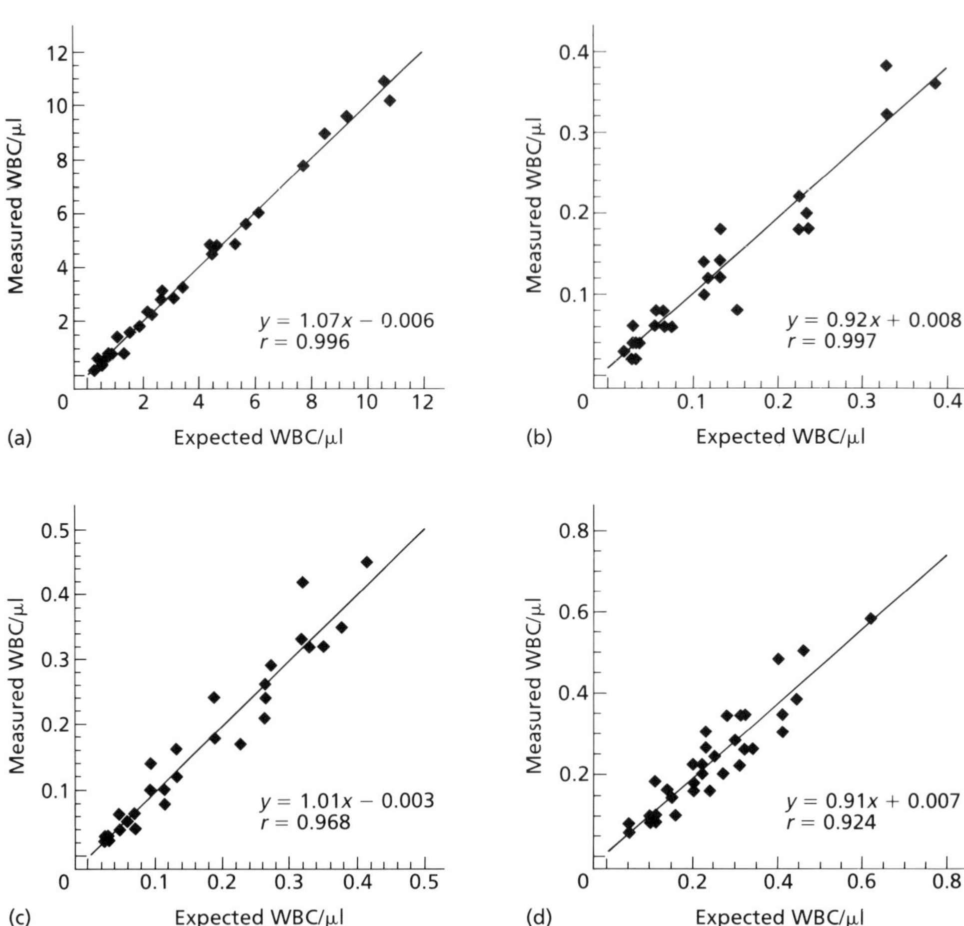

Fig. 5.2 Validation of the Nageotte chamber white blood cell (WBC) counting method. (a) 0.2–12 WBC/μl; (b) 0.02–0.4 WBC/μl; (c) 0.01–0.5 WBC/μl; (d) 0.02–0.8 WBC/μl. See text for details.

the values of WBC concentration measured by the Nageotte chamber are plotted as a function of the expected values. It can be seen in all four groups that there is a linear relationship between the measured and expected values, with excellent correlation coefficients ranging from 0.996 to 0.929. The slopes of this curves are nearly equal to 1.

Table 5.5 shows that we should not expect more than 25% accuracy. Indeed, with Group a, in 90% of cases, the differences between measured and expected values were less than 25%. In Group c, in 70% of cases the differences were less than 25%. Thus, increasing the sensitivity to 0.01 WBC/μl, by concentrating the sample, makes it possible to detect a minimal number of about 2.5×10^3 residual leukocytes per transfused unit, which corresponds to a more than 5 log depletion. These results

Table 5.5 Accuracy of the counting method: difference (%) between measured and expected values

	Difference <25%	Difference <10%
Group a:	25/28	21/28
(0.2–12 WBC/µl)	(90%)	(80%)
Group b:	21/30	9/30
(0.01–0.5 WBC/µl)	(70%)	(30%)

WBC, white blood cell.

substantiate the use of a Nageotte chamber to quantitate precisely low levels of residual WBCs — between 0.01 and 10 WBCs/µl in RBC and platelet suspensions.

Summary

Efficient removal of contaminating leukocytes from red cell or platelet suspensions is currently obtained by filtration. Systematic BC removal from RBCs [20], together with preparation of partially purified platelets, such as platelets obtained from BC or from the new apheresis procedure [21], is particularly beneficial for filtration, especially if we refer to clinical studies describing thresholds of HLA alloimmunization [22], refractoriness to platelets [23], and virus transmission [24,25], approaching 1×10^6 WBC per transfused unit. But the interpretation of results concerning filtration-induced leukocyte depletion depends greatly on the accuracy of the method used to perform WBC counts [26]. The ever-improving performances of filters, leading to a more than 3 $\log_{10}$ depletion, make it necessary to use a sufficiently sensitive counting method which is able to detect less than 0.1 WBC/µl [27–32]. General publications demonstrate interest in the flow cytometric technique [33–35], even though the concentration levels seem to be currently limited to 0.1 WBC/µl.

We chose to count and validate our assays on a Nageotte chamber using variable volumes of RBC or platelet samples. In these studies, the theoretic limit of detection was 0.2 WBC/µl. The interlaboratory controls carried out demonstrate the reliability limit: 2.5 WBCs/µl with a CV equal to 25%. This observation makes it necessary to give a prudent interpretation of the results. We are convinced that the 0.2 WBC/µl absolute sensitivity is insufficient with regard to future improvements in filtration. Therefore a concentration step of the sample is necessary. We developed a simple and reproducible counting method using the Nageotte chamber, able to detect leukocyte concentrations as low as 0.01 WBC/µl in RBC suspensions and 0.02 WBC/µl in platelet suspensions. The results we obtained show a good correlation coefficient through different reference ranges (from 0.01 to 12 WBCs/µl). Now, by this modified counting method, we are able to measure a nearly 6 log depletion. This counting method can easily be implemented in routine use and must include periodic validaton.

These studies confirm that the current efficiency of filtration is opening the way for new products, adapted to new therapeutic indications. Analysis of the results of red cell filtration shows that the efficiency of filtration, expressed in log depletion (log (pre-WBC) – log (post-WBC)) is almost identical for both groups: 3.18 log for filtration of regular RBCs versus 3.41 log for BC-poor RBCs. Nevertheless, the final result, in terms of residual WBCs, is better after BC removal: 78% of filtered BC-depleted RBC concentrates contain less than 1×10^6 leukocytes versus only 43% of regular RBC concentrates. This improvement is obtained at the expense of a greater hemoglobin loss: 79% of filtered RBC concentrates contain more than 40 g of hemoglobin versus only 62% of filtered BC-poor RBC concentrates. Thus a compromise must be found between great leukocyte removal and great red cell loss.

Differences between filters with regard to hemoglobin loss are significant, and can be accounted for mainly by differences in size and filtration procedures, and to a much lesser extent, by a degree of inaccuracy in measuring. We think that RBC filtration should not generate a more than 10% loss, i.e. approximately 6 g of hemoglobin. This is most important when this method is applied to BC-poor RBC concentrates, since BC removal alone results in a hemoglobin loss of 4 g. Improvements are expected if filter sizes diminish, or if bypass tubing is used, thus permitting air rinsing. It should be noted that this new procedure, which was used successfully at the end of this study, on a Sepacell filter, reduced hemoglobin loss. Further improvements are still to be made.

As for red cell filtration, this study on platelet suspensions proved that leukocyte-depletion by filtration allows most blood centers to reach a high level of platelet purification: about 90% of filtered PC or APC1 contained less than 5×10^6 WBCs, while about 95–99% of filtered BC-PC and APC2 contained less than 1×10^6 WBCs. This improvement is obtained through using new equipment and procedures. At this point, we have to remember that our objective is to prevent HLA immunization, refractory state and CMV, HTLV-I infections, using leukocyte-depleted blood components.

RBC and platelet filtration is becoming necessary to offer patients the best products with the minimal deleterious effects. Finally, the studies of the PSL group show the necessity of regular and rigorous quality controls to establish the performances of commercially available filters and to consolidate the important role of labile blood product quality control laboratories in blood transfusion centers.

Acknowledgments

The authors wish to express their thanks to Ms N. Michel for her active participation in data presentation, the laboratory assistants in the different blood transfusion centers for their technical cooperation, and Ms N. Sarron for her help in preparing this document.

References

1 Payne R. The association of febrile transfusion reactions with leukoaglutinins. *Vox Sang* 1957;2: 233–241.

2 Perkins HA, Payne R, Ferguson J, Wood M. Non-haemolytic febrile transfusion reactions. Quantitative effects of blood components with emphasis on isoantigenic incompatibility of leukocytes. *Vox Sang* 1966;11:578–600.

3 Van Marwijk Kooy M, Van Proojnen HC, Moes M, Bosma Stants I, Akkerman JWN. Use of leukocyte-depleted platelet concentrates for the prevention of refractoriness and primary HLA alloimmunisation: a prospective, randomized trial. *Blood* 1991;77:201–205.

4 Andreu G, Dewailly J, Leberre C *et al*. Prevention of HLA immunization with leukocyte-poor packed red cells and platelet concentrates obtained by filtration. *Blood* 1988;72:964–969.

5 De Graan Hentzen YCE, Gratama JW, Mudde GC *et al*. Prevention of primary cytomegalovirus infection in patients with hematologic malignancies by intensive white cell depletion of blood products. *Transfusion* 1989;29:757–760.

6 Sekiguchi S, Takahashi TA. Leukocyte-depleted blood products and their clinical usefulness. In Brozovic B, ed. *The Role of Leukocyte Depletion in Blood Transfusion Practice*. Oxford: Blackwell Scientific Publications, 1988:26–34.

7 Friedman LI, Sadoff BJ, Stromberg RR. White cell counting in red cells and platelets: how few can we count? *Transfusion* 1990;30:387–389.

8 Pikul FJ, Farrar RP, Boris MB *et al*. Effectiveness of two synthetic fiber filters for removing white cells from AS-1 red cells. *Transfusion* 1989;29:590–595.

9 Reverberi R, Menini C. Clinical efficacy of five filters specific for leukocyte removal. *Vox Sang* 1990;58:188–191.

10 Sadoff BJ, Miller K, Stromberg RR. Methods for measuring a six log 10 leukocyte depletion in red cells. *Transfusion* 1991;31:150–154.

11 Wenz B, Burns ER, Lee V, Miller WK. A rare-event analysis model for quantifying white cells in white cell-depleted blood. *Transfusion* 1991;31:156–159.

12 Rawal BD, Schwadron R, Busch MP, Endow R, Vyas GN. Evaluation of leukocyte removal filters modelled by use of HIV infected cells and DNA amplification. *Blood* 1990;76:2159–2161.

13 Leng B, Garcez R, Chong C, Furuzawa R, Carmen R. Leukocyte counting by microscope: a methods evaluation. *The 1990 ISBT/AABB Book of Abstracts* S57:17. Presented at the ISBT/AABB joint meeting, Los Angeles, Nov 1990.

14 Wenz B, Besso N. Quality control and evaluation of leucocyte depleting filters. *Transfusion* 1989;29:186–187.

15 Reesink HW, Veldman H, Henrichs HJ, Prins HK. Removal of leukocyte from blood by filtration. A comparison study on the performance of two commercially available filters. *Vox Sang* 1982;42: 281–288.

16 Koermer K, Sahlmen P, Zimmermann B, Kubaneck B. Preparation of leukocyte-poor red cell concentrates: comparison of five different filters. *Vox Sang* 1991;60:61–62.

17 Kickler TS, Bell W, Ness PM, Drew H, Pall D. Depletion of white cells platelet concentrate with a new adsorption filter. *Transfusion* 1989;29:411–414.

18 Bock M, Heim MU, Weindler R *et al*. White cell depletion of single-donor platelet preparations by a new adsorption filter. *Transfusion* 1991;31:333–334.

19 Freedman J, Blanchette V, Hornstein A *et al*. White cell depletion of red cell and pooled random-donor platelet concentrates by filtration and residual lymphocyte subset analysis. *Transfusion* 1991;31:433–440.

20 Hogman CF, Eriksson L, Hedlund K, Wallvik J. The bottom and top system: a new technique for blood component preparation and storage. *Vox Sang* 1988;55:211–217.

21 Simon TL, Sierra ER, Ferdinando B, Moore R. Collection of platelets with a new cell separator and their storage in a citrate-plasticized container. *Transfusion* 1991;31:335–339.

22 Sniecinski I, O'Donnell MR, Nowicki B, Hill LR. Prevention of refractoriness and HLA alloimmunization using filtered blood products. *Blood* 1988;71:1402–1407.

23 Saarinen UM, Kekomäki R, Siimes MA, Myllylä G. Effective prophylaxis against platelet refractoriness in multitransfused patients by the use of leukocyte-free blood components. *Blood* 1990;75: 512–517.

24 Gilbert FL, Hayes K, Hudson IL, James J and the neonatal cytomegalovirus infection study group. Prevention of transfusion-acquired cytomegalovirus infection in infants by blood filtration to remove leucocytes. *Lancet* 1989;3:1228–1231.

25 Rawal B, Yen TSB, Vyas GN, Bush M. Leukocyte filtration removes infectious particulate debris but not free virus derived from experimentally lysed HIV-infected cells. *Vox Sang* 1991;60:214–218.

26 Dumont LJ. Sampling errors and the precision associated with counting very low numbers of white cells in blood components. *Transfusion* 1991;31:428–432.

27 Greenwalt TJ, Allen CM. A method for counting leukocytes in filtered components. *Transfusion* 1990;30:377–379.

28 Kao KJ, Scornik JC. Accurate quantitation of the low number of white cells in white cell-depleted blood components. *Transfusion* 1989;29:774–777.

29 Takahasi TA, Hosada M, Sekiguchi S. Cytospin method: new method for the determination of residual leukocytes in leukocyte-depleted platelet concentrates. *Jpn J Transfus Med* 1989;35:497–503.

30 Vakkila J, Myllyla G. Amount and type of leukocytes in "leukocyte-free" red cell and platelet concentrates. *Vox Sang* 1987;53:76–82.

31 Wester MR, Prins HK, Huisman JG. A new radioimmunoassay for the detection of small amounts of white cells and platelets in red cell concentrates: implications for blood transfusion. *Transfusion* 1990;30:117–125.

32 Curtis BR, Silva VA, Marlo DJ, Chaplin H. A simple method for counting blood cells (WBC) in low WBC platelet products. *The 1990 ISBT/AABB Book of Abstracts* S231:58. Presented at ISBT/AABB joint meeting, Los Angeles, Nov 1990.

33 Bodensteiner DC. A flow cytometric technique to accurately measure postfiltration white blood cell counts. *Transfusion* 1989;29:651–653.

34 Dzik WH, Ragosta AA, Cusak WF. Flow cytometric method for counting very low numbers of leukocytes in platelet products. *Vox Sang* 1990;59:153–159.

35 Takahashi TA, Hosada M, Sekiguchi S. A flow cytometric method to detect residual leukocytes in platelet and red cell concentrates. *J Jpn Soc Blood Transfus* 1990;36:429–437.

Discussion

MERYMAN: Do you have any information regarding the differential after filtration? That is, the differential count of the remaining white cells, such as granulocytes and monocytes?

MASSE: No, we have none. They are different for different kinds of cells.

CULLIS: I can tell you from an independent study that the cells which go through initially are predominantly granulocytes with the Asahi 200 or 500 filters but I don't know about the others.

STIENSTRA: I see that you used the most sensitive method of counting leukocytes in

Group D and also acetic acid in your staining fluid or in your buffer. Aren't you afraid that the acetic acid may lyse some leukocytes, so that you count fewer leukocytes than are in your preparation? I have the experience with normal Fuchs-Rosenthal staining solution that when I have normal Schiff's acetic acid in the staining solution, I lose some leukocytes, so normally with microscopic methods, which I have used in the past, I leave the acetic acid out of the staining. What's your comment on that?

MASSE: We have changed the lysing solution from plaxan to acetic acid at 3% for the platelets to avoid the formation of microaggregates after the centrifugation step and to increase the dissolution of platelets. But we tested the damage to leukocytes with a known concentration of leukocyte suspension and did not find a difference or any important loss. We think that, to be sure of our method for concentration of the sample, we must recover more than 90% of initial white cells. It is our minimum level to recover the white cells. We can tolerate a loss of 10%.

WHYTE: What method do you use for your preliminary concentration of leukocytes before counting? Are you using the Ficoll-Hypaque method or a different method?

MASSE: No, we don't use the Ficoll-Hypaque concentration. We use only lysing solution and then centrifugation. We remove the supernatant really gently, and then to wash the suspended pellet we use a part of the lysing solution, the volume of which is precisely measured.

TAKAHASHI: I was very impressed by your beautiful work. As you know, we are using a flow cytometer to count residual leukocytes. Today you showed us the super Nageotte techniques and the sensitivity is at least equal to that of our method and sometimes much better. I know you also have experience using a flow cytometer. Which method do you recommend to use for the quality control of leukocyte-depleted blood components in blood banks or blood centers?

MASSE: Thank you very much for your comment and your question. I would like to say that a good counting method must be transferable from one center to another one and from one country to another country. You know that we are ready to cooperate with different centers, including Japanese centers. We recommend the simplest method and most inexpensive method. We tried to use different methods with flow cytometers such as the Cytoron and with another cytometer. But for quality control we think that we have to check a large part of the samples very often every day to make sure that the objective is reached in the great majority of filtered products. I think that this kind of study is indispensable as the first step before carrying out clinical study to measure the clinical effect of filtration to be sure that the present objective will be reached.

SNIECINSKI: What about the quality control of the filtered blood products? Is there a consensus of the French cooperative study group regarding the frequency of the testing? How many filtered blood components should be tested in routine transfusion, each component or a certain percentage of components?

MASSE: Presently we control more than 30%. When we are changing some aspect of the procedure, we check about 100% for 1 week, 2 weeks, or 1 month. And then, when there are no changes, we check more than 30%.

BROZOVIĆ: It is admirable that you have managed to get 21 centers to cooperate and use the same kind of technique and to get results which are so uniform. When we tried this several years ago in England we managed to get six centers to cooperate and they could not get sufficiently close together to have joint results. What about the quality control of filtration which is now taking place at the bedside? What are your views and what would be your recommendation in terms of quality control for all of the filtration procedures carried out at the bedside as opposed to those which are carried out in laboratories in the other centers?

MASSE: As to your first comment, it was not so difficult to manage 21 blood centers in France because we have got the same objective concerning quality production. About your question, I think the interests and maybe the advantages of this kind of national study rest for a large part on a large number of controls and the strict application of standardized protocols including different parameters, such as temperature, initial count of white cells, and so on. We cannot imagine a search evaluation from the bedside filters, which we consider to be too late.

STIENSTRA: Like Dr Brozović, I was also astonished at the uniformity of the counting you had in the 21 blood centers. I think that means there are very good medical technicians in France. But those measurements last at least a quarter of an hour and a maximum of 30 min. And when I ask my medical technician manually to count leukocytes officially, she panics a bit. How do you manage it? Are there medical technologists counting leukocytes the whole day? How many people do you have counting, and are you counting all products going out of the blood bank to the clinicians or are you only doing some of them to gain a general impression of the quality of the products you deliver?

MASSE: We think filtration is a new procedure that we have to make a great effort to test now. A lot of centers in France make an effort to evaluate the efficiency of this filtration. Thank you for your comment about the technicians. I think maybe we are not such good technicians. But more important is the training of the technicians and to organize meetings with technicians one day with the same microscope with the same method. In this way the technicians do good work. For about 5 or 6 years, we have developed the policy of quality control for blood component production in different centers and we try to use the same techniques for the filtration.

STIENSTRA: But still the method is subjective; it is not an objective method. Flow cytometry methods like Dr Takahashi mentioned are objective, using an instrument. I love instruments, and I think methods using them are more precise and their results are more reproducible compared to subjective methods.

6 · Quality control of leukocyte depletion in blood banking with a flow cytometer: flow cytometry to determine low concentrations of white cells in leukocyte-poor platelet concentrates

S. Stienstra and D. de Vos

Red Cross Blood Bank Nijmegen, Greet Grooteplein Zuid 10, 6525 GA Nijmegen, The Netherlands

Abstract

In patients who receive periodic blood transfusions, white blood cells (WBCs) in blood bank cell products may initiate alloantibodies against human leukocyte antigens (HLA). These antibodies may be the cause of refractoriness of platelets and other transfusion complications such as febrile reactions and pulmonary edema. Therefore, a demand exists for quantitative information on even small amounts of WBCs in blood cell products. The particle-counting techniques of modern hematologic routine cell counters are found to be insufficiently sensitive in detecting low levels of WBCs in leukocyte-depleted products. Other previously proposed techniques, such as cytospin [1] or hemacytometer procedures [2], take too much time.

A very fast and simple technique for accurate quantification of low concentrations of white cells and red cells simultaneously in leukocyte-poor platelet concentrates has been developed with the use of a flow cytometer.

Introduction

WBCs in platelet concentrates may initiate alloantibodies against HLA. In particular, cancer patients undergoing chemotherapy, who periodically receive platelet transfusions, are at risk for allosensitization to Class I HLA antigens. These antibodies may be the cause of refractoriness of platelets and other transfusion complications such as febrile reactions.

Contaminating WBCs may adversely affect platelet function and posttransfusion recovery of stored platelet concentrates. This loss of platelet function is mainly due to lowering of plasma pH as a result of the accumulation of lactic acid, a product of anaerobic metabolism of both WBCs and platelets [3,4]. High concentrations of contaminating WBCs aggravate the fall in pH [5,6]. The third adverse effect of WBCs contaminating platelet concentrates is the release of proteolytic enzymes from these

63

cells; this may cause proteolysis of platelet membrane glycoproteins, thereby affecting membrane composition and platelet function [7].

For these reasons we produce our platelet concentrates under extremely optimized and reproducible conditions.

Materials and methods

Development of the method

Leukocyte-poor platelet concentrates are produced by an optimized buffy coat method, originally developed by Pietersz *et al.* [3]. Platelet suspensions from usually six donors are pooled. The total volume of a platelet concentrate, made up of six donor platelet suspensions, is approximately 300 ml. This method of counting leukocytes in platelet concentrates is also suitable for single donor cytapheresis platelet concentrates.

Flow cytometric WBC counting is done using a Coulter Epics Profile II flow cytometer equipped with a 488 nm argon laser. This technique is based upon difference in granularity of the different cell types in platelet concentrates. To obtain a better discrimination in granularity (side scatter), the platelets have their shape changed artificially with Triton X-100. Neither aggregation nor degranulation takes place. The concentration is checked in every new charge of this solution. Triton X-100 decreases the side scatter of the platelets (Fig. 6.1). Due to the Triton X-100 in this critical concentration, the platelets swell and round out (Fig. 6.2). The treatment does not affect the side scatter signal from erythrocytes and leukocytes (Fig. 6.3). The platelet peak shifts to the left and moves from the erythrocyte and leukocyte peak in the log side scatter (LSS) histogram (Fig. 6.4).

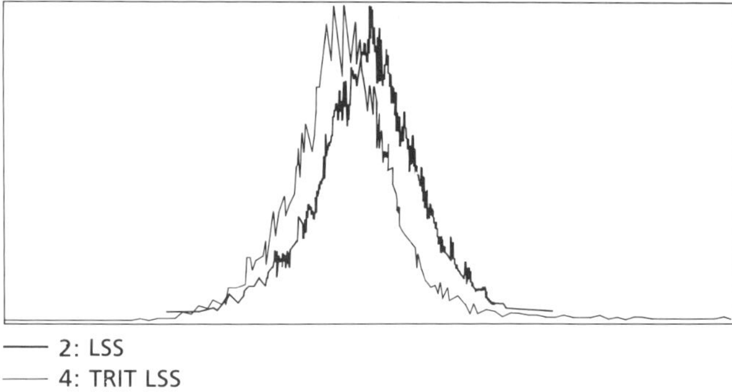

Fig. 6.1 Due to the Triton X-100 (TRIT) treatment, the side scatter of the platelets decreases a reproducible amount of channel numbers in log side scatter (LSS). Before: line 2 LSS; after: line 4 TRIT LSS.

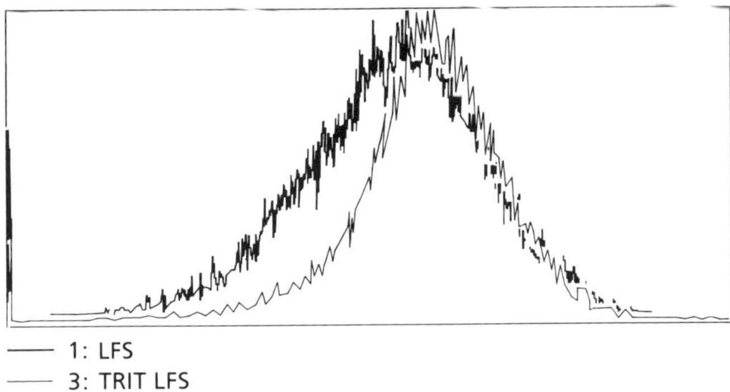

Fig. 6.2 Due to the Triton X-100 (TRIT) in this critical concentration, the platelets swell and round out. In log forward scatter (LFS), a more uniform population of platelets whose shape has been changed artificially comes into existence. Before: line 1 LFS; after: line 3 TRIT LFS.

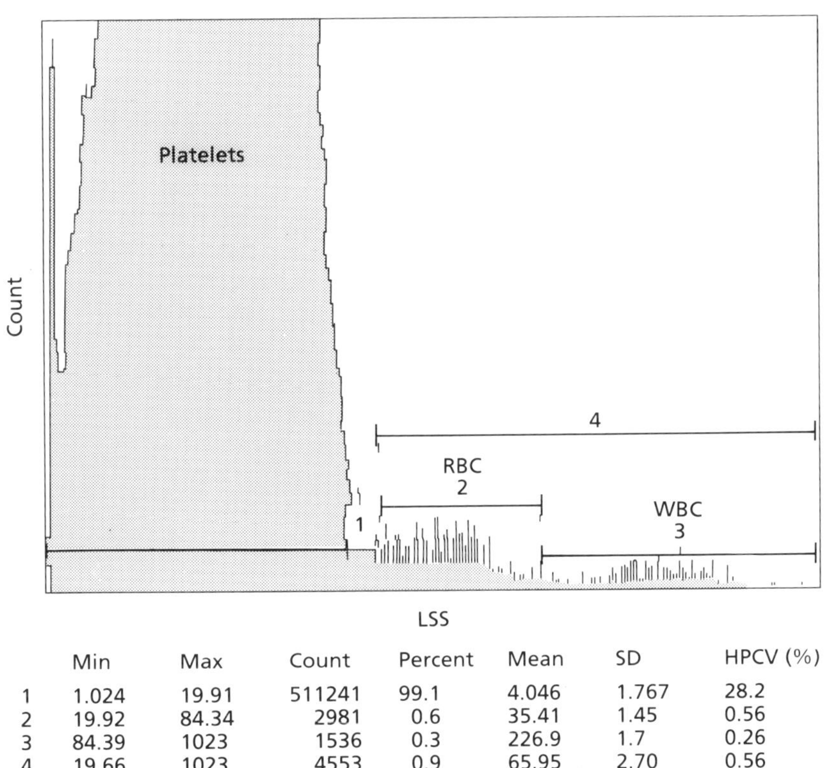

	Min	Max	Count	Percent	Mean	SD	HPCV (%)
1	1.024	19.91	511241	99.1	4.046	1.767	28.2
2	19.92	84.34	2981	0.6	35.41	1.45	0.56
3	84.39	1023	1536	0.3	226.9	1.7	0.26
4	19.66	1023	4553	0.9	65.95	2.70	0.56

Fig. 6.3 The artificial shape change with Triton X-100 moves the platelet peak (1) in the log side scatter (LSS) histogram to the left and the erythrocyte peak (2) and leukocyte peak (3) no longer overlap with the platelet peak.

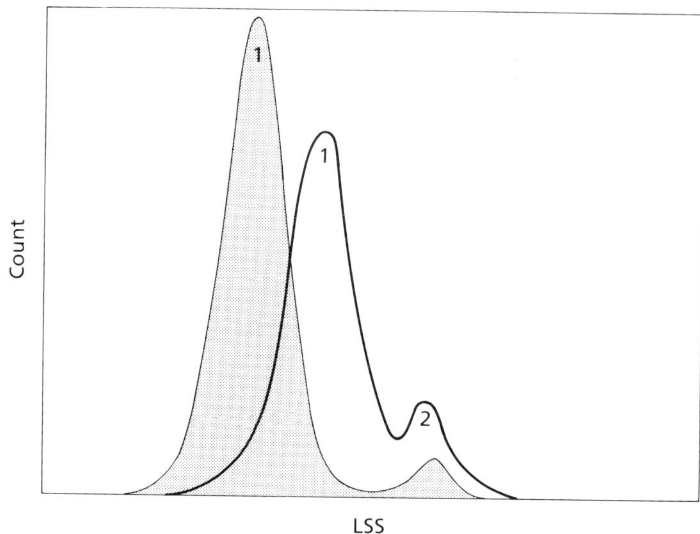

Fig. 6.4 After Triton X-100 treatment the platelet peak (1) moves to the left and gets higher, as the platelets become more uniform. Red cells (2) and white cells (2) do not change position.

Streptokinase is used to avoid contamination of the flow cytometer by fibrin and blockage of the cell flow in the flow-chamber by activated platelets.

The tubes and reagent solution are kept in the freezer ($-20°C$). The reagent solution contains 25 µl streptokinase (1 u/ml, Streptase, Behringwerke Marburg, Germany), 250 µl Triton X-100 (0.01 g/l Sigma, St Louis, USA) and 725 µl saline. Before measurement a tube is thawed and 200 µl of sample is added. After gently mixing, and after the swirling effect has vanished, the sample is ready for analysis. The flow cytometer takes 50 µl from the diluted reaction mixture for its measurement. When very low concentrations of leukocytes are expected, this volume can be increased. The WBCs are distinguished in a 1-parameter LSS histogram from the erythrocytes and platelets.

In the flow cytometer Coulter Isoton II is used as sheath buffer. This contains 7.93 g/l sodium chloride, 0.38 g/l disodium ethylenediaminetetraacetic acid, 0.40 g/l potassium chloride, 0.19 g/l sodium dihydrogen phosphate, 1.95 g/l disodium hydrogen phosphate and 0.30 g/l sodium fluoride.

The location of the leukocytes in the histogram has been checked with propidium iodide DNA-staining of the WBCs (50 µg/l propidium iodide and 20 µg/l RNase). The WBCs can be detected with the red fluorescence due to the propidium iodide staining and the cluster of events from the white cells can be located in the forward scatter (FS) to LSS histogram. By creating a bitmap in the red fluorescence histogram, the position of the leukocytes in the LSS is determined. These experiments are done on a Bruker

ACR-1000 flow cytometer. The performance of this instrument conforms to the Epics Profile II.

As a fixed and known flow rate is used and the period of time is tuned, the exact volume of sample can be calculated. The flow rate is constant as the flow cytometer pushes the sample with a syringe in the measuring chamber. In this way the exact number of leukocytes in the sample can be determined, as the amount of events within the histogram area of interest in which all leukocytes in the platelet concentrate appear.

The number of red cells can be calculated using the same method. In another bitmap without overlap with the bitmap for white cells, the exact number of red cells can be measured.

With the data obtained, the concentrations of WBCs and red cells can be calculated in relation to the volume of platelet concentrate.

The discriminator and amplifier settings are set on a level that makes it impossible to count the total number of platelets with this protocol. To calculate the fraction of WBCs or red cells in relation to the total amount of cells, the total amount of platelets in the sample must be known. This can be done with a routine hematologic cell counter or with the flow cytometer using another protocol.

In correlation studies the leukocytes in platelet concentrates were measured electronically using a Coulter type cell counter, Analys Instruments 134 ($r = 0.7$), or Technicon H-1 cell counter with flowcytometric principle ($r = 0.6982$), and manually with a Fuchs-Rosenthal hemocytometer using a dilution of $1 : 10$ in gentian-violet saline ($r = 0.6$). As the flow cytometer is a much more sensitive instrument with far better coefficient of variation, we had to choose another method of validation in this domain of low concentrations of leukocytes in blood bank products.

Validation of the method

Counting the amount of red and white cells in leukocyte-poor platelet concentrates can be compared with rare cell detection. As it is impossible to get a sample of a platelet concentrate which is absolutely free of red or white cells, linearity studies cannot be done with original samples. Linearity studies in which normal samples are diluted with concentrates which were filtered many times to eliminate the white cells are described. In the low concentration range, which is the normal measuring range, optimal linearity was not attained. This might be due to debris which came into existence during filtering. After filtering a unit, debris is detected due to this filtering in almost all our samples.

Therefore we have chosen to simulate the rare cell event detections with beads which have the same scatter pattern as platelets, and other beads which have the same pattern as white cells in the histograms on the flow cytometer. The test samples for those experiments consisted of two populations of standard beads for flow cytometry with different scatter signals. A population of blank beads (no fluorescence,

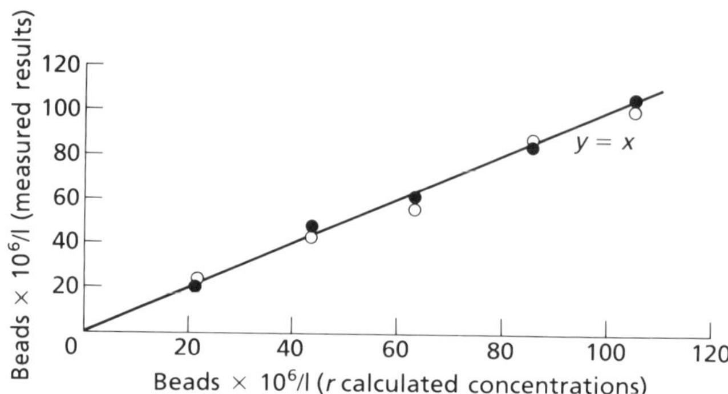

Fig. 6.5 Validation of the method used to count very low numbers of leukocytes in platelet concentrates with standard beads. The range from 20 to 100×10^6 leukocyte-like beads per liter in a concentration of approximately 8×10^{12} beads with a platelet-like scatter pattern is used. ● side scatter ($r = 0.9971$); ○ red fluorescence ($r = 0.9981$).

diameter 2 µm; Flow Cytometry Standards) represented the platelets. The concentration of these beads is kept constant during the performance of the test.

Immuno-brite red fluorescent level II beads, diameter 10 µm (Coulter) represented the leukocytes. The concentration of these beads varied from 1 to 100×10^6/l.

The same protocol as for the WBC count in platelet concentrates was used to set up the flow cytometer. An extra 1 parameter histogram was created for the logarithmic red fluorescence signal. The linearity and the deviation from the perfect curve ($y = x$) were determined.

In the linearity studies for measurements in platelet concentrates, leukocyte-like beads were used in the range from 20 to 100×10^6 leukocyte-like beads per liter in a concentration of approximately 8×10^{12} beads with a platelet-like scatter pattern.

The coefficient of regression is determined by the parameter side scatter and red fluorescence (control). The regression coefficient r is 0.9971 with side scatter and 0.9981 with red fluorescence as test parameter (Fig. 6.5).

The coefficient of regression is determined by the parameter side scatter and red fluorescence as shown in Figure 6.5 ($r = 0.9986$ and $r = 0.9983$, respectively).

Daily quality control

To establish quality control of our routine blood bank cell counters and the flow cytometer, we developed with Analytics (Delfzijl, The Netherlands) a standard material containing fixed platelets produced from human buffy coats. This material has the same concentration of WBCs and platelets as routine platelet concentrates.

A standard preparation of platelets prepared from buffy coats and containing approximately 10^{12} stabilized platelets per liter and 0.08×10^9 stabilized leukocytes per liter was found to be stable for over 1 month. A coefficient of variation of 1.9% was determined over a period of 40 days.

Results

With this newly developed technique of flow cytometric counting of leukocytes in platelet concentrates without any staining, we counted in 1989 in our routine donor platelet concentrates approximately 600×10^9 platelets per liter. We measured about 260×10^6 red cells per liter and 60×10^6 WBCs per liter. This corresponds with 200×10^9 platelets, 85×10^6 red blood cells, and 20×10^6 WBCs per six donor unit. Acquainted with the new precise counting method we optimized the production of platelet concentrates and in 1991 we measured routinely approximately 45×10^6 WBCs per liter in platelet concentrates. This corresponds to 15×10^6 WBCs per six donor unit. The amounts of platelets and red cells in the platelet suspension were about the same (Fig. 6.6).

Summary

After a period in which we studied the possibilities of several types of blood cell counters we decided that it was impossible to find a blood cell counter suitable for the detection of very small numbers of WBCs in platelet concentrates.

The particle-counting techniques of modern hematologic routine cell counters are insufficiently sensitive in detecting low levels of WBCs in blood bank cell products. So, there is a demand for an instrument for quality control of WBC-depleted blood bank products.

We changed our search for measuring instruments to flow cytometers. We compared three flow cytometers (Facscan; Becton Dickinson, Bruker ACR-1000, Coulter Epics II) with two protocols we had developed. We agree with Kao and Scornik [8] that adding solutions to lyse red cells gives debris which interferes with the identification of white blood cells, so we did not lyse cells.

Platelets are a problem in flow cytometric measurements, as we found with the development of our technique measuring WBCs in platelet concentrates. Artificially changing the shape of the platelets and adding streptokinase solve these problems.

The linearity studies indicated that the precision and sensitivity of the flow cytometric measurements of white blood cells in both erythrocyte and platelet concentrates were superior to the time-consuming hemocytometric methods and to common measurements with sophisticated clinical blood cell counters. Therefore it is not realistic to correlate the newly developed method with these conventional methods. At higher concentrations of leukocytes it is possible and we can get good correlations, but that is not our domain of interest.

The experiments with the stabilized platelet concentrate standard solution indicated the high reproducibility of the developed method. Together with the results of the linearity studies we have the impression that whenever we can count and interpret more than 1 200 000 events on the instrument, we can count even lower concentrations of WBCs in blood bank cell products.

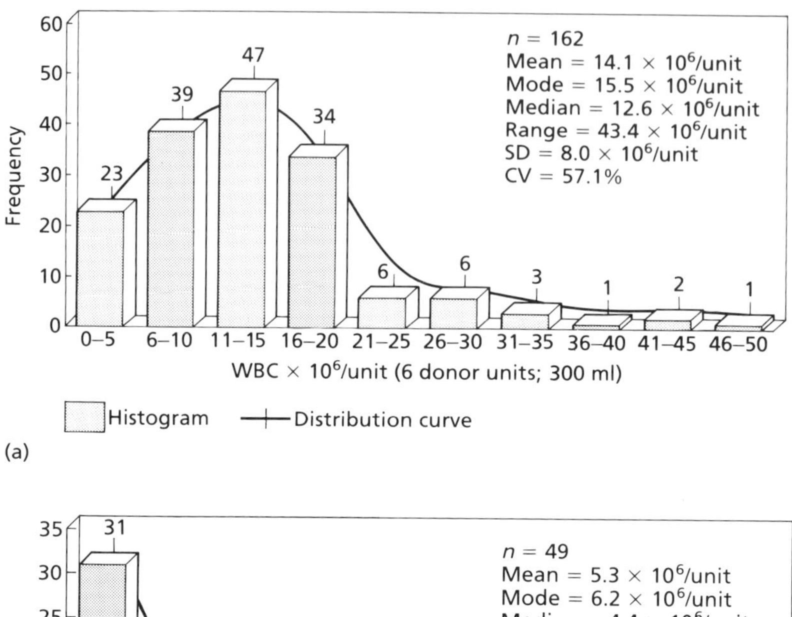

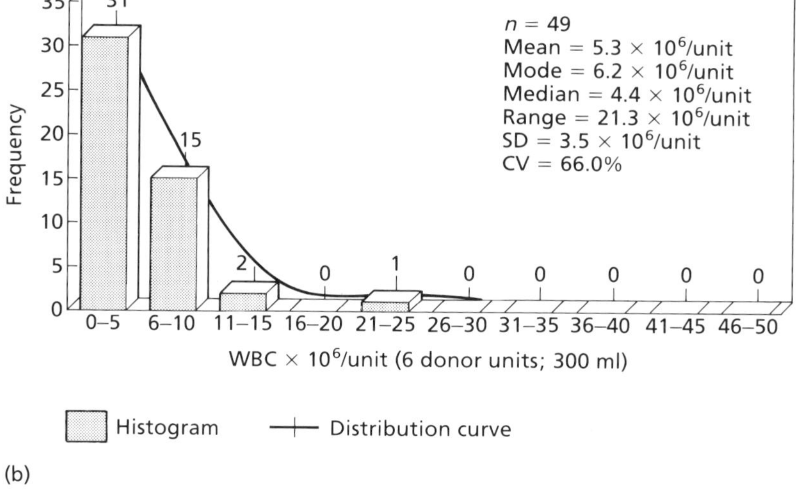

Fig. 6.6 The newly developed method of daily quality control procedures: distribution of the number of white blood cells (WBCs) in platelet concentrates. (a) Preceding results; (b) new results.

The lymphocytes are both potent stimulators of alloimmunization reactions and potential carriers of blood-borne retroviruses, like human immunodeficiency virus. New procedures, as described in this article, will be useful not only in the evaluation of the techniques for preparing WBC-depleted blood products, but also in the further investigation of the maximal number of WBCs that can be allowed in blood components for the prevention of primary allosensitization of HLA antigens and to prevent transfection of retroviruses by blood bank products (Fig. 6.7). With this well-reproducible and sensitive counting method, we have already optimized the fine tuning in our production of leukocyte-poor platelet concentrates to get better products with lower numbers of white cells.

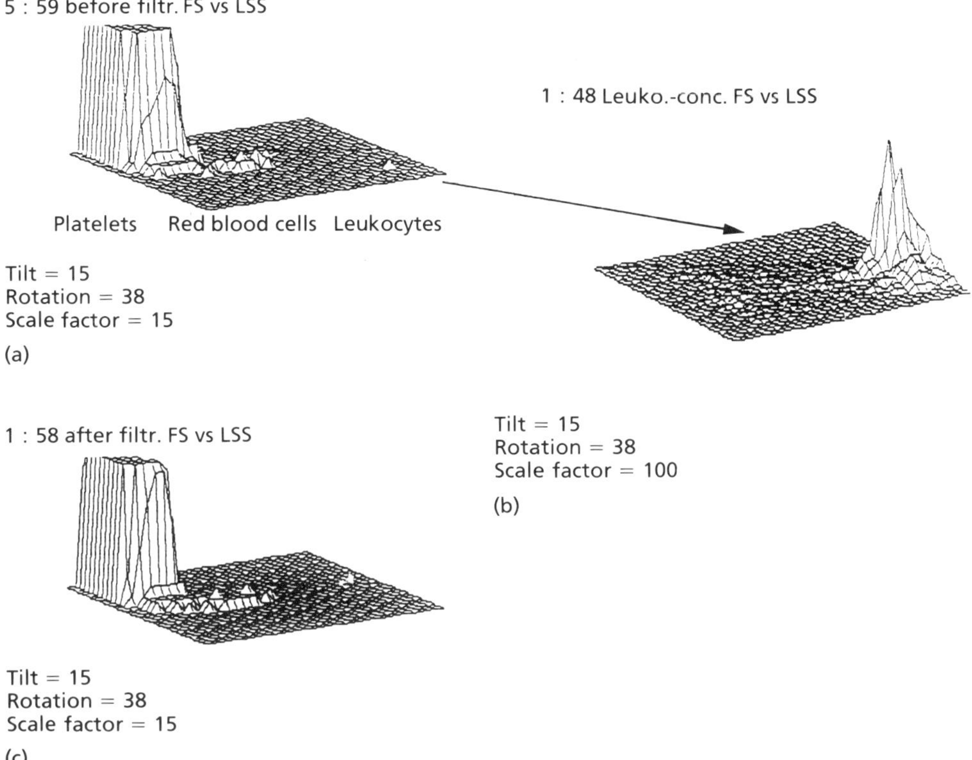

Fig. 6.7 Results of leukocyte depletion by filtration. (a) Platelet concentrate before filtration; (b) amplification of the leukocyte section; (c) after filtration with the Pall PL-100 filter.

Flow cytometry to determine low concentrations of white cells in red cell concentrates

We count the white cells in red blood cell concentrates with a technique which is similar to the technique of Bodensteiner [9,10]. We have one major difference. Bodensteiner uses a concentration of 1 g/l Triton X-100 to lyse the red cells. The white cells stay intact but they get leaky at this concentration and are red-fluorescent-stained with propidium iodide (50 mg/ml; Molecular Probes, Eugene, USA). The propidum iodide enter the white cell and stains specifically the DNA and RNA. To prevent reticulocytes staining, 20 µg/l RNase (Sigma, St Louis, USA) is added.

We use 0.2 g/l Triton X-100, a concentration which is five times lower than the technique of Bodensteiner. At this concentration the red cells do not lyse: lysing gives too much debris. Debris from red cells interferes in the measurement and limits the counting of very low concentrations of white cells within the red cells. At this lower Triton X-100 concentration, the white cells still get punctured. We select the stained white cells within the red cells with the flow cytometer. Therefore we have to select

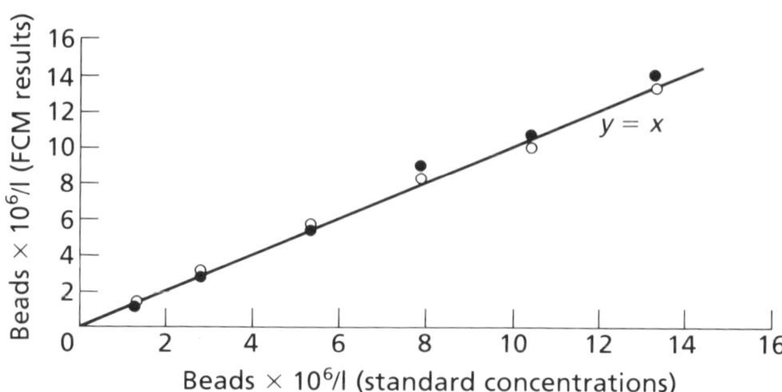

Fig. 6.8 Validation of the method used to count very low numbers of leukocytes in red cell concentrates with standard beads. The range from 1 to 14×10^6 leukocyte-like beads per liter in a concentration of approximately 600×10^9 beads with an erythrocyte-like scatter pattern is used. ● side scatter ($r = 0.9986$); ○ red fluorescence ($r = 0.9983$).

a bitmap in which all stained cells appear and we have to count more events. The total number of events is not a strict limitation as the Coulter Epics II flow cytometer can count 1 200 000 events in a reasonable time.

The problem with the remaining platelets that Kao and Scornik [8] noted in their counting of leukocytes in red blood cell concentrates was not experienced by us as filtered blood contains a very small amount of platelets.

The validation is done like the validation of counting low numbers of leukocytes in platelet concentrates. In linearity studies for measurements in red cell concentrates, we used the range from 1 to 14×10^6 leukocyte-like beads per liter in a concentration of approximately 600×10^9 beads with an erythrocyte-like scatter pattern (Fig. 6.8).

Correlation studies with common hematologic cell counters give reasonable results, but as already mentioned, these instruments are not designed for this purpose and do not give optimal results (Fig. 6.9).

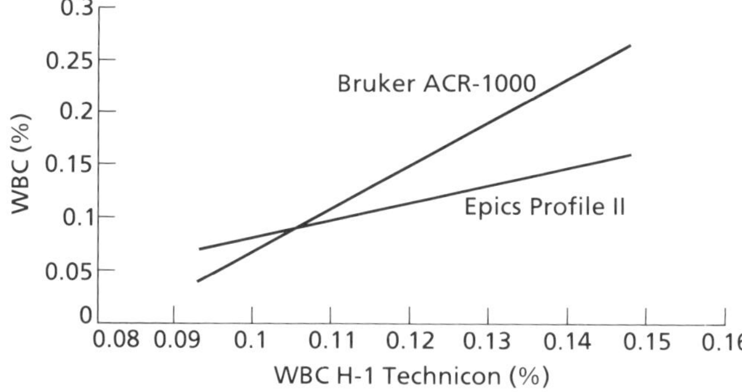

Fig. 6.9 Correlation studies with other instruments, together with the validation results, indicate that the flow cytometric method has better reproducibility and sensitivity. Comparison of Epics Profile II ($r = 0.8435$) and Bruker ACR-1000 ($r = 0.7021$) with H-1 Technicon, in white blood cell (WBC) count-filtered erythrocytes.

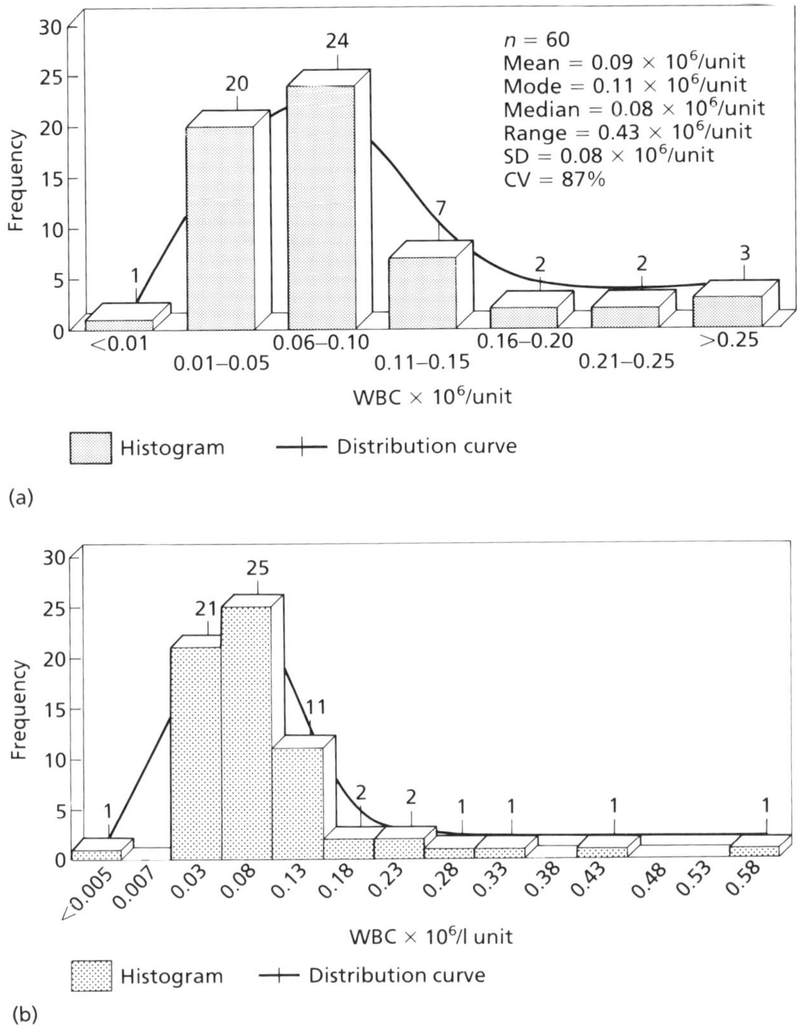

(a)

(b)

Fig. 6.10 Preceding (a) and new (b) results obtained with the flow cytometric method in routine production. Distribution of the number of white blood cells (WBCs) in filtered erythrocytes.

The results in our blood bank in counting the low numbers of leukocytes in filtered red cell concentrates are given in Figure 6.10. The technique for counting the low numbers of leukocytes remaining after filtering with a flow cytometer has already proven its value in routine production in our blood bank.

References

1 Takahashi TA, Hosoda M, Sekiguchi S. Cytospin method for the determination of residual leukocytes in leukocyte-depleted platelet concentrates. *Jpn J Transfus Med* 1989; 35:497–503.

2 Greenwalt TJ, Allen CM. A method for counting leukocytes in filtered components. *Transfusion* 1990;30:377–379.

3 Pietersz R, Loos J, Reesink H. Platelet concentrates stored in plasma for 72 hours at 22°C prepared buffy coats of citrate-phosphate-dextrose blood collected in a quadruple bag saline-adenine-glucose-mannitol system. *Vox Sang* 1985;49:81–85.

4 Murphy S, Kahn RA, Holme S *et al.* Improved storage of platelets for transfusion in a new container. *Blood* 1982;60:194–200.

5 Kilkson H, Holme S, Murphy S. Platelet metabolism during storage of platelet concentrates at 22°C. *Blood* 1984;64:406–414.

6 Ellis P, Champion A. Effect of white cells and platelet size on pH in platelet concentrates (PC). *Transfusion* 1983;23:415 (abstract).

7 Sloand EM, Klein HG. Effect of white cells on platelets during storage. *Transfusion* 1990;30:333–338.

8 Kao KJ, Scornik JC. Accurate quantitation of the low number of white cells in white cell-depleted blood components. *Transfusion* 1989;29:774–777.

9 Bodensteiner DC. A flow cytometric technique to accurately measure post-filtration white blood cell counts. *Transfusion* 1989;29:651–653.

10 Bodensteiner DC. Leucocyte depletion filters: a comparison of efficiency. *Am J Hematol* 1990;35:184–186.

Discussion

SNIECINSKI: If I understood correctly, you stated that you do not issue any platelet products that have white cell counts above 1×10^7 to clinicians. Does this mean that every platelet product is evaluated for the white cell content before being issued for transfusion?

STIENSTRA: That depends on the department to which we deliver the platelets. When we deliver platelets to departments which need leukocyte-depleted blood bank products, we always use platelets below that margin of 2×10^6 WBC/unit.

SNIECINSKI: Which means you test every platelet product?

STIENSTRA: We test every platelet concentrate. This method is simple and cheap, as it does not use any staining, and is also very fast. We can do the measurement within 2 minutes.

SNIECINSKI: Do you do this measurement just before issuing for transfusion?

STIENSTRA: Yes, of course. We do this measurement before we deliver the products to the clinicians, as when we have delivered the product, it is out of our sight and then we do not know what is happening with it. So when we deliver the platelet concentrate, the level of white cells is written on the label. We guarantee it is lower than that. Some other department which need platelets for severe bleeding or something like that get platelets which might have a slightly higher amount of white blood cells in the platelet concentrates. But that is the smaller part of our production. So we select and do not filter.

BROZOVIĆ: Do you discard any platelet concentrates on the basis of a high leukocyte count?

STIENSTRA: We do not discard platelets as, in the routine with the buffy coat method, we always have platelet concentrates which are sufficient for the surgical departments. Sometimes when the platelets are not viable enough or there are far too many white cells, it is mainly because of problems with the automated instruments which we use for the buffy coat method; we use the Compomat. Then we discard the whole unit, also the red cells, because there are problems there as well.

WHYTE: Has the selection of low white cell count platelets for your hematology and oncology patients reduced the number of platelet concentrates that you have to make in your center by reducing refractoriness?

STIENSTRA: I cannot say that. We are now busy collecting and looking at the data of the hematologic and oncologic departments. I do not have enough data yet. I'll be prepared to give you an answer in about 3 months, and then I can also give an answer on the types of leukocytes left in the preparation. (All I know now is that it is about 80% granulocytes and a few lymphocytes and monocytes.)

CULLIS: Will the solutions that you used to cause the differentiation of the cells be commercially available so that we could all use them in our work?

STIENSTRA: The method is rather simple. I like simple methods, and it could easily be commercialized. I think, like a normal hemocytometer, everyone can do it, but there are some things you need, and the most important thing is a dedicated flow cytometer. The problem is instrumentation. You need a real blood bank-dedicated flow cytometer. This has to have first, very good sensitivity and cytoscatter, a high flow rate because a lot of cells have to go through the measurement chamber, and then it needs to have a big computer with a huge memory. As I prefer to count and interpret all events and electronically to select by computer which cells I want to count, the computer must be big. But computers are so cheap that it can easily be developed, so I think we need a blood bank-dedicated flow cytometer in the future for the quality control of the cell products which we deliver.

SNIECINSKI: I'm a little bit confused about the issue of the granulocyte content in the filtered platelet concentrates. Are those platelet concentrates evaluated immediately after collection or after storage?

STIENSTRA: We routinely prepare platelet concentrates with the buffy coat method. We keep these concentrates on a horizontal shaker and when the request for them comes, we mix six single-donor platelet concentrates together, we do flow cytometry, and then we deliver the 6 donor units to the clinicians.

SNIECINSKI: Then you deal with platelets of different ages. You would not expect to see granulocytes in platelets that have been stored for several days.

BROZOVIĆ: Is there any possibility that platelet duplets, triplets, and quadruplets are recognized by the flow cytometer as granulocytes?

STIENSTRA: I think there is another answer to that question. In general, in Europe and also in the States, they keep platelet concentrates for 4 or 5 days. But our maximum is 3 days. Most of the platelet concentrates are only 1 or 2 days old, and most experiments are done with platelet concentrates produced from single-donor concentrates only 24 h old.

MERYMAN: What is the total volume of concentrate that passes through the flow cytometer in your routine assay?

STIENSTRA: We have a 200 µl sample. We add 1 ml of reagent and the cytometer takes 50 µl samples. This is added by a syringe, so the flow rate is constant and the volume is exactly known. You have probably heard from users of Becton-Dickinson flowcytometers. This instrument is working on pressure so that you are never sure of the amount of sample. As we use a syringe we are quite sure of the right volume.

MERYMAN: So you are looking then at less than 50 µl of the original platelet suspension, is that correct? That's not very much.

STIENSTRA: Yes, that's correct. Sometimes we count more but that is the newest differentiation we have made on our instrument. We have doubled the volume as we have changed the syringe from 2.5 to 5 ml, and this gives more information to the computer. But it does not matter because we focus only on that area where you expect to find the white cells and you neglect a lot of the other cells during the measurement so you can save a lot of work for the computer at that moment.

7 · Comparison of highly sensitive methods used to count residual leukocytes in filtered red cell and platelet concentrates

T.A. Takahashi, M. Hosoda, H. Abe, and S. Sekiguchi

Hokkaido Red Cross Blood Center, Yamanote 2-2, Nishi-ku, Sapporo 063, Japan

Abstract

A new generation of leukocyte removal filters has made it difficult to count the few remaining leukocytes in the filtered platelet concentrates (PC) and red cell concentrates (RCC) using automated electronic cell counters or visual counts in hemocytometers. Also new hemapheresis systems, such as the Cobe Spectra and CS-3000 Plus, produce plateletpheresis with very low contamination of leukocytes. We have developed a flow cytometric method (FCM) able to measure the small number of leukocytes remaining in both filtered PC and RCC. The Orthocytoron flow cytometer was used for FCM, and one part of pre- and postfiltered PC and RCC were added to 7.5 parts of propidium iodide (PI) solution containing RNase, sodium citrate, and Triton X-100. When RCC and PC had been filtered with leukocyte removal filters (Pall, Sepacell, and Imugard), the automated electronic cell counter or hemocytometer frequently failed to detect leukocytes in the filtrate, whereas the FCM could detect leukocytes to concentrations as low as 1.77×10^{-1} cells/µl. The limit of sensitivity was improved to 1.77×10^{-2} cells/µl by concentrating samples 10-fold before PI staining.

We have also applied the polymerase chain reaction (PCR) for amplification of a single copy cellular gene (β-globin) to detect the extremely low number of contaminating leukocytes. Using the serial dilution of leukocytes as standard for the PCR, amplified DNA was detected in the samples containing less than 2 cells/ml. The combined use of these techniques should be helpful for the quality control of leukocyte-depleted blood components.

Introduction

The recent improvement in leukocyte removal filters has made it difficult to count the few remaining leukocytes in platelet concentrates using automated electronic cell counters or visual counts in hemocytometers. In addition, new hemapheresis systems, such as the Cobe Spectra, produce hemapheresis platelets with extremely low contamination of leukocytes. The need for reliable techniques for the determination of small amounts of leukocytes in filtered blood components for the quality control of leukocyte-poor components and for the evaluation of new filters is increasing. Here we describe three methods (flow cytometry [1], cytospin [2], and polymerase chain reaction (PCR) [3]) which we have developed to measure small numbers of leukocytes remaining in the hemapheresis platelet concentrates prepared by the COBE Spectra and the new model of the Fenwal CS-3000 (Baxter Healthcare, Deerfield, IL, USA), and in both filtered PC and RCC, including those filtered by 6 log leukocyte removal filters. Various techniques have been developed quite intensively in the last 6 months, each method having both advantages and disadvantages. However, the combined use of these techniques should be helpful for the evaluation of new filters and for the quality control of leukocyte-poor blood components.

Materials and methods

Flow cytometry

For flow cytometry, different apparatuses were used: an Ortho Cytoron (Ortho Diagnostic Systems, Tokyo, Japan), a Facscan (Becton Dickinson, Mountain View, CA, USA) and an Epics Profile II (Coulter Electronics, Hialeah, FL, USA). However, we chose to use the Ortho Cytoron flow cytometer, as this instrument incorporates a sample delivery system which delivers a defined volume of sample to the flow cells. The Epics Profile II, which incorporates a delivery system similar to the Ortho Cytoron, can be used for the same purpose, and so far we have gotten good results. For the flow cytometric measurement, nuclei of leukocytes in PC and RCC were stained with propidium iodide. The propidium iodide solution contains propidium iodide, ribonuclease, sodium citrate, and Triton X-100 in phosphate-buffered saline (Table 7.1). We filtered the solution through a Millipore filter, and then froze and stored it at $-80\,^{\circ}$C until use. For staining, 100 µl of pre- and postfiltered RCC and PC was mixed with 750 µl of the staining solution, and incubated for 10 min at room temperature. The stained samples were then analyzed in the Ortho Cytoron flow cytometer. The number of red fluorescent nuclei in the leukocyte region was counted.

Table 7.1 Composition of propidium iodide solution

Propidium iodide	5 mg/100 ml
Ribonuclease A	100 mg/100 ml
Sodium citrate, monobasic	100 mg/100 ml
Triton X-100	100 µl/100 ml

In phosphate-buffered saline (pH 7.4)

Staining with propidium iodide solution
100 µl of pre- and postfilter platelet concentrate or red cell concentrate + 750 µl of propidium iodide solution incubated at $25\,^{\circ}$C for 10 min

Figure 7.1 shows the cytogram and histogram of the propidium iodide-stained platelet concentrates before and after filtration with a Sepacell PL filter. The number beneath each figure indicates the number of cells in 60 μl of stained sample. To determine the accuracy of the flow cytometric measurements, the leukocytes in 1 u of red cell concentrate were exclusively removed by repeating filtration five to six times with Sepacell R-500 [4] filters. Isolated mononuclear cells from another unit of red cell concentrate were counted, and a specific number of mononuclear cells was added to the leukocyte-free RCC. This mononuclear cell-loaded RCC was then serially diluted

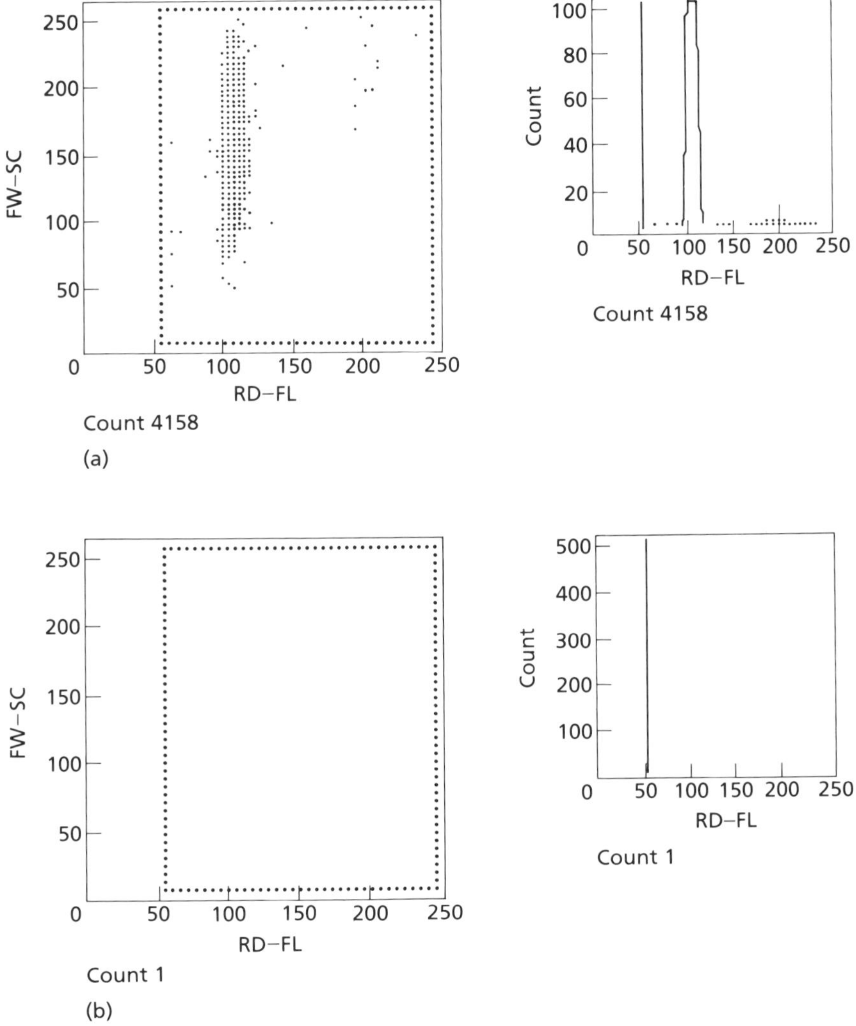

Fig. 7.1 Cytogram and histogram of propidium iodide-stained platelet concentrate by Sepacell PL (5N) (a) before filtration and (b) after filtration. FW-SC, forward scatter; RD-FL, red fluorescence.

with the leukocyte-free RCC. The extent of correlation between concentrations of leukocytes as measured with the Cytoron and the concentrations expected from the hemocytometer counts were determined. The same "spike" experiment was performed using PC. The correlation between the measurement of the Cytoron and the cell number expected by hemocytometer was expressed by the regression line.

Cytospin method

We have applied a cytocentrifuge method to count the residual leukocytes in leukocyte-depleted platelet concentrates (LDPC) using a Shandon Cytospin 2 (Shandon Southern Products, Runcorn, Cheshire, UK). The procedure for the cytospin technique is shown in Figure 7.2. Optimal conditions of cytocentrifugation were investigated for the centrifugation speed and period, for the volume of the sample, for the effects of RCC and PC, and so on. After the blood filtration, it took an average of 30 min to complete the whole procedure. Cells adhering to the slide glass within a

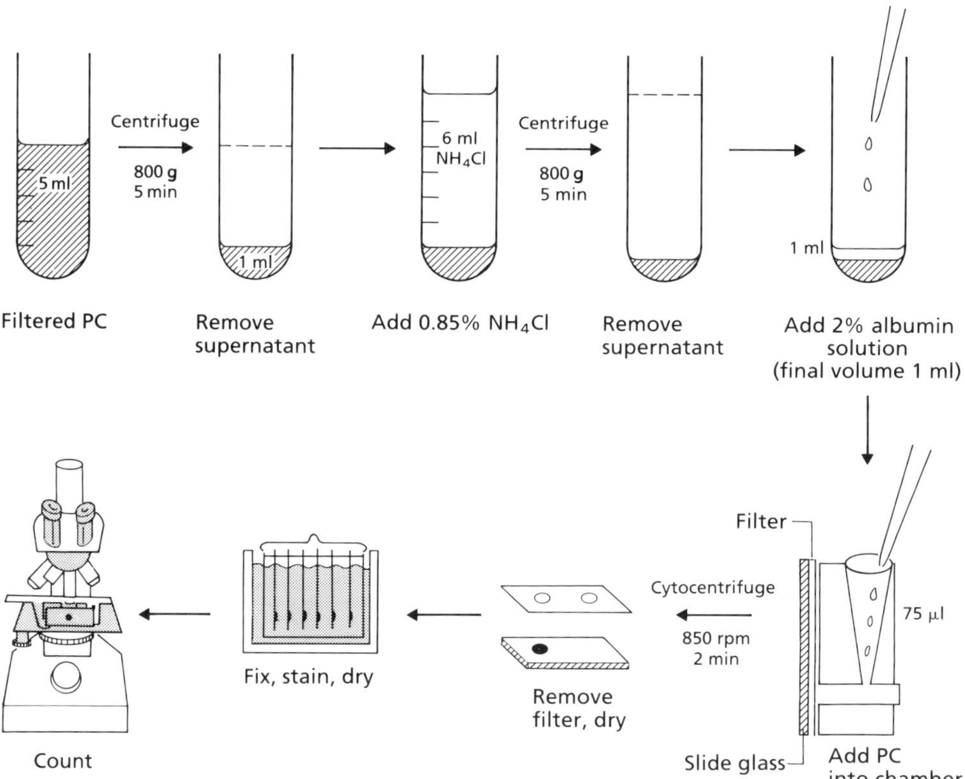

Fig. 7.2 Procedure for the cytospin method. PC, platelet concentrate.

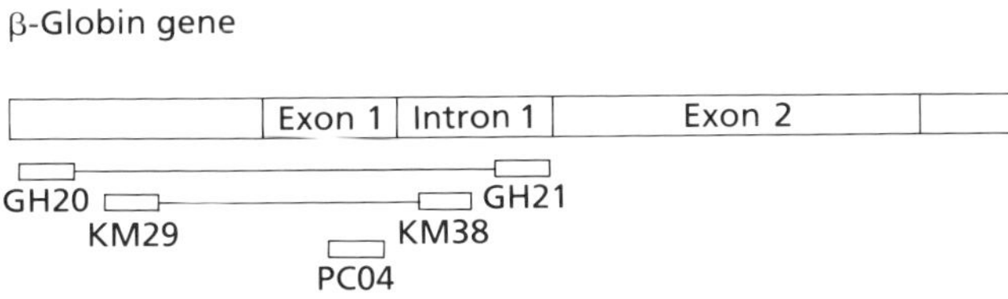

Fig. 7.3 Position of the primers and the probe for amplifying and detecting β-globin gene.

circle (diameter: 6 mm) were counted under a light microscope. Each step in the process, i.e. the 5-fold concentration of PC, the hemolysis of contaminating red cells with 0.85% NH_4Cl solution and the small volume of PC applied in the Cytospin chamber, should be considered to obtain a constant recovery of cells on the slide.

Polymerase chain reaction method

We chose β-globin gene to be amplified, because this gene is already well characterized and the primers are on the market (Takara, Kyoto, Japan). To obtain the number of leukocytes, the sample is first serially diluted 10-fold, and then five tubes at each dilution point are applied to the PCR. PCR was carried out using GH20 and GH21 primers (Fig. 7.3) and cycled 35 times at 95°C, 30 s; 55°C, 30 s; 72°C, 90 s; by a thermal cycler (model 9600; Perkin Elmer Cetus, USA). PCR products were separated on 2% agarose gel electrophoresis and then analyzed by Southern hybridization using ^{32}P-labeled probe, PCO_4. To avoid the use of radioactive materials, we developed a double PCR method in which β-globin gene was reamplified using the

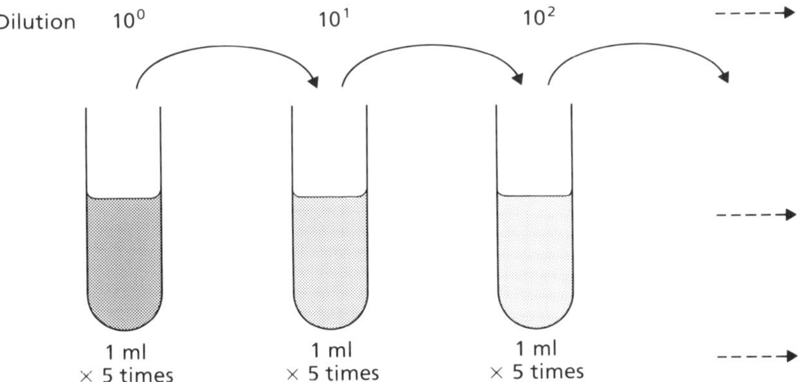

Fig. 7.4 Evaluation of the results from polymerase chain reaction. Filtered red cell concentrate was serial diluted with Hanks' balanced salt solution (HBSS). DNA was extracted from 1 ml of each diluent and applied on polymerase chain reaction five times.

primers of KM29 and KM38 following its amplification using primers of GH20 and GH21. The end-point at which all five tubes are positive is accepted as the order of residual leukocytes (Fig. 7.4).

Results

Flow cytometry

The number of leukocytes measured on the Cytoron as a function of cell number expected from the hemocytometer count can be expressed by the regression lines: $y = 0.801x + 0.672$ ($r = 0.999$) for PC and $y = 0.823x - 0.454$ ($r = 0.999$) for RCC (Fig. 7.5). From the slope of the line, we found the measurements with the Cytoron to be about 20% below the expected cell counts.

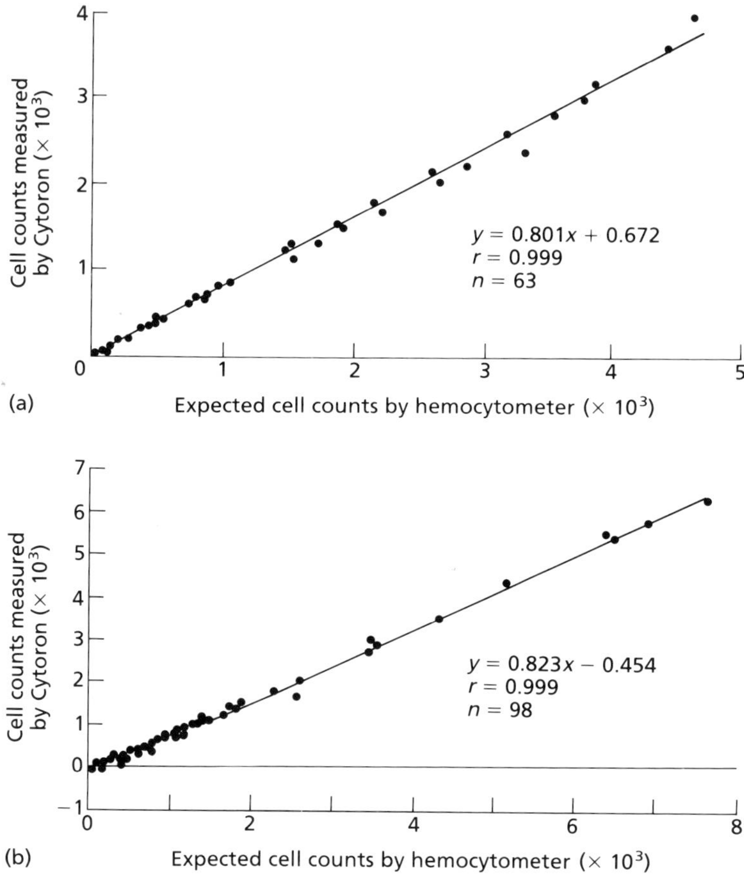

Fig. 7.5 Correlation between measurement of leukocytes by Cytoron and cell number expected by hemocytometer counts. (a) Platelet concentrate; (b) red cell concentrate.

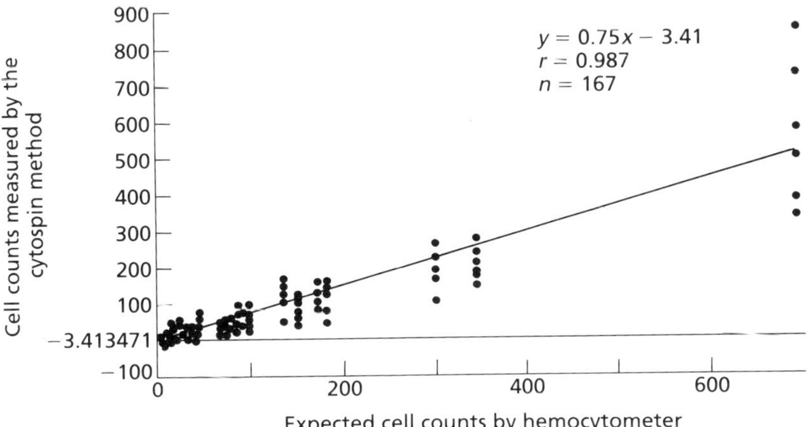

Fig. 7.6 Correlation between measurements of leukocytes in platelet concentrate by the cytospin method and cell number expected by hemocytometer counts.

Cytospin

The correlation of measurements by the cytospin technique and number of cells expected by hemocytometer count was expressed by a regression line, $y = 0.75x - 3.41$ ($r = 0.987$, $n = 167$), as shown in Figure 7.6. The cytospin method could detect leukocytes at concentrations as low as 1.2×10^{-2} cells/μl, which means that this technique is about 10 times more sensitive than the flow cytometric method.

Polymerase chain reaction method

As shown in Figure 7.7, this PCR method could successfully detect 2.4 cells in 1 ml. This sensitivity is 10 to 100-fold superior to that of the flow cytometric method. The double PCR method showed sensitivity similar to that of radioisotopic PCR (data not shown). Since the double PCR method could detect leukocytes of the order of 10^0/ml,

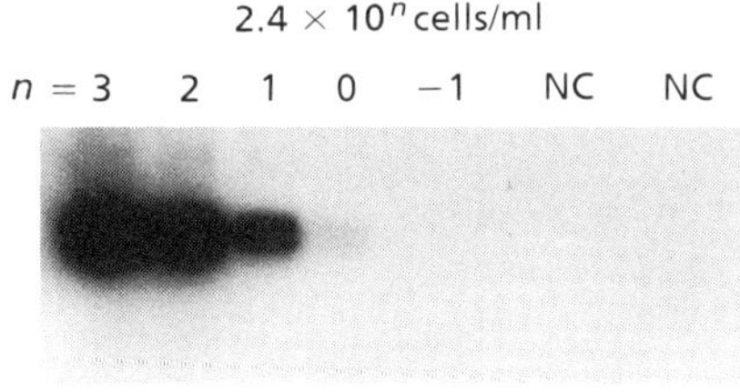

Fig. 7.7 The lower detection limit of polymerase chain reaction (PCR) using primers for β-globin gene and mononuclear cells. Southern blot analysis was carried out after PCR using mononuclear cells which were purified from peripheral blood using Ficoll gradient and serial diluted with Hanks' balanced salt solution. Water was used as the negative control of PCR.

Table 7.2 Measurement of leukocytes in filtered red cell concentrate (RCC) with 6 $\log_{10}$ leukocyte-removal filter

	Number of leukocytes (cells/ml)			
Experiment no.	Cytoron	(CV%)	PCR	$(10^0\ 10^1\ 10^2\ 10^3)*$
1	3.54×10^0	(220)	10^0	(5/5 2/5 0/5 NT)†
2	7.08×10^0	(158)	10^1	(5/5 5/5 2/5 NT)†
3	3.54×10^0	(220)	10^0	(5/5 0/5 0/5 NT)†
4	$< 3.54 \times 10^0$	(ND)	10^1	(5/5 5/5 0/5 NT)†
5	1.06×10^0	(129)	10^2	(5/5 5/5 5/5 0/5)†

* Dilution ratio of filtered RCC.
† Times sample was polymerase chain reaction-positive in five measurements.
CV, coefficient of variation; ND, not determined; NT, not tested.

we applied this method to count residual leukocytes following the method described in the section on materials and methods, above. We compared the results from the flow cytometric method, Cytoron, and PCR. The sample to be measured was RCC-filtered with a new filter which can obtain 6 log reduction. As shown in Table 7.2, PCR could detect leukocytes of the order of 10^0–10^2/ml.

Discussion and Conclusion

For the flow cytometric method, a dilution of 20% is caused by the sheath fluid in a sip tube when blood cells are drawn into the fluidic line of the Cytoron (Fig. 7.8). However, the coefficient of variation indicated that the degree of dilution was quite constant. After correction of the Cytoron measurements using these regression equations, there was a significant correlation between the measurement of leukocytes in PC and RCC by the Cytoron and hemocytometer in the range of 1×10^5–10^7 cells/ml ($r = 0.99$).

The efficacies of leukocyte removal filters were compared using the flow cytometric method. We filtered RCC with three types of filters, then counted the leukocytes in the filtrates with a Coulter counter S Plus IV, Neubauer hemocytometer, and Cytoron (Table 7.3). Measurements by Coulter counter and Neubauer hemocytometer, which are commonly used at laboratories, frequently failed to detect leukocytes in the filtrates. On the other hand, measurements by the Cytoron could detect leukocytes in all the filtrates. The same comparative experiments were done for platelet concentrate using Sepacell PL and Pall PL filters (Table 7.4). The flow cytometric technique could detect residual leukocytes in three filtrates at a level which was less than the detection sensitivity of the flow cytometer, which is 0.177 cells/µl. For these cases, we concentrated the samples 10 times by centrifugation, and stained them with propidium iodide. Then, to increase the sensitivity of the flow cytometric method, we concentrated the sample before flow cytometric analysis. Table 7.5 shows the

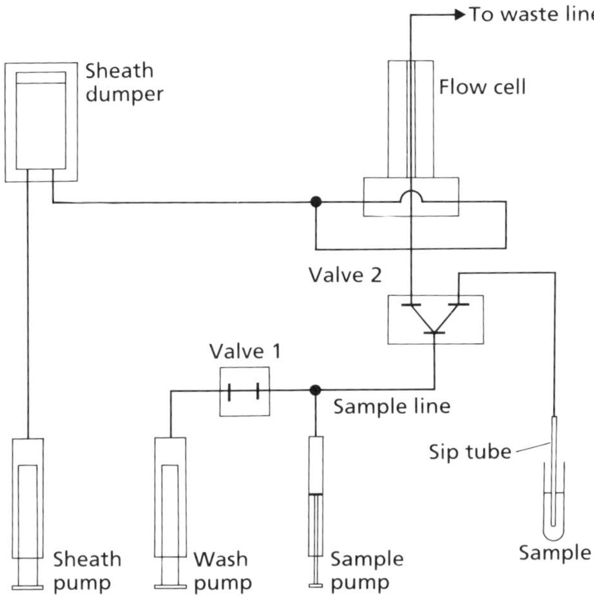

Fig. 7.8 Schematic diagram of the fluidic line in the Ortho Cytoron.

Table 7.3 Residual leukocytes in the filtered red cell concentrates*

| Filter | Experiment no. | Measurements ($\times 10^6$) | | | Removal rate (%) |
		Coulter counter	Hemocytometer	Flow cytometry	
Sepacell R-500†	1	0.00	0.00	0.80	99.97
	2	0.00	1.76	4.64	99.85
	3	0.00	0.00	0.11	99.99
	4	3.09	1.71	1.38	99.95
	5	0.00	0.00	0.88	99.96
Imugard E†	1	0.00	0.00	3.26	99.94
	2	0.00	0.00	2.06	99.94
	3	0.00	0.00	1.59	99.95
	4	4.40	4.90	2.06	99.92
	5	0.00	5.35	3.26	99.83
Pall RC-100‡	1	0.00	0.97	1.53	99.91
	2	0.00	0.00	1.01	99.96
	3	6.14	2.73	2.22	99.83
	4	0.00	2.86	0.75	99.98
	5	7.63	2.83	1.96	99.88

* Red cell concentrates prepared from 400 ml of whole blood.
† Preserved at 4°C for 3 days.
‡ Preserved at 4°C for 1 day.

Table 7.4 Residual leukocytes in the filtered platelet concentrates

		Measurements				
Filter	Experiment no.	Coulter counter $\times 10^6$	Hemocytometer $\times 10^6$	Flow cytometry $\times 10^4$	Cytospin $\times 10^4$	Removal rate (%)
Sepacell PL (5N)*	1	0.00	0.00	6.04		99.972
	2	1.96	0.00	3.61		99.970
	3	0.92	0.00	3.39		99.972
	4	2.75	0.00	0.00	1.05	99.990
	5	0.00	0.00	0.00	0.98	99.992
Sepacell PL (10N)†	1	0.00	0.00	3.39		99.990
	2	11.17	0.00	21.10		99.940
	3	1.92	0.00	7.24		99.973
	4	0.00	0.00	5.54		99.991
	5	0.00	0.00	28.23		99.934
Pall PL-50‡	1	0.00	0.00	0.00	1.28	99.994
	2	0.00	0.00	2.18		99.991
	3	0.00	0.00	2.09		99.990
	4	0.00	0.00	2.11		99.983
	5	0.00	0.00	4.05		99.984

*10 units of PC were stored at 22°C for 1 day.
† 20 units.
‡ 12 units, stored for 1 day.

Table 7.5 Increments of coefficient variation (CV) by centrifugal concentration

		CV (%)		
Products	Cell number (cell/µl)	Without concentration		With concentration
Platelet concentrate	0.195	82.2	→	32.4
	0.585	38.9	→	20.6
	0.975	35.8	→	13.5
	1.470	35.0	→	12.1
Red cell concentrate	0.195	84.0	→	36.8
	0.319	46.2	→	30.3
	0.797	41.0	→	20.4
	1.576	20.4	→	16.8

Coefficient variation: (s.d./mean) × 100%.

increment of coefficient variation when the sample was concentrated 10-fold. The coefficient of variation value was improved significantly by the concentration of both the RCC and PC samples, that is, the accuracy of the measurement was improved. This modification makes it possible to determine the efficacy of newly developed high

Table 7.6 Efficiency of Sepacell R-S350 (whole blood)

Storage period	Leukocyte removal rate (–log)	Total residual leukocytes ($\times 10^4$)	Platelet removal rate (–log)	Red cell recovery (%)
0 day	4.60 ± 0.28	5.61 ± 2.95	2.79 ± 0.15	89.63 ± 1.62
1 day	4.88 ± 0.22	3.32 ± 1.59	2.41 ± 0.42	85.67 ± 7.61

Mean ± 1 s.d. ($n = 9$).

performance filters, such as the R-S350 [5] (Asahi Medical, Tokyo, Japan) and Pall BPF-4 [6] (Pall Biomedical Products, East Hills, NY, USA; Tables 7.6 and 7.7) and to count the number of leukocytes in platelet concentrates prepared by the Cobe Spectra and CS-3000 Plus (Fig. 7.9).

The cytospin method could detect leukocytes at concentrations as low as 0.012 cells/µl. Another advantage of the cytospin technique is that the differential counts of leukocytes can be determined by staining the cells with Guimsa. Knowing the population of residual leukocytes in filtered blood products is as important as knowing the number of leukocytes. We concentrated the residual leukocytes in the filtered red cell concentrate and platelet concentrates by centrifugation with Ficoll or Percoll, and looked at the differential population of leukocytes using a flow cytometer [7]. Among leukocytes collected from the filtered PCs, monocytes were most effectively removed by all of the filters tested. When using the filters made for the RCC, monocytes are also most effectively removed. One must be careful because granulocytes tend to escape from filters made of nonwoven polyester fibers such as the Sepacell R-500 if RCC is fresh and filtered at above 4°C.

Concerning the removal rate of T and B cells, B cells are removed more effectively by filters made for RCCs. A similar tendency was also observed with the filters made for PCs but the specificity to B cells of filters was much less than that observed using filters made for RCCs. CD8-positive cells are more specifically removed by the filters made for PCs than CD4-positive cells. Among the filters, the Imugard RC filter [4], which is made of microporous polyvinyl alcohol, could remove CD8-positive cells. This type of study should help to clarify the mechanism of alloimmunization or viral infection transmitted by specific leukocytes and also to elucidate the mechanism of leukocyte depletion by filters, which are not perfectly understood at present [8].

Table 7.7 Efficiency of Pall BPF-4 (RCC)

Storage period	Leukocyte removal rate (–log)	Total residual leukocytes ($\times 10^4$)	Platelet removal rate (–log)	Red cell recovery (%)
0 day	3.93 ± 0.27	41.2 ± 31.4	2.24 ± 0.10	88.59 ± 0.88
3 days	4.61 ± 0.18	6.85 ± 2.12	2.35 ± 0.25	88.49 ± 0.96
5 days	4.79 ± 0.26	3.76 ± 1.47	1.91 ± 0.20	88.28 ± 1.27

– log (post/pre); mean ± 1 s.d. ($n = 3$).

                                   Chapter 7

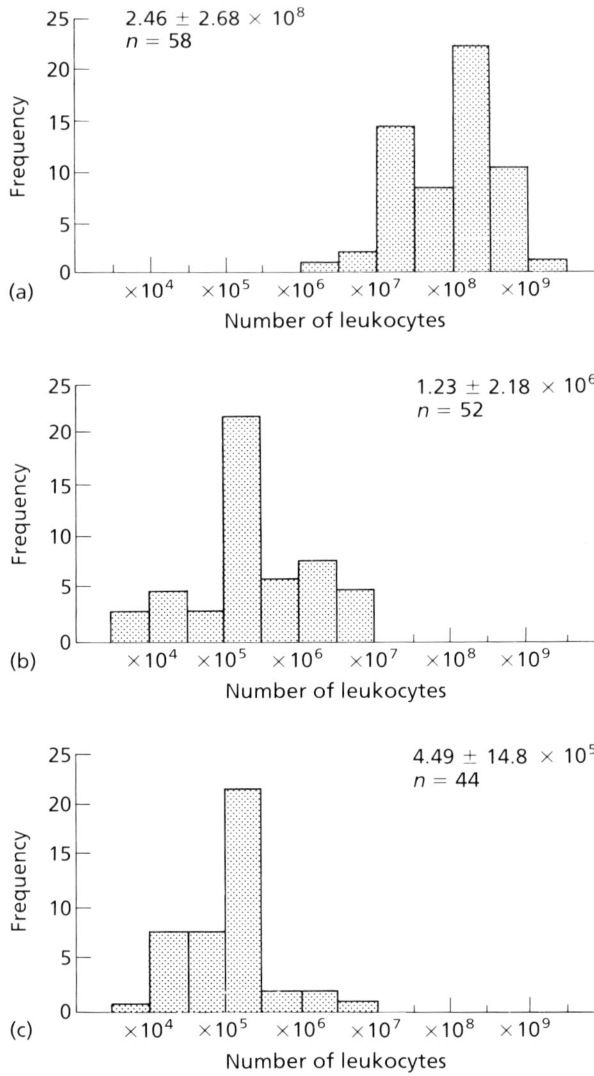

Fig. 7.9 Contaminated leukocytes in the products prepared by three different hemapheresis machines: (a) CS-3000; (b) CS-3000 Plus; (c) Cobe Spectra.

Table 7.8 [9] and Figure 7.10 summarize the limits of detection sensitivity of several counting methods and the numbers of residual leukocytes in RCC and PC filtered with currently available filters. The limit of sensitivity of the Cytoron was 177 cells/ml and concentrating samples 10-fold before propidium iodide staining improved this to 17 cells/ml, while that of the cytospin method was 12 cells/ml. The Nageotte chamber [10], which is a hemocytometer with a high-volume counting area (50 μl) and is popularly used among French researchers, shows high sensitivity, but the

Table 7.8 Sensitivity limit of different counting methods

Counting method	Limit of counting sensitivity (number of leukocytes) (µl)
Coulter counter (S Plus IV)	100*
Technicon H-1	50*
Neubauer hemocytometer 36 large squares	2.8
Nageotte hemocytometer	0.170
Flow cytometery	0.177
× 10 concentration	0.017
Cytospin	0.012

* From Wenz and Besso [9].

counting in the chamber is time-consuming. The limit which the Cytoron can detect is 17 cells or more per milliliter. If the same sample was measured by this method repeatedly, the coefficient of variance was slightly high (Table 7.2). This seems to indicate that the Cytoron is less reliable. On the other hand, PCR shows good reproducibility and higher sensitivity. In conclusion, the PCR method can cope with the new filters which will be developed soon to remove more leukocytes to prevent viral infections, such as human immunodeficiency virus and human T cell leukemia virus I [11].

Though various techniques have been developed quite intensively in the last months, each method has both advantages and disadvantages. The flow cytometric

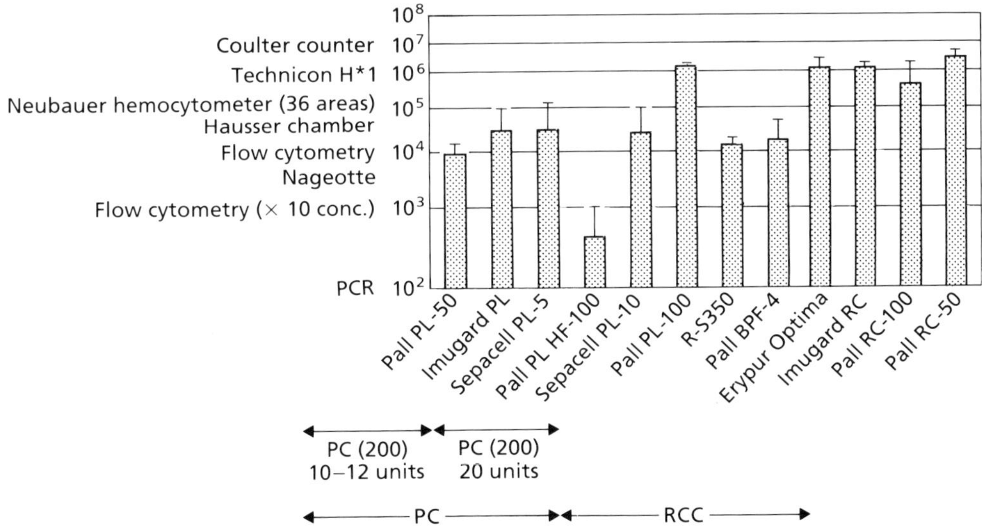

Fig. 7.10 Concentration of residual leukocytes in 100 ml of filtered red cell concentrate (RCC) or platelet concentrate (PC) and the sensitivity of counting methods. PCR, polymerase chain reaction.

method using the Ortho Cytoron flow cytometer has the advantages of easy operation, speed, and high sensitivity. The cytospin method would be helpful when the flow cytometer is not available and has the advantage of defining the population of leukocytes in the filtered blood products. The PCR method may be a promising method of detecting extremely low numbers of contaminating leukocytes. The combined use of these techniques should be helpful for the evaluation of new filters and the quality control of leukocyte-poor blood components.

References

1 Takahashi TA, Hosoda M, Sekiguchi S. A flow cytometric method to detect residual leukocytes in platelet and red cell concentrates. *Jpn J Transfus Med* 1990;36:429–437.

2 Takahashi TA, Hosoda M, Sekiguchi S. Cytospin method for the determination of residual leukocytes in leukocyte-depleted platelet concentrates. *Jpn J Transfus Med* 1989;35:497–503.

3 Abe H, Mogi Y, Hosoda M, Takashi TA, Sekiguchi S. Detection of a small number of residual leukocytes in filtered blood products by polymerase chain reaction. *J C Exp Med* 1992;160:887–888.

4 Segawa K, Hasegawa H, Hosoda M, Takahashi TA, Sekiguchi S. A new leukocyte removal filter — Imugard E for red cell concentrates — comparison of the efficacy with Sepacell R-500N. *Jpn J Transfus Med* 1990;36:497–503.

5 Takahashi TA, Oka S, Nishimura T *et al.* Evaluation of a new leukocyte removal filter, the R-350, in a closed system. *Jpn J Transfus Med* 1992;38:17–23.

6 Takahashi TA, Hosoda M, Sekiguchi S. Leukocyte depletion from red cell concentrates with the Pall RC100, PC50 and BPF4 filters. *Jpn J Med Instr* 1992;62:68–77.

7 Mogi Y, Hosoda M, Takahashi TA, Sekiguchi S. Flow cytometric analysis of residual leukocytes in filtered blood components. *Jpn J Transfus Med* 1991;37:617–626.

8 Freedman J, Blanchette V, Hornstein A *et al.* White cell depletion of red cell and pooled random-donor platelet concentrates by filtration and residual lymphocyte subset analysis. *Transfusion* 1991;31:433–440.

9 Wenz B, Besso N. Quality control and evaluation of leukocyte-depleting filters. *Transfusion* 1989;29:186–187.

10 Masse M, Andreu G, Angue M *et al.* A multicenter study on the efficiency of white cell reduction by filtration of red cells. *Transfusion* 1991;31:729–797.

11 Kobayashi M, Yano M, Kwon KW, Takahashi TA, Ikeda H, Sekiguchi S. Leukocyte depletion of HTLV-I carrier red cell concentrates by filters — the viral infectivity of residual leukocytes in the filtered red cell concentrates. *Jpn J Transfus Med* 1992;38:408–416.

Discussion

SNIECINSKI: In regard to the new Sepacell filter, after collection is any waiting period required before you can filter a fresh unit of blood?

TAKAHASHI: No, it is not necessary to wait. We can immediately proceed with filtration and preparation of blood components.

STIENSTRA: I like the data you presented on the differentiation of the leukocytes left after filtration. Did you do that with monoclonal antibodies with fluorescent staining?

TAKAHASHI: Yes.

STIENSTRA: Using those monoclonal antibodies could you always identify the monocytes, lymphocytes, and granulocytes?

TAKAHASHI: No. To identify monocytes, granulocytes, and lymphocytes, we used forward scatter and side scatter. For subpopulations such as T, B, and CD4 or CD8 cells, we used monoclonal antibodies.

MAEDA: When we measure the number of leukocytes, do we need to select the type of flow cytometer? Can we fit any flow cytometer to this measurement by modifying the machine?

HOSODA: We examined Facscan, but in vain, for the machine was not made to absorb a steady volume of samples in each measurement. There are some reports on the application of other types of machines, but they seem to be difficult to operate. In the case of the Cytoron, whereas this machine can adjust the sample volume with a syringe pump, it was very easy to count the residual leukocytes.

MAEDA: Thus, we have to select a flow cytometer to perform your method, don't we?

HOSODA: As I said before, some people were actually using Facscan or Epics. It is not impossible but may be rather difficult.

8 · Flow cytometric analysis of residual leukocytes in filtered blood components

Y. Mogi, T.A. Takahashi, M. Hosoda, and S. Sekiguchi

Hokkaido Red Cross Blood Center, Yamanote 2-2, Nishi-ku, Sapporo 063, Japan

Abstract

Red cell concentrates (RCCs) and platelet concentrates (PCs) were filtered by Imugard IG-400Y, Pall RC-100, Sepacell R-500N, Imugard RC, Pall PL-100, Sepacell PL-5N, and Imugard PL filters, and the residual leukocytes in the filtered RCCs and PCs were analyzed by flow cytometry.

For both RCCs and PCs monocytes were most effectively removed by leukocyte depletion filters. Among the filters made for RCC, the Imugard RC removed B, NK, and CD8$^+$ cells specifically. CD8$^+$ cells were more effectively removed than CD4$^+$ cells by the filters made for PCs but specificity to B and NK cells was not shown, except by the Imugard IG-400Y.

Introduction

Blood products contain 10^7–10^9 leukocytes per unit [1]. These leukocytes are known to induce the nonhemolytic febrile transfusion reaction (NHFTR), transfusion-associated human leukocyte antigen (HLA) alloimmunization, and to carry disease, causing the transfusion of transmitted viruses such as human T lymphotropic virus I (HTLV-I) and cytomegalovirus (CMV), and to cause graft-versus-host disease (GvHD) [1,2]. The number of leukocytes which induce each side-effect varies, for example, leukocytes need to be reduced to below 1–5×10^6 cells to prevent HLA alloimmunization [2–5]. It is also known that these side-effects are caused by different types of leukocytes [6,7]. The removal rates of leukocyte-depletion filters have been improved in recent years [8–12], while methods for counting very low numbers of residual leukocytes have been devised [13–18]. However, to prevent side-effects and to elucidate further the mechanisms by which these side-effects are caused by contaminated leukocytes, the populations and subpopulations of lymphocytes in filtered blood products should be studied as well as the number of leukocytes.

In this study, the numbers and populations of leukocytes, and the subpopulations and subsets of lymphocytes in filtered RCCs and PCs, were analyzed by the flow cytometric method.

Materials and methods

Blood products

Respectively, RCCs and PCs were made from 400 and 200 ml donations of whole blood (WB) from healthy donors. The blood was collected in triple bags with 56 ml of citrate phosphate dextrose (CPD). PC was stored at room temperature with horizontal agitation (60 rpm, 20–22 °C).

Filtration procedure

One unit of RCC was filtered with a Pall RC-100 (Pall, Glen Cove, NY, USA) or Sepacell R-500N (Asahi Medical, Tokyo, Japan), consisting of nonwoven polyester fibers, an Imugard RC (Terumo, Tokyo, Japan) composed of microporous polyvinyl alcohol, or an Imugard IG-400Y (Terumo) made of cotton wool.

PC 20 u was filtered through a Pall PL-100 made of nonwoven polyester fibers or Imugard IG-400Y and 10 u of PC through a Sepacell PL-5N made of nonwoven polyester fibers coated with polymer or an Imugard PL made of microporous polyurethane.

Leukocyte separation and concentration in postfiltration samples

To analyze the subpopulations of lymphocytes in filtered blood components the leukocytes in them were separated out and concentrated. Filtered RCC 2 or 3 u was pooled and diluted with an equal volume of Hanks' balanced salt solution without Ca^{2+} and Mg^{2+} (HBSS). A 30 ml aliquot of the diluted filtered RCC was layered on 20 ml of Ficoll-Paque (1.0777 g/ml, Pharmacia, Piscataway, NJ, USA) and centrifuged at 380 g for 30 min at room temperature. Mononuclear cells were harvested from the interface and washed first in HBSS then twice in HBSS with albumin (2% w/v). The cells were resuspended in 2 ml of HBSS with 2% albumin and used for analysis of subpopulations of lymphocytes.

In addition, 20 ml aliquots of 20 u of filtered PC were layered on to 20 ml of 33% Percoll (1.04 g/ml, Pharmacia, Uppsala, Sweden). After centrifugation at 127 g for 15 min at room temperature, the pellets were washed three times with phosphate-buffered saline (PBS) containing 1 : 10 volume of ACD. Finally, 2 ml of concentrated residual cells was used for analysis.

Subpopulation and subset analysis

Two milliliters of the lysing reagent (Ortho Diagnostic Systems, Tokyo) was added to 100 µl of sample and incubated for 15 min at room temperature. The population of leukocytes was analyzed using an Ortho Cytoron flow cytometer (Ortho Diagnostic

Systems, Tokyo). Granulocytes, monocytes, and lymphocytes were detected by forward and side-scattering. The samples for measurement of subpopulations were centrifuged at 300 **g** for 10 min at 4°C, had the supernatant removed and were then washed twice with 4 ml of PBS. PBS was added to the pellet and the total volume adjusted to 100 µl. Then the sample with 10 µl of monoclonal antibodies labeled with fluorescein isothiocyanate (FITC) or phycoerythrin (PE) or 10 µl of a negative control (FITC-conjugated murine immunoglobulin) added was incubated in an ice bath for 30 min. After washing with 4 ml of PBS, we removed the supernatant and resuspended the pellet in 1 ml of PBS. This cell suspension was analyzed by flow cytometer and we determined the positive rate of green (FITC) or red (PE) fluorescence about the cells indicated in the lymphocyte region.

Monoclonal antibody

We used Ortho-mune OK series (Ortho) monoclonal antibodies. OKT3 (CD3) is an antibody against human T lymphocytes and OKT4 (CD4) and OKT8 (CD8) mainly react with human helper/inducer T lymphocytes and suppressor/cytotoxic T lymphocytes, respectively. OKB20 (CD20) identifies human B lymphocytes and OKNK (CD16) reacts with natural killer (NK)/killer (K) cells, including large granular lymphocytes (LGL) and granulocytes.

Leukocyte counting

A 100 µl sample was added to 750 µl of propidium iodide (PI) solution. After incubation for 10 min at room temperature the cells were detected on the two-dimensional dot plot of forward-scatter and red fluorescence by flow cytometry and the number of leukocytes was calculated [14].

Statistical analysis

We used the two-tailed paired *t*-test to determine the differences between the subpopulations and the subsets of lymphocytes before and after filtration and judged differences to be significant when the P value was less than 0.05.

Results

Removal rate by filtration and the number of residual leukocytes

Figure 8.1 shows the removal rates of leukocytes and the number of residual leukocytes when fresh or 1-day-stored RCCs were filtered. Generally the removal rate of monocytes was highest in populations of leukocytes and more granulocytes were removed than lymphocytes. When fresh RCCs were filtered using a Sepacell R-500N,

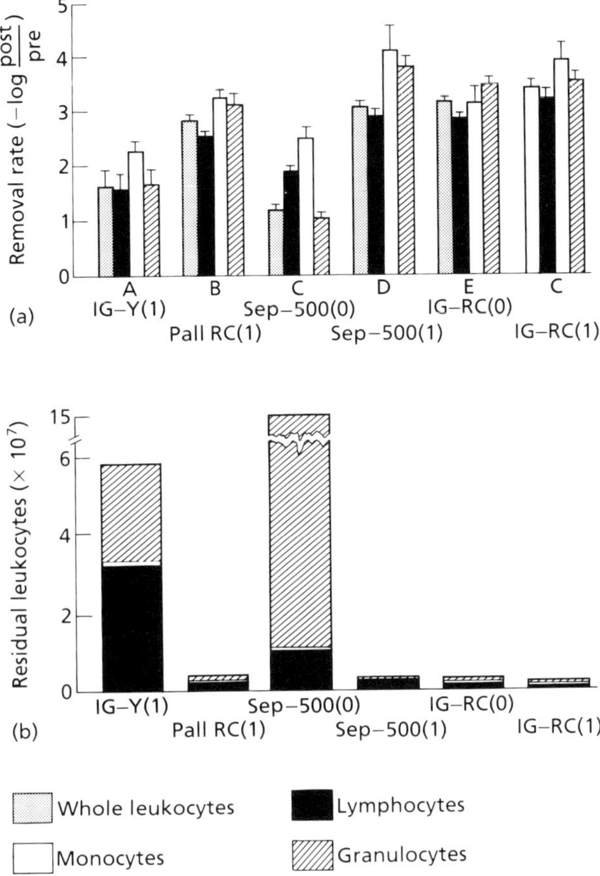

Fig. 8.1 (a) The removal rate of leukocytes and (b) the number of residual leukocytes per bag in filtered red cell concentrate (RCC). The removal rate is shown as mean $\pm$ 1 s.e. (0) and (1) indicate fresh and 1-day-stored RCC, respectively. (A) $n = 3$; (B) $n = 4$; (C) $n = 5$; (D) $n = 7$; (E) $n = 6$. IG-RC, Imugard RC; IG-Y, Imugard IG-400Y; Pall RC, Pall RC-100; Sep-500, Sepacell R-500N.

the removal rate of leukocytes was only 93.2% because many granulocytes came out. But when RCC was stored for 1 day the result was as good as those with other filters. The Imugard RC removed leukocytes very well from both fresh and stored RCC. The total number of residual leukocytes was $1.5 \pm 0.4 \times 10^8$ cells with the Sepacell R-500N (fresh RCC), $5.8 \pm 2.9 \times 10^7$ cells for the Imugard IG-400Y and below 4×10^6 cells for the other filters ($n = 4$).

The leukocyte removal rates of four kinds of filters for PC and the numbers of residual leukocytes are shown in Figure 8.2. All filters depleted monocytes most effectively. The Imugard PL removed 99.91% (3.07 $\log_{10}$) of leukocytes and the number of residual leukocytes was $2.5 \pm 0.8 \times 10^5$ cells for this filter, but $7-8 \times 10^5$ cells were left by the other filters.

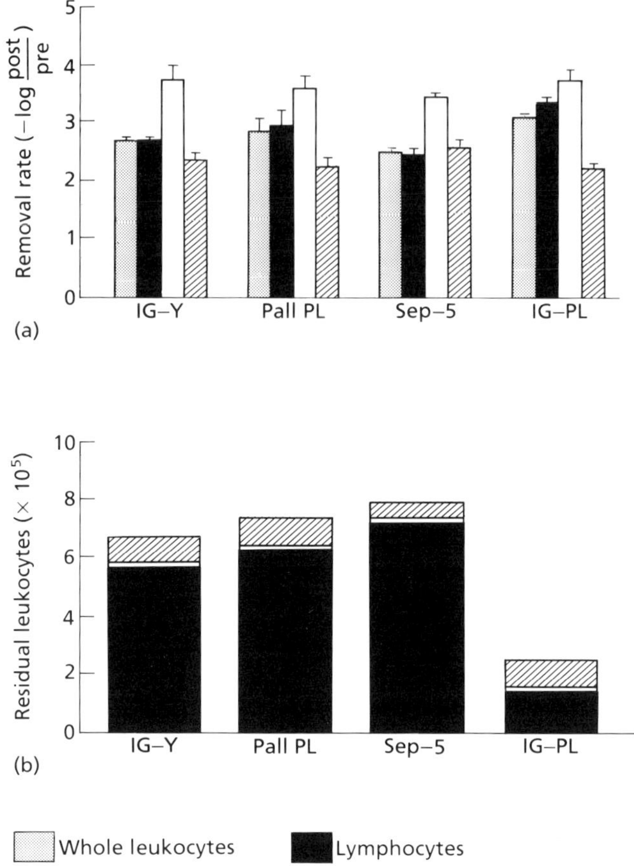

Fig. 8.2 (a) The removal rate of leukocytes and (b) the number of residual leukocytes per 20 u in filtered PC. The removal rate is shown as mean $\pm$ 1 s.e. $n = 4$. IG-PL, Imugard PL; IG-Y, Imugard IG-400Y; Pall PL, Pall PL-100; Sep-5, Sepacell PL-5N.

Subpopulations and subsets of lymphocytes in filtered blood products

T and B lymphocytes

The ratio of T lymphocytes to B lymphocytes after filtration was significantly higher than that before filtration with all filters for RCC except the Pall RC-100 (Fig. 8.3). When using the Imugard RC there was a marked difference, especially in fresh RCC (T/B in prefiltration 6.50 $\pm$ 1.05; in postfiltration 225.56 $\pm$ 72.38), and in stored RCC (pre: 7.13 $\pm$ 0.26; post: 33.16 $\pm$ 10.67). This suggested that B cells were removed

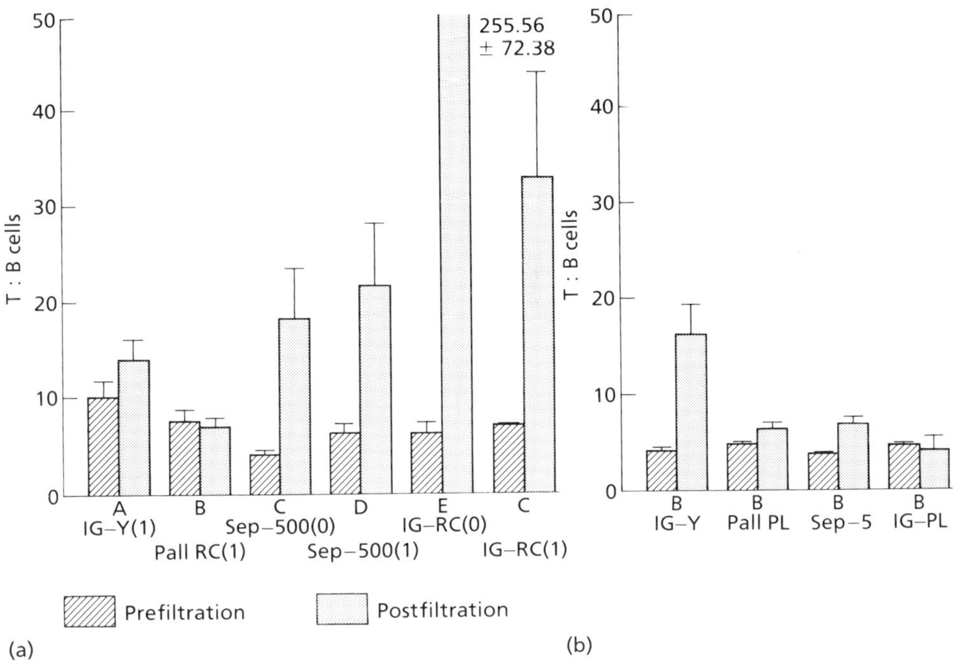

Fig. 8.3. The ratio of T cells to B cells in filtered (a) red cell concentrate (RCC) and (b) platelet concentrate (PC). The ratio is shown as mean ± 1 s.e. (0) and (1) indicate fresh and 1-day-stored RCC, respectively. (A) $n = 3$; (B) $n = 4$; (C) $n = 5$; (D) $n = 7$; (E) $n = 6$. IG-PL, Imugard PL; IG-RC, Imugard RC; IG-Y, Imugard IG-400Y; Pall PL, Pall PL-100; Pall RC, Pall RC-100; Sep-5, Sepacell PL-5N; Sep-500, Sepacell R-500N.

more effectively than T cells by filters for RCC. A significantly high value of the ratio of T cells to B cells was obtained after PC filtration by the Imugard IG-400Y, while the ratio of T cells to B cells also tended to be higher after filtration by the Sepacell PL-5N and Pall PL-100, though there was no difference when using the Imugard PL.

Natural killer cells

The Sepacell R-500N and Imugard RC had a tendency to remove NK cells more effectively than T cells (Fig. 8.4). When using the Sepacell R-500N, the ratio of T cells to NK cells was larger in stored RCC (21.81 ± 6.60) than in fresh RCC (9.35 ± 2.54). In contrast to this, when using the Imugard RC it was smaller in stored RCC (13.10 ± 3.54) than in fresh RCC (47.65 ± 16.16). The Pall RC-100 also tended to remove NK cells more effectively than T cells, though a significant difference was not observed.

No filters made for PC showed specificity to NK cells.

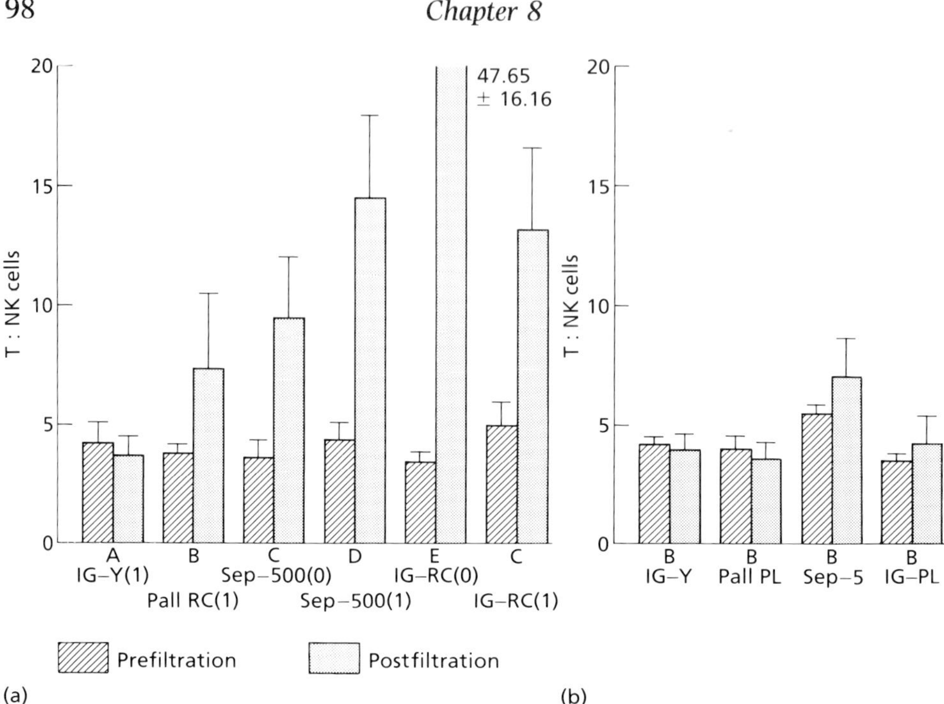

Fig. 8.4 The ratio of T cells to natural killer (NK) cells in filtered (a) red cell concentrate (RCC) and (b) platelet concentrate (PC). The ratio is shown as mean ± 1 s.e. (0) and (1) indicate fresh and 1-day-stored RCC, respectively. (A) $n = 3$; (B) $n = 4$; (C) $n = 5$; (D) $n = 7$; (E) $n = 6$. IG-PL, Imugard PL; IG-RC, Imugard RC; IG-Y, Imugard IG-400Y; Pall PL, Pall PL-100; Pall RC, Pall RC-100; Sep-5, Sepacell PL-5N; Sep-500, Sepacell R-500N.

CD4-positive and CD8-positive T cells

When fresh RCCs were filtered by the Sepacell R-500N and both fresh and stored RCC were filtered by the Imugard RC, the ratio of CD4$^+$ to CD8$^+$ in residual T lymphocytes was larger than in prefiltration T cells (Fig. 8.5). Particularly when using the Imugard RC for fresh RCC filtration the postfiltration ratio was 5.55 ± 1.41 — about four times that at prefiltration (1.44 ± 0.15).

CD8$^+$ cells were more specifically removed by the filters for PC. The ratio of CD8$^+$ to CD4$^+$ at postfiltration was 5.25 ± 0.75 for the Imugard PL and 3.05–3.46 for other filters, which was more than twice that at prefiltration.

Summary

When fresh RCCs were filtered by the Sepacell R-500N, granulocytes came out of the filters, and the total removal rate of leukocytes was lower (Fig. 8.1). This tendency toward granulocyte leakage in fresh RCC filtration [9,19] was also present when using

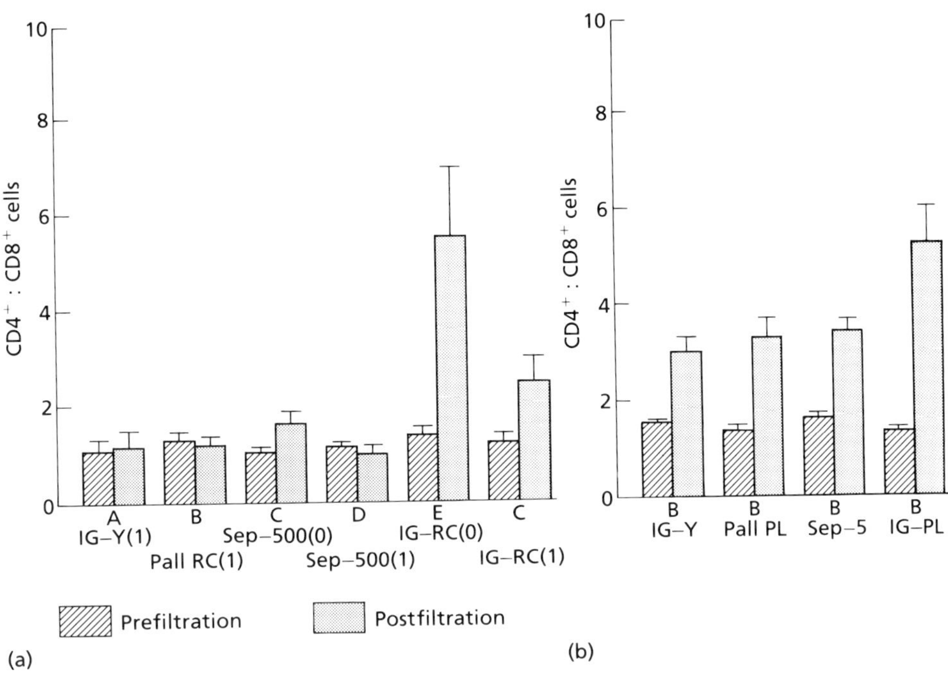

Fig. 8.5. The ratio of CD4$^+$ cells to CD8$^+$ cells in filtered (a) red cell concentrate (RCC) and (b) platelet concentrate (PC). The ratio is shown as mean $\pm$ 1 s.e. (0) and (1) indicate fresh and 1-day-stored RCC, respectively. (A) n = 3; (B) n = 4; (C) n = 5; (D) n = 7; (E) n = 6. IG-PL, Imugard PL; IG-RC, Imugard RC; IG-Y, Imugard IG-400Y; Pall PL, Pall PL-100; Pall RC, Pall RC-100; Sep-5, Sepacell PL-5N; Sep-500, Sepacell R-500N.

the Pall RC-50 (Pall), which is also made of nonwoven polyester fibers (authors' unpublished data), but not with the Imugard RC, made of microporous polyvinyl alcohol. This apparently reflects the difference of materials used in the filters. However, when fresh RCCs were filtered at room temperature with the Sepacell R-500N after refrigeration at 4°C for 2–3 h, the granulocyte leakage was reduced considerably [9]. Nor did granulocytes come out of the experimental R-S350 filter, which was composed of high-density nonwoven fibers [20]. Thus, the granulocyte leakage might be caused by active passage through the filters.

The residual leukocytes in filtered PC were composed of greater numbers of lymphocytes than in filtered RCC (Fig. 8.2). This result probably reflects the fact that most leukocytes in PC before filtration were lymphocytes.

Up to this time the Imugard IG-400Y, made of cotton wool, has generally been used as the second-generation filter for leukocyte depletion from RCC and PC, but the removal rate of leukocytes was not good enough to prevent alloimmunization, and many red blood cells were lost. Moreover, platelets adhered to the fibers. Among third-generation filters, the Sepacell R-500N and Pall RC, made of micropolyester fibers in nonwoven cloth, raised the removal rate of leukocytes and contributed to the decrease of filter volume. Leukocyte depletion in nonwoven polyester fibers is first due to passive adhesion on fibers; second, to capture in close contact with the fibers (trapping), and third, to active adhesion [21]. On the other hand, it was considered that the Imugard RC, made of microporous polyvinyl alcohol, depleted leukocytes by trapping in addition to adhesion.

Steneker and Biewenga [22] identified the populations of residual leukocytes in each polyester layer of three filters made of nonwoven polyester fibers and studied the mechanisms of leukocyte depletion. They described how granulocytes and monocytes were mainly captured by adherence, whereas lymphocyte depletion depended on either trapping (Pall RC-100) or adhesion (Sepacell R-500). In most cases of RCC or PC filtration monocytes were most effectively removed (except for fresh RCC filtration by the Imugard RC). This suggests that monocytes are larger than other cells, and have stronger adherence. That monocytes and B cells were more specifically removed by the filters is consistent with the report of Vakkila and Myllylä [23]. From the tendency for the removal rate of monocytes to be high and for B cells and CD8$^+$ cells to be removed more easily than T cells and CD4$^+$ cells, respectively, we deduce that in addition to trapping depending on the cell size, cell adhesion is an important factor in the mechanism of leukocyte depletion, regardless of the material. Yoshida *et al.* evaluated the lymphocyte depletion of specific subsets by filtration when using a Sepacell R-500 and an Imugard IG-500 (cotton wool) for lymphocyte-rich plasma collected by hemapheresis [24]. Their samples included a greater number of lympho-cytes and the removal rate was less than that in this study, so it is difficult to compare the results, though the more effective removal of B cells and CD8$^+$ cells is consistent with our results.

Both the Pall RC-100 and Sepacell R-500N are made of nonwoven polyester fibers, but there are some differences in their removal specificities, especially for B cells. The filter surface of the Pall RC is coated with a radiation graft, in contrast to the fibers in Sepacell R-500N, which are not. The results of this study may help in the investigation of the relation of the surface electric charge of fibers to cell adhesion.

Since the surface of the fibers in the filters made of nonwoven polyester fibers is treated for prevention of platelet adhesion, the tendency to specific cell depletion was expected to be reduced in comparison with RCC filters. Certainly the specificity to B cells decreased (Fig. 8.3) and, when using Pall and Sepacell filters for PC, the removal rate of NK cells was less than when using the filters for RCC (Fig. 8.4). However, the filters for PC tend to remove CD8$^+$ cells more effectively than CD4$^+$ cells (Fig. 8.5). As yet, no evidence that the size or adherence of CD4$^+$ cells is different from that of CD8$^+$ cells has been obtained, so to explain this result it is necessary to study in detail the cells and the filter materials.

Imugard RC and Imugard PL filters composed of micropores are made of different materials and have differently shaped micropores, so it is difficult to infer the mechanisms of leukocyte depletion from our results. However, we can hypothesize that the difference of adherence rather than cell size is probably the reason why the Imugard RC made of microporous polyvinyl alcohol showed stronger specificity to B and NK cells than not only the Imugard PL but also the filters made of nonwoven polyester fibers.

As described above, the populations of residual leukocytes in filtered blood products differ according to the kind of filter and the storage period of RCC, but are similar under similar conditions. It is important to consider again the *in vivo* experiments reported up to the present on prevention of alloimmunization using leukocyte-depletion filters. That B cells expressing major histocompatibility complex class II antigen are removed specifically is very important for prevention of alloimmunization, because class II antigen-positive cells are said to be the main immunogen. Further specific removal of CD8$^+$ cells may influence the occurrence of GvHD and be effective for prevention of transfusion–transmission of viruses in specific leukocytes.

It will be necessary to investigate in detail the characters of the lymphocytes which leak from each type of filter.

References

1 Sekiguchi S. Blood transfusion in organ transplantation. *Transplant Now* 1989;2:357–365.

2 Meryman HT. Cleaning up red cells and platelets: alloimmunization, immunosuppression and disease transmission. In: McCarthy LJ, Baldwin ML, eds. *Controversies of Leukocyte-poor Blood and Components*. Arlington: American Association of Blood Banks, 1989:1–26.

3 Fisher M, Chapman JR, Ting A, Morris PJ. Alloimmunization to HLA antigens following transfusion with leucocyte-poor and purified platelet suspensions. *Vox Sang* 1985;49:331–335.

4 Myllylä G. Leukco-depletion: the Finnish experience. Presented at the Meeting of British Blood Transfusion Society on the Aspects of Blood Filtration, Birmingham, UK, 1990.

5 Saarinen UM, Kekomäki R, Siimes MA, Myllylä G. Effective prophylaxis against platelet refractoriness in multitransfused patients by use of leukocyte-free blood components. *Blood* 1990;75:512–517.

6 Sekiguchi S, Takahashi TA. Leucocyte-depleted blood products and their clinical usefulness. In: Brozović B, ed. *The Role of Leucocyte Depletion in Blood Transfusion Practice*. Oxford: Blackwell Scientific Publications, 1989:26–34.

7 Ikeda Y, Handa M. Leukocyte depletion from blood products. *Immunohaematology* 1989;11:145–152.

8 Takebe M, Hatomi S, Tsubokura M. The preparation of leukocyte-poor concentrated red cells for transfusion by Imugard E leukocyte removal filter. *Jpn J Transfus Med* 1989;35:622–626.

9 Segawa K, Hasegawa H, Hosoda M, Takahashi TA, Sekiguchi S. A new leukocyte removal filter Imugard E for red cell concentrates: comparison of the efficacy with Sepacell R-500N. *Jpn J Transfus* 1990;36:497–503.

10 Miyamoto M, Sasakawa S, Ishikawa Y, Ogawa A, Nishimura T, Kuroda T. Development of a new filter for preparation of leukocyte-poor platelet concentrates at the bedside. *Jpn J Transfus Med* 1989;35:370–374.

11 Takahashi TA, Hosoda M, Mogi Y *et al.* A new porous polyurethane filter to remove leukocytes from platelet concentrates. *Jpn J Transfus Med* 1991;37:24–31.

12 Takahashi TA, Hosoda M, Sekiguchi S. Leukocyte depletion from platelet concentrates with new filters: the Pall PL100 and PL50. *Jp J Med Instr* 1990;60:351–357.

13 Takahashi TA, Hosoda M, Sekiguchi S. Cytospin method for the determination of residual leukocytes in leukocyte-depleted platelet concentrates. *Jpn J Transfus Med* 1989;35:497–503.

14 Takahashi TA, Hosoda M, Sekiguchi S. A flow cytometric method to detect residual leukocytes in platelet and red cell concentrates. *Jpn J Transfus Med* 1990;36:429–437.

15 Bodensteiner DC. A flow cytometric technique to accurately measure postfiltration white blood cell counts. *Transfusion* 1989;29:651–653.

16 Dzik WH, Ragosta A, Cusack WF. Flow-cytometric method for counting very low numbers of leukocytes in platelet products. *Vox Sang* 1990;59:153–159.

17 Wenz B, Burns ER, Lee V, Miller WK. A rare-event analysis model for quantifying white cells in white cell-depleted blood. *Transfusion* 1991;31:156–159.

18 Sadoff BJ, Dooley DC, Kapoor V, Law P, Friedman LI, Stromberg RR. Methods for measuring a 6 $\log_{10}$ white cell depletion in red cells. *Transfusion* 1991;31:150–155.

19 Miyamoto M, Shiba M, Mura T, Sasakawa S. The preparation of leukocyte-poor concentrated red cells (CRC) by Sepacell R-500 filter. *Jpn J Transfus Med* 1990;36:567–573.

20 Takahashi TA, Oka S, Nishimura T, *et al.* Evaluation of a new high-performance leukocyte removal filter, the R-S350, in a closed system. *Jpn J Transfus Med* 1992;38:401–407.

21 Takahashi TA, Hosoda M, Mogi Y, Sekiguchi S. Preparation of leukocyte-depleted blood products by filtration. *Blood Programme* 1991;14:311–316.

22 Steneker I, Biewenga J. Histologic and immunohistochemical studies on the preparation of white cell-poor red cell concentrates: the filtration process using three different polyester filters. *Transfusion* 1991;31:40–46.

23 Vakkila J, Myllylä G. Amount and type of leukocytes in 'leukocyte-free' red cell and platelet concentrates. *Vox Sang* 1987;53:76–82.

24 Yoshida H, Ito K, Uchino H. Preliminary study for therapeutic filtration lymphocytapheresis. *Jpn J Transfus Med* 1986;32:389–393.

Discussion

KOMURO (Japan NIH): What do you think is the meaning of lymphocyte subpopulations?

MOGI: It is well known that HLA-DR antigens are expressed on monocytes and B cells. We can safely say that DR-expressing cells tend to be removed effectively, according to our experimental result that these cells were ready to be removed. But in the case of T cells, only activated T cells express DR-antigens and I'm not sure whether activated T cells can be easily removed or not from only these results. Further analysis seems to be required.

Part 3
Basic Aspects

9·Mechanism of leukocyte removal with fibers

S. Oka, K. Maeda, T. Nishimura, and N. Yamawaki

Research and Development Laboratory, Asahi Medical Co. Ltd,
2111–2 Oaza-Sato, Oita City, Oita 870–03, Japan

Abstract

The mechanism of leukocyte removal with fibers was studied using polyester nonwoven fabric, and followings were found. Leukocytes are removed at a constant ratio against thickness of the nonwoven fabric, and this ratio of removal varies with changes in average fiber diameters and chemical properties of the fiber surface of nonwoven fabrics. Increasing the amount of leukocytes to be treated causes a dose-dependent reduction in the removal rate at the upper stream of the nonwoven fabric.

These observations strongly suggest that the mechanism of leukocyte removal is mainly an adsorption. It was also observed that an adhesion mechanism removed granulocytes throughout the experiment using a metabolism inhibitor.

Taking account of these results, a new higher-performance leukocyte removal filter R-S350 was developed and its basic performance was evaluated. It was confirmed that this filter could assure a 4 log depletion of leukocytes in actual use.

Introduction

Medical needs with regard to leukocyte removal filters can be divided into two main categories. One is an improvement of leukocyte removal rate in order to prevent alloimmunization. The other is development of new technology which enables the selective removal of some kinds of leukocytes in order to carry out selective cytapheresis treatment, such as removal of helper T cells for autoimmune diseases and removal of suppressor T cells for cancers.

These needs can be arranged according to the following technical subjects for those engaged in the development of leukocyte removal filters:

1 Making clear the effects of the physical structure of nonwoven fabric and chemical properties of fiber surface on the leukocyte removal rate or selectivity of leukocyte removal in order to design suitable filter materials for individual purposes.

2 Combining findings from **1** with the quality assurance of filters and supplying safe products.

In our present study, selecting polyester nonwoven fabrics as a filter material, we tried to clarify the leukocyte-removing mechanism through consideration on the relationship between the physicochemical structure of the filter material and leuko-cyte removal performance and on a possible relationship between leukocyte removal and leukocyte metabolism. We developed a new high-performance filter R-S350, based on the findings of the above-mentioned study and investigated the feasibility of quality assurance. In addition, we would like to introduce our recent trials giving selective removability to the filter material by a polymer-coating technique.

Materials and methods

Study of the leukocyte-removing mechanism

Filter material

Polyester nonwoven fabrics manufactured by a melt-blown process (average fiber dia-meter; 1.7 and 1.2 μm) and the same coated with poly(2-hydroxyethylmethacrylate; polyHEMA) were used.

Preparation of red cell concentrate

Red cell concentrate (RCC) derived and prepared in accordance with the Japanese Red Cross standard operation procedure and stored at 4°C for 3 days was used.

In a part of the experiments, RCC with 0.1% (w/v) sodium azide added as metabolism inhibitor was used.

Filtration

To examine the relationship between the thickness of the filter material and the concentration of residual leukocytes and residual platelets, the RCC was filtered at a flow rate of 2 ml/min through filter units assembled by filling containers having an effective filtering area of 9 cm^2 with the above-mentioned filter material so as to adjust the packing density to 0.14 g/cm^3.

In some experiments, plastic particles having the same diameter with leukocytes or platelets (STADEX SS-021-P and SS-071-P, Japan Synthetic Regin, Tokyo, Japan; Uniform Latex Particles, diameter 6.4 μm, Dow Chemical Company, IN, USA; Coulter calibration standard diameter 13.7 μm, Coulter Electronics, Hialeath, FL, USA) were filtered in the same manner, and the removal behavior was compared with blood cells.

Measurement of concentration of leukocytes, platelets, and plastic particles

The concentration of leukocytes before filtration was measured with a hemacytometer after having stained leukocytes with Türk's solution. The concentration of leukocytes after filtration was measured with a hemacytometer under epifluorescence microscope after hemolyzing recovered blood with ammonium oxalate and staining the leukocyte nucleus with fluorescent dye, acridine orange. The concentration of platelets before and after filtration was measured with an automatic blood cell counter (Sysmex microcell counter F-800, Toa Medical Electronics, Kobe, Japan). The concentration of plastic particles was measured with a particle counter (Coulter multisizer, Coulter Electronics, Hialeath, FL, USA).

Analysis of the residual leukocyte subset in filtered red cell concentrate

The RCC after filtration was concentrated five times by centrifugation, then the cells were adhered to a slide with cytospin (Cytospin2. Shandon Southern Products, Runcorn, Cheshire, UK) and stained with Diff-Quick (Harleco, Gibbstown, NJ, USA). Then the ratio of lymphocytes, monocytes, and granulocytes was measured under microscope.

Evaluation of the R-S350 filter

The R-S350 was assembled by filling a container having an effective filtering area of 45 cm^2 with polyester nonwoven fabrics so as to adjust the packing density to 0.28 g/cm^3 and layer thickness of 5.1 mm.

RCC 350 ml (stored 1–2 days), of which the hematocrit value was adjusted to 55% in estimation of the mean hematocrit value of RCC with preservatives such as AS-1 by adding physiologic saline, was filtered through a R-S350 filter by a head-distance of 1.5 m. The leukocyte removal rate, red cell recovery, and filtration time were evaluated. In this experiment, leukocytes after filtration were counted by the fluorescence/hemacytometer technique developed by Sadoff *et al.* [1].

Results

Study of the leukocyte-removing mechanism

Relation between leukocyte-removing behavior and thickness or average fiber diameter of polyester nonwoven fabric

Nonwoven fabrics of average fiber diameter 1.7 or 1.2 μm were assembled into three types of housing of differing thickness. The concentration of residual leukocytes in 2 ml of RCC emerging first from each filter assembly was examined. As a result, it was confirmed that the leukocyte concentration decreased exponentially against the thickness of the nonwoven fabric. Therefore, the logarithmic residual rate of leukocytes was reduced in proportion to the thickness of the fabric (Fig. 9.1). This indicates that leukocytes are removed at a constant rate against the unit thickness of nonwoven fabric. This phenomenon can be explained by the following mathematical

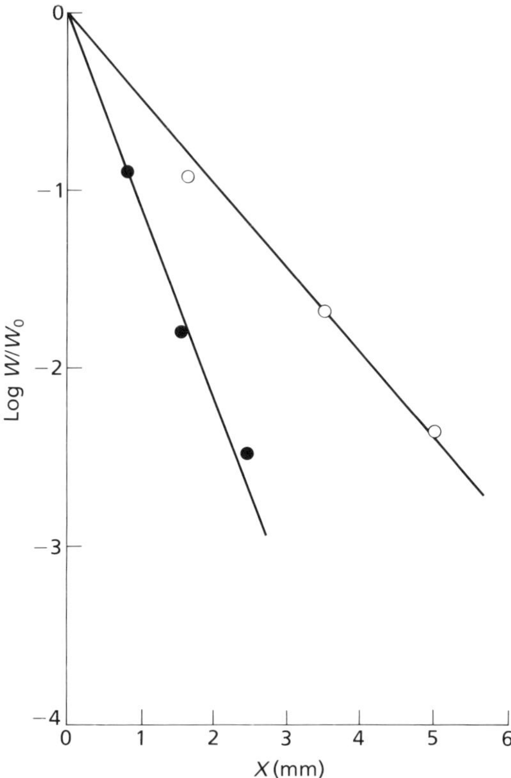

Fig. 9.1 Logarithmic residual rate of leukocytes after filtration plotted against the thickness of the nonwoven fabrics. W/W_0, residual rate of leukocytes; X, thickness of the nonwoven fabric; ● nonwoven fabric of average fiber diameter 1.2 μm; ○ nonwoven fabric of average fiber diameter 1.7 μm.

formula:

$$-dW = Wnp\,dx$$

where $-dW$ is the decrease in leukocyte concentration after filtration through the fabric having a thickness of dx; W is the concentration of leukocytes before filtration; n is the contact time of leukocytes to the adsorption points per unit thickness; p is the probability of removal per contact; and dx is the differential thickness of the fabric.

The integral of this equation for $x = 0$ to $x = x$, $w = W_0$ to $w = W$ is as follows:

$$\int_{W_0}^{W} dW/W = -\int_{0}^{X} np\,dx$$

which gives:

$$\log_{10}(W/W_0) = -(npx)/2.303$$

This equation explains the phenomenon we observed. As shown in Figure 9.1, the slope of the nonwoven fabric of average fiber diameter 1.2 μm is twice as great as that of 1.7 μm. According to the above model, it is speculated that the difference in slope of the nonwoven fabrics is due to the difference in the n value of each fabric. Since both fabrics are used in the same packing density in this experiment, the length of fibers contained in the unit volume of fabric of 1.2 μm is calculated to be twice as great as that of 1.7 μm.

Scanning electron microphotographs of leukocytes captured by nonwoven fabric (Fig. 9.2) show that leukocytes are caught in a fiber network where two or more fibers have contact with each other; this can be expressed as the crossover point.

Such crossover point of fibers seems to be a substantial site of adsorption. The number of crossover points in a unit volume of the nonwoven fabric of average fiber diameter 1.2 μm, which is calculated on the hypothesis that fibers are straight and arranged randomly in the fabric, is 2.8 times more than that of 1.7 μm. Though this does not accurately meet the experimental number that we observed, it is not far from the possibility of explaining the results. It is necessary in the future to refine the above crossover point model as well as to make clear the true nature of the adsorption points.

Dependence of leukocyte removal on its metabolism

To examine whether the leukocyte metabolism takes the role in the removal of leukocytes — in other words, whether leukocytes are passively removed by the fabric or actively adhere to the fabric — similar experiments were carried out by adding 0.1% sodium azide as a metabolism inhibitor. The contents of the residual leukocyte subset were also analyzed in order to determine if there is any difference between granulocytes and lymphocytes.

As shown in Figure 9.3, the addition of sodium azide showed no difference in lymphocyte removal by nonwoven fabric and it was observed that lymphocytes were passively removed. In contrast, the residual rate of granulocytes was increased by the addition of sodium azide, suggesting the contribution of active adhesion.

However, the effect of sodium azide on the granulocyte removal rate was small and the passive removal mechanism mainly contributed to the removal of granulocytes.

Which is the passive removal mechanism — adsorption or sieving?

It has been observed in the above experiments that the passive removal mechanism mainly contributed to leukocyte removal. In other words, the adsorption model as a passive removal mechanism well matches the phenomenon we observed. To investigate the possibility of a sieving mechanism as the passive removal mechanism, we further examined the effect on the removal rate if we chemically modified the fiber surface or if we changed the amount of leukocytes applied. Plastic particles with

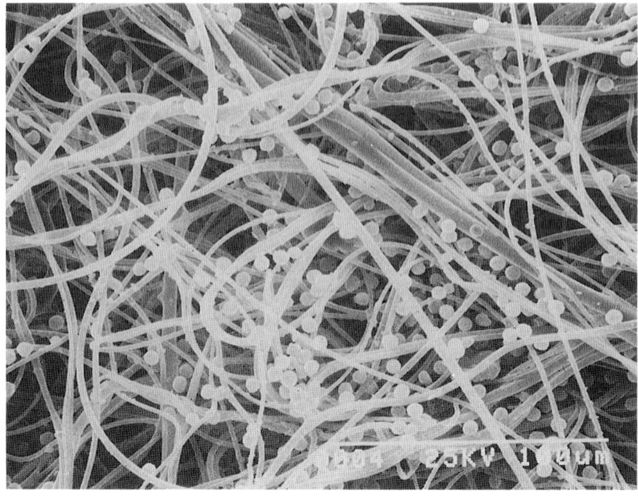

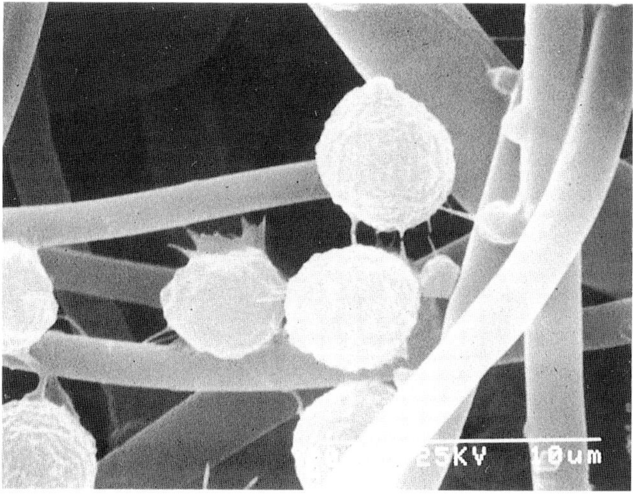

Fig. 9.2 Scanning electron microphotographs of leukocytes captured by nonwoven fabric with a diameter of 1.8 μm.

similar diameters to those of leukocytes or platelets were filtered in the same manner and their removal behavior was compared with those of blood cells.

As stated above, leukocytes were removed in a constant proportion to the thickness of nonwoven fabric, while the removal of platelets and plastic particles was found to be unrelated to the thickness of the fabric (Fig. 9.4).

This suggests that platelets and plastic particles are mainly removed at the upper stream in the nonwoven fabric and not removed during passing through the

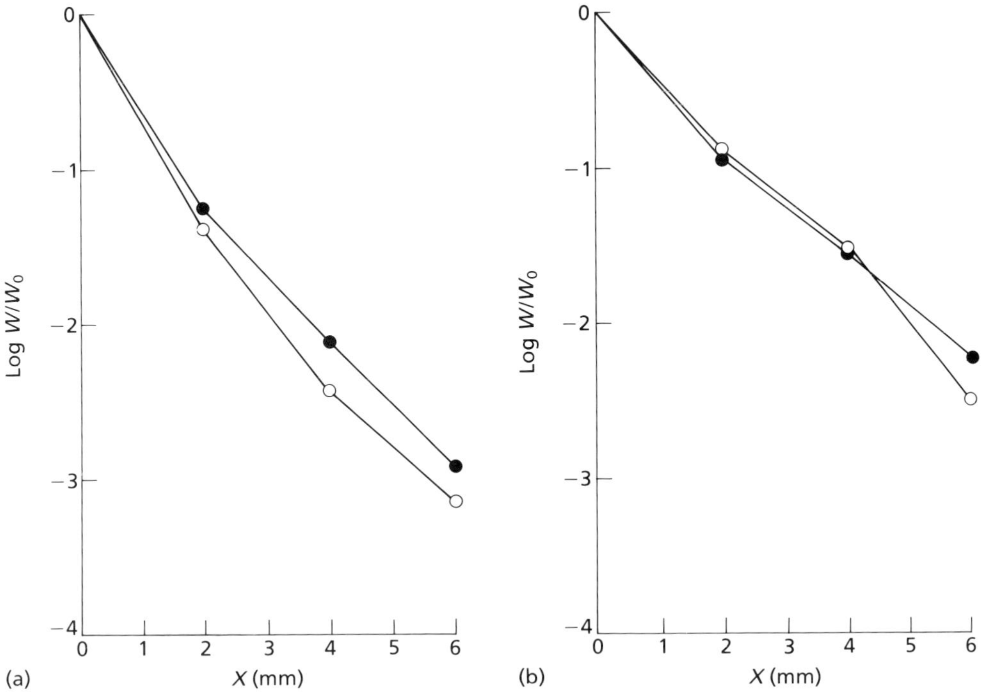

Fig. 9.3 Effect of 0.1% sodium azide on the logarithmic residual rate of leukocytes.
(a) Granulocytes; (b) lymphocytes. Red cell concentrates were filtered through nonwoven fabric of average fiber diameter of 1.7 µm at 25 °C. W/W_0, residual rate of leukocytes; X, thickness of the nonwoven fabric; o without sodium azide (control); ● with 0.1% sodium azide (NaN$_3$).

remaining part of the fabric, and they must be removed with the different mechanism from the case of leukocytes.

As a next step, we carried out a similar experiment using the nonwoven fabric which was coated with polyHEMA to change the chemical properties of the fiber surface. In this experiment, the leukocyte removal rate was apparently decreased, while the removal rate for plastic particles remained unchanged (Fig. 9.5).

Considering the above model, it can be interpreted that the reduction in the leukocyte removal rate can be attributed to the reduction in the adsorption probability per contact P, due to the coating with polyHEMA. The reason for no change in removal rate of plastic particles is supposed to be that the particles are removed not by adsorption but by sieving.

Then, we investigated how the removal rate varied when we increased the amount of leukocytes or plastic particles applied to the nonwoven fabric (Fig. 9.6).

In the case of leukocytes, the logarithmic residual rate of leukocytes in the upper stream part of the fabric increased due to the amount of leukocytes applied.

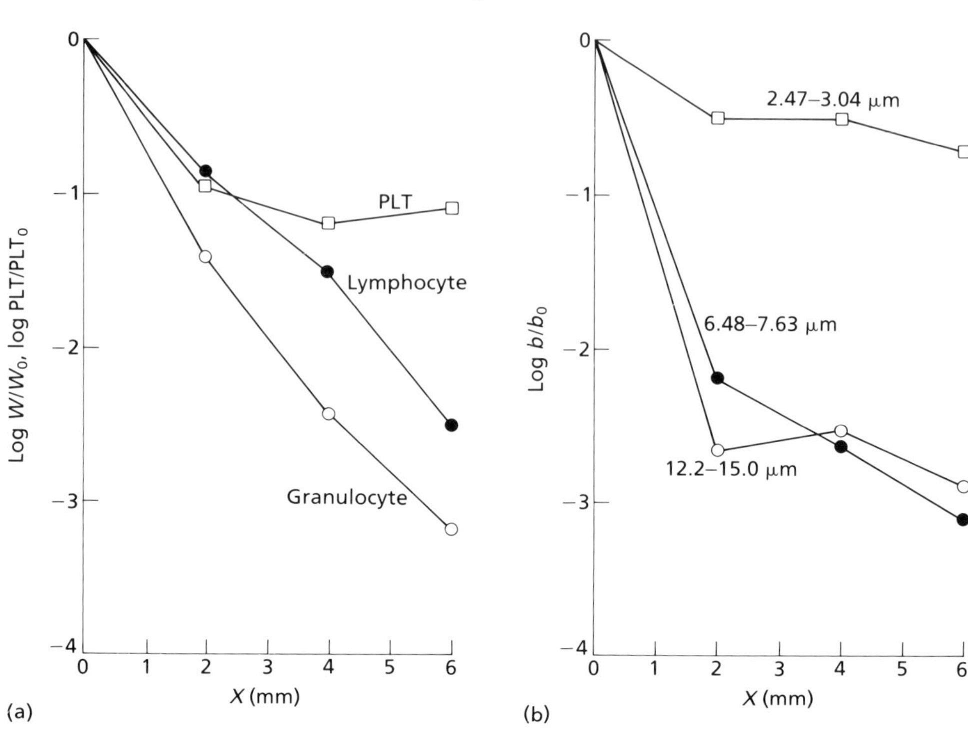

Fig. 9.4 Comparison of the removal behavior between (a) blood cells and (b) plastic particles. Red cell concentrates and particles were filtered through nonwoven fabric of average fiber diameter 1.7 μm at 25°C. b/b_0, residual rate of plastic particles; X, thickness of the nonwoven fabric; PLT/PLT$_0$, residual rate of platelets; W/W_0, residual rate of leukocytes.

This suggests that most of the adsorption points in the upper stream part of the fabric have been already filled with leukocytes. This causes the decrease in the amount of remaining adsorption points in the fabric which is to be observed as a decrease in leukocyte removal capacity in the upper stream part of the fabric.

On the other hand, such a phenomenon was not observed with plastic particles, and this suggests again that the removal mechanism is the sieving.

Evaluation of the R-S350

Based on the above findings obtained from our experiments, we developed a new high-performance filter, the R-S350. The nonwoven fabric used in this filter is of smaller diameter and is packed with a higher density than filters commercially available in order to have higher leukocyte removal efficiency. The effective filtration area and thickness of the filter are designed taking into account the reduction in leukocyte removal performance due to the increase in the amount of treated leukocytes.

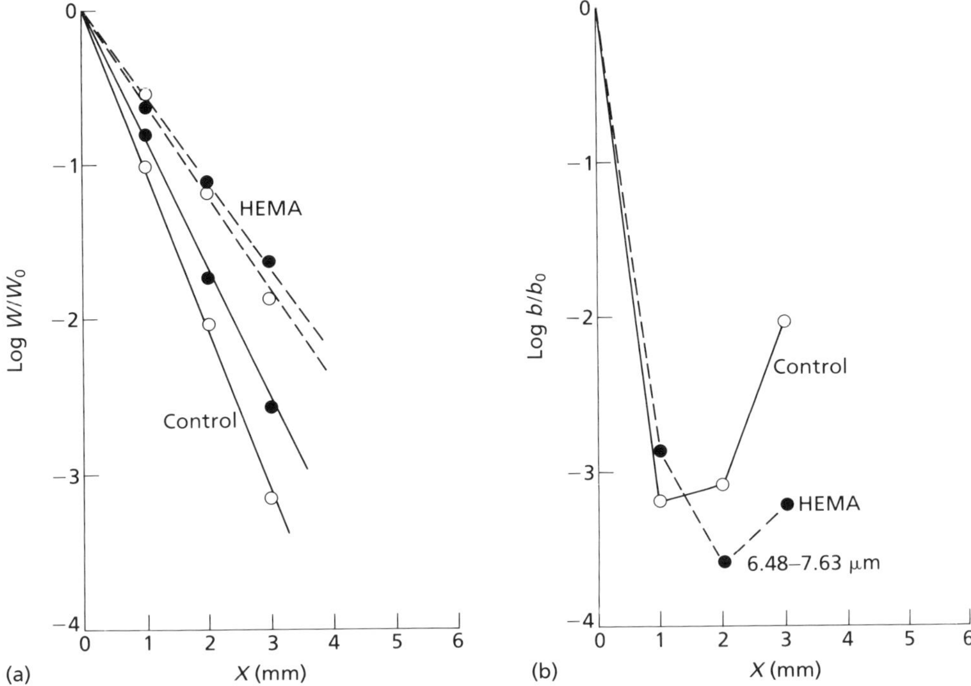

Fig. 9.5 The effect of change in the chemical properties of fiber surface on removal behavior of (a) leukocytes and (b) plastic particles. Red cell concentrate and particles were filtered through nonwoven fabric of average fiber diameter 1.2 μm at 25 °C. b/b_0, residual rate of plastic particles; HEMA, poly(2-hydroxyethylmethacrylate); W/W_0, residual rate of leukocytes; X, thickness of the nonwoven fabric; ○ granulocyte; ● lymphocyte.

Assuming that this filter is used for prestorage filtration, we evaluated the filter using blood preserved within 2 days (Table 9.1).

The residual leukocyte number was 4.56×10^4 on average, 3.5×10^5 maximum, and 1.7×10^3 minimum. In a total of 25 cases, all counts were of the order of 10^3–10^4 except two cases where the count exceeded 10^5. The leukocyte removal rate was 4.87 log average and the standard deviation was 0.44 log. The probability of obtaining a leukocyte removal rate not reaching 4 log calculated from the above values is slightly lower than 3%, and thus we can state that this filter can assure 4 log depletion of leukocytes in actual use.

Summary

Mechanism of leukocyte removal

It was strongly suggested from a series of experiments that the leukocyte-removing mechanism by the nonwoven fabric is mainly adsorption and active adhesion takes an

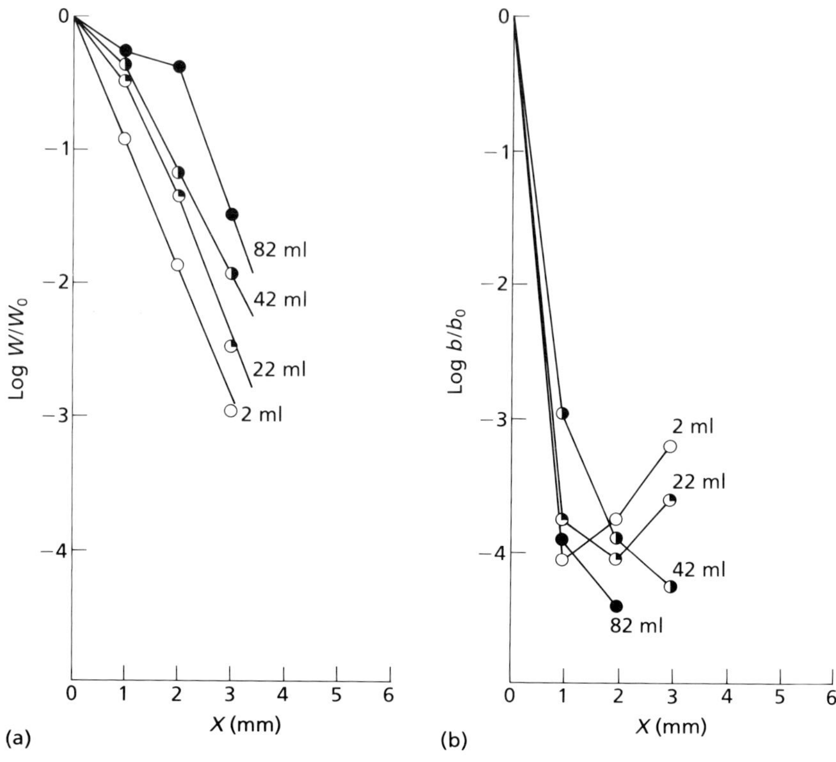

Fig. 9.6 Changes in residual rate of (a) leukocytes and (b) plastic particles with increasing filtered volume of blood or particle suspension. Red cell concentrate and particles were filtered through nonwoven fabric of average fiber diameter 1.2 μm at 25 °C. b/b_0, residual rate of plastic particles; W/W_0, residual rate of leukocytes; X, thickness of the nonwoven fabric.

Table 9.1 The filtration performance of the R-S350 filter (mean ± 1 s.d.)

Blood age (days)	n	WBC removal (logs)*	Residual WBCs ($\times 10^4$)	RBC recovery (%)	Filtration time (min)
1	6	5.08 ± 0.75	6.86 ± 13.67	87.2 ± 1.0	14.6 ± 1.1
2	19	4.80 ± 0.29	3.84 ± 2.52	86.3 ± 1.9	16.2 ± 3.6
Average	25	4.87 ± 0.44	4.56 ± 6.74	86.4 ± 1.8	15.5 ± 3.1

* $^-$log W/W_0.
RBC, red blood cell; WBC, white blood cell.

additional role in removal of granulocytes. The reason why platelets showed similar behavior to plastic particles is unknown. Since the blood used in the experiment had been stored at 4 °C for 3 days before use, it is supposed that the function of platelets might have been lost during preservation and this is why the platelets behaved as abiotic particles.

Steneker and Biewenga [2] investigated the mechanism of leukocyte depletion in Sepacell R-500 and two other filters, and reported that 40% of lymphocytes could not be washed out from Sepacell R-500, and supposed that these lymphocytes might have been captured by adhesion. The nonwoven fabrics we used in the present study are identical with those used in Sepacell, but we obtained different results, as mentioned above. As the blood employed for their experiments was fresh (stored at 20°C within 24 h), and the timing of washing out was 5–10 min after the completion of filtration, it can be assumed that the lymphocytes may have been captured by adsorption mechanism and thereafter activated during the time before washing. We think further minute studies will be necessary to clarify the influences of blood conditions, such as age or temperature at filtration, on the leukocyte removal mechanism and what the adsorption force originates in.

If leukocytes are removed by an adsorption mechanism, changes in chemical properties of fiber surface may be able to modify the leukocyte removal rate. Figure 9.7 shows such a case, where fresh whole blood was filtered by the polyester nonwoven fabric coated with the copolymer of poly(HEMA-co-diethylamino-ethylmethacryrate; HE-x: x is a content (mol%) of diethylaminoethylmethacryrate in the copolymer [3].

Here, the pass ratio of leukocytes and platelets varies greatly according to the HE composition. In a particular composition, the pass ratio of platelets was high, while

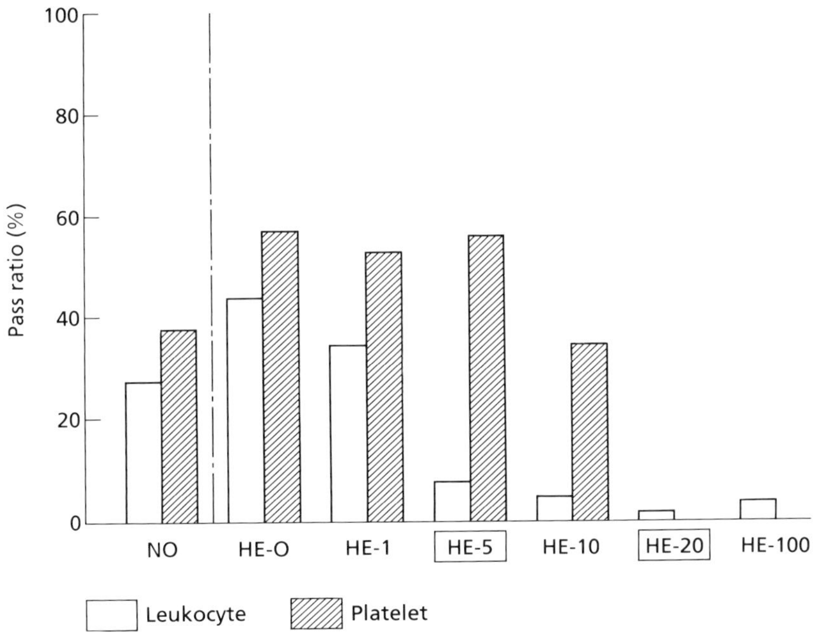

Fig. 9.7 Effects of HE-x coating (see text). The pass ratio of leukocytes and platelets varies according to the composition of HE-x, HE-5 can remove leukocyte selectively.

that of leukocytes was low; thus the selective removal of leukocytes was achieved when platelets were least removed and this coated material was applied to the Sepacell PL.

Figure 9.8 shows a flow cytometric analysis of immunoglobulin-bearing cells in lymphocyte suspension before and after the selective removal of B cells from mouse spleen cells by means of a column packed with glass beads coated with poly-(HEMA-copolyamine macromer) [4,5].

Selective removal of B cells is still at the research stage and further investigations are required before it can be available commercially for medical applications. However, it shows the possibility of selective removal of various cells, if the chemical properties of the material surface are well designed. We also think that it is possible to improve the leukocyte removal efficiency by changing the chemical properties of the fiber surface. We would like to expand this study more in these directions in the future.

Evaluation of R-S350

The R-S350 is developed as a high-performance filter for the prevention of alloimmunization, which attracts some of the greatest attention among the transfusion-associated complications. According to previous reports, residual leukocyte number needs to be less than $1-5 \times 10^6$ per transfusion to prevent alloimmunization [6,7].

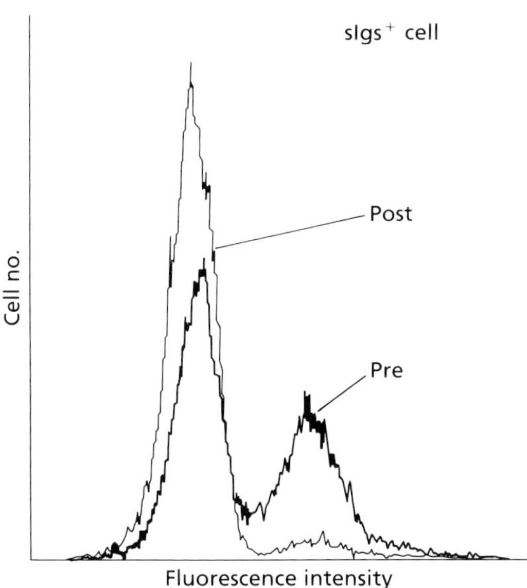

Fig. 9.8 Flowcytometric analysis of B cells separated from T cells using poly(HEMA-copolyamine macromer). sIgs+, surface immunoglobulin-positive.

As a result of our present evaluation, the residual leukocyte number was 4.56×10^4 on average, 3.5×10^5 maximum, and 1.7×10^3 minimum. Of a total of 25 cases, all counts were of the order of 10^3–10^4, except two cases where the count exceeded 10^5, which satisfies the above-mentioned criteria. On the other hand, from a viewpoint of quality assurance, the stability of leukocyte removal rate is an important issue. The leukocyte removal rate in our present study was 4.87 log on average and the standard deviation was 0.44 log. The probability of obtaining a leukocyte removal rate not reaching 4 log calculated from the above values is slightly lower than 3%; this filter is considered to be able to assure the substantial 4 log depletion within the scope of blood conditions applied in our evaluation. We think it is essential to make further studies of the effects of blood conditions on leukocyte removal rate, such as age of blood, hematocrit, temperature, and type of preservatives used, in order to consider the quality assurance of the filter from a wider angle.

References

1 Sadoff BJ, Dooley DC, Kapoor V, Law P, Friedman LI, Stromberg RR. Methods for measuring a 6 $\log_{10}$ white cell depletion in red cells. *Transfusion* 1991;31:150–155.

2 Steneker I, Biewenga J. Histologic and immunohistochemical studies on the preparation of white cell-poor red cell concentrates: the filtration process using three different polyester filters. *Transfusion* 1991;31:40–46.

3 Nishimura T, Kuroda T, Mizoguchi Y, Watanabe H, Rikumaru H, Umegae M. Advanced methods for leucocyte removal by blood filtration. In: Brozović B, ed. *The Role of Leucocyte Depletion in Blood Transfusion Practice.* Oxford: Blackwell Scientific Publications, 1989:35–40.

4 Maruyama A, Senda E, Tsuruta T, Kataoka K. Synthesis and characterization of polyamine graft copolymers with a poly(2-hydroxyethyl methacrylate) backbone. *Macromol Chem* 1986;187:1895–1906.

5 Oka S, Yoshida M, Yamamizu T *et al.* A new separation method of T cells from B cells. In: *Abstract, Third World Biomaterials Congress.* Kyoto, 1988, 4P-06.

6 Fisher M, Chapman JR, Ting A, Morris PJ. Alloimmunization to HLA antigens following transfusion with leucocyte-poor and purified platelet suspensions. *Vox Sang* 1985; 49:331–335.

7 Sarrinen UM, Kekomaki R, Siimes MA, Myllyla G. Effective prophylaxis against platelet refractoriness in multitransfused patients by use of leukocyte-free blood components. *Blood* 1990;75:512–517.

Discussion

IKEDA: In your presentation, the platelets seemed to behave as if they were an inorganic substance. What is the reason that the removal characteristics of platelets are different from that of leukocytes in Sepacell filtration?

OKA: I think it depends on the state of blood products. I suppose, the platelets showed the same behavior as inorganic particles because the blood used in this study had been stored at 4°C for 3 days and the platelets had almost lost their function as platelets. That's why they behaved just like inorganic particles.

ITO (Kyoto University Medical School): When the leukocytes present sparsely and there is no competition among leukocytes, it is considered to depend on the frequency of collision between one leukocyte and one location for adhesion on nonwoven filters that the one leukocyte can occupy the location. What about the leukocytes in peripheral blood?

OKA: Although I have no quantitative model, I think, leukocytes compete several scores with the adhesion location when they are passing through the non-woven fiber of 1 mm in depth, resulting in one chance or none for adhesion. These phenomena may control the removal characteristics. As I have not examined it in detail, I cannot answer as to whether the leukocytes compete for the location for adhesion or not. In RCC, leukocytes are surrounded by an overwhelming majority of red blood cells (RBCs) and some kinds of interactions may occur between RBCs and leukocytes. Leukocytes might be driven away from the location by a chain of RBCs. I think that an examination from the viewpoint of hydromechanical study is required.

TAKAHASHI: It is a common phenomenon that the granulocytes tend to come out when a quite fresh blood unit is filtered with the filters made of nonwoven polyester fibers such as Sepacell R-500 and Pall RC-100. Also more granulocytes leak as the temperature rises. How can you explicate this phenomenon according to your explanation that the mechanism of filtration is due to the difference of ability of adhesion?

OKA: We did it with 2- to 3-day-old blood. If more fresh blood could be used, the results would be changed. It is reported that granulocytes may come out from a 1.7 μm type. On the other hand, no problem occurred in the case of 1.2 μm type. Regarding the R-S350, no effect was reported even if fresh blood was used. I think that the possibility of the leakage of granulocytes in fresh blood is likely related to the softness and the transformability of the granulocyte membrane. This is also suggested from the facts that we could not see this phenomenon if it was done at 4°C or performed with a filter made of fine fibers of 1.2 μm in a mean diameter.

SEKIGUCHI: It is true that granulocytes come out when we filter fresh blood. I think this phenomenon does depend not on the characters of each granulocyte but on the formation of microaggregates. I am presupposing a mechanism as follows. When the blood is fresh, there are no microaggregates, namely each granulocyte behaves separately to pass through the filter or absorb on it. On the other hand, when the blood is stored for 3 or 4 days, very small microaggregates appear and they stick to fibrin etc., thus they are easily removed. What is your comment on this?

OKA: I think that there also exists such a mechanism for removal. Leukocytes may stick to microaggregates or are involved with the microaggregates. I think your hypotheses may contribute much, especially in old blood stored for 1–2 weeks.

10 · Mechanism of leukocyte removal by porous material

S. Kora, H. Kuroki, T. Kido, N. Katsurada, and M. Sado

*Terumo Corporation Research and Development Center, 1500 Inokuchi, Nakai-machi,
Ashigarakami-gun, Kanagawa 250–01, Japan*

Abstract

We tried to specify the mechanism of leukocyte removal from blood products by porous material using a porous polyurethane sheet. We found a linear relationship between the thickness of porous material and $\log_{10}$ reduction rate for leukocytes. As this behavior of leukocytes in porous material is not at all different from that of nonbiologic particles, particular biologic interaction is not suggested as taking part in the trapping mechanism.

We also found that the deformability of cells plays an important role in their evacuation from the capture sites. It is suggested that the difference in deformability between leukocytes and erythrocytes is a major reason for the selective removal of leukocytes by porous filter material.

Introduction

To reduce the risk of transfusion reactions caused by contaminating leukocytes, such as graft-versus-host disease and alloimmunization, a simple and inexpensive method for leukocyte removal from blood products has been awaited. Recently, we have developed two types of leukocyte removal filters, Imugard RC and Imugard PL, which are made of sponge-like porous sheets.

During development, we have tested the applicability of many kinds of porous material to leukocyte removal filters and specified some major factors involving the removal mechanism. In this report, we express the results of our latest study, that imply the mechanism of leukocyte removal by porous material.

Materials and methods

The porous filter material

Porous polyurethane sheets were punched to disks of 47 mm diameter. Each disk was introduced into a holder (Swinnex-47, Nihon Millipore, Tokyo, Japan) and submitted for the blood filtration experiment. In some cases, we intentionally used filter material of low performance in leukocyte removal, because the leukocyte reduction rate of the material of normal performance is too high for an accurate count of leukocytes in filtered blood.

Blood collection and filtration

About 400 ml of blood was collected from healthy volunteer donors in triple blood bags containing 56 ml of citrate phosphate dextrose (CPD) as an anticoagulant (Teruflex TC-400; Terumo, Tokyo, Japan). Concentrated red cell units (CRCs) were separated by centrifugation at 375 **g** for 20 min at 22°C in a centrifuge (CR-7B3, Hitachi, Japan) equipped with a rotor (RR5S2). The hematocrits of the CRCs were about 65%. Unless otherwise stated, CRCs were stored for 7–14 days at 4 ± 2°C before filtration. The average number of contaminating leukocytes in a CRC unit was approximately 5×10^9. CRC 40 ml was passed through a filter by gravity. The flow rate was about 8 ml/min.

Leukocyte count

The number of leukocytes in initial and filtered CRCs was counted with an automated blood cell counter (Sysmex NE-6000; TOA, Kobe, Japan) and, in part, with a Neubauer hemacytometer [1].

The $\log_{10}$ reduction rate was calculated with the following formula:

$$\log_{10} \text{reduction} = -\log_{10}(N/N_0)$$

where N is number of leukocytes passed through the filter and N_0 is the total number of leukocytes applied to the filter.

Scanning electron microscopy

Observations of filter material and trapped leukocytes were performed with a scanning electron microscope (JSM-840; JEOL, Tokyo, Japan) [1].

Results

A longitudinal section of a porous polyurethane sheet used in this study was observed with a scanning electron microscope (SEM). As shown in Figure 10.1, pores were connected to each other to form three-dimensional maze-like fluid paths in the porous sheet.

We observed filter material after filtration with a SEM to know where and how leukocytes are trapped in it. A typical view is shown in Figure 10.2. Most trapped leukocytes were found in small depressions or in narrow channels whose dimensions were nearly equal to or smaller than their sizes. Almost all the trapped leukocytes were of normal spherical shape. Highly deformed cells were not found.

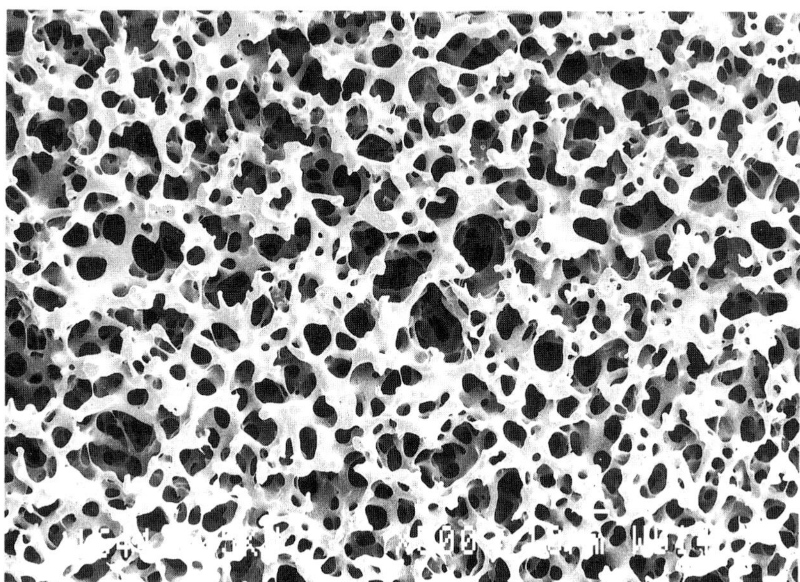

Fig. 10.1 A longitudinal section of a porous polyurethane sheet used in this study. A porous polyurethane sheet was observed with a scanning electron microscope. Magnification × 295.

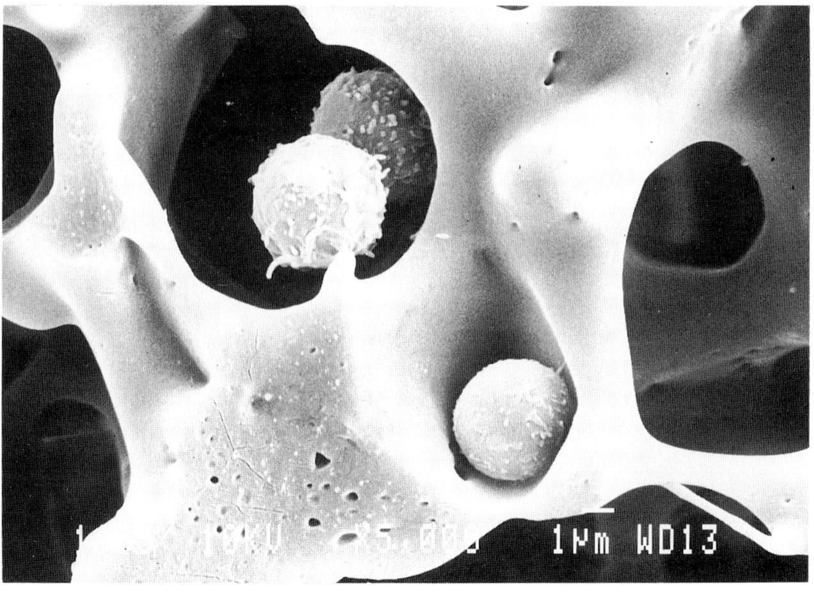

Fig. 10.2 Leukocytes trapped in a porous filter material. After filtration, the porous polyurethane sheet was fixed with 1% glutaraldehyde for 1 h at room temperature, dehydrated with ethanol, and observed with a scanning electron microscope. Magnification × 2950.

A longitudinal section of filter material after filtration from the blood-entering side through the blood-leaving side is shown in Figure 10.3. Larger numbers of trapped cells were found in the neighborhood of the blood-entering side of the porous sheet. We divided this photograph into seven sections from the entering side to the leaving side; we counted the trapped leukocytes in each section, and plotted the numbers of trapped cells against the distance from the entering-side of the filter. The results show a roughly linear relationship between the logarithm of numbers of leukocytes trapped in each section and the distance from the blood-entering surface of the filter to each section (Fig. 10.4). This relationship, as will be discussed later, means that the probability of leukocytes being trapped when they pass through a unit volume of the porous sheet is equal everywhere in the filter. In other words, the postulated capture sites for leukocytes are distributed uniformly throughout the filter material.

To ensure the homogeneity of distribution of the postulated capture sites in the porous material, we performed two series of experiments. First, we sliced a 0.9 mm thick porous polyurethane sheet into three 0.3 mm thick sheets and compared their ability to trap leukocytes with that of the original sheets. As shown in Figure 10.5, the leukocyte removal rate of three pieces of 0.3 mm thick porous material was similar to that of one 0.9 mm thick original sheet. Second, we varied the thickness of the porous sheet by stacking up to five pieces and measured the $\log_{10}$ reduction rate. The results,

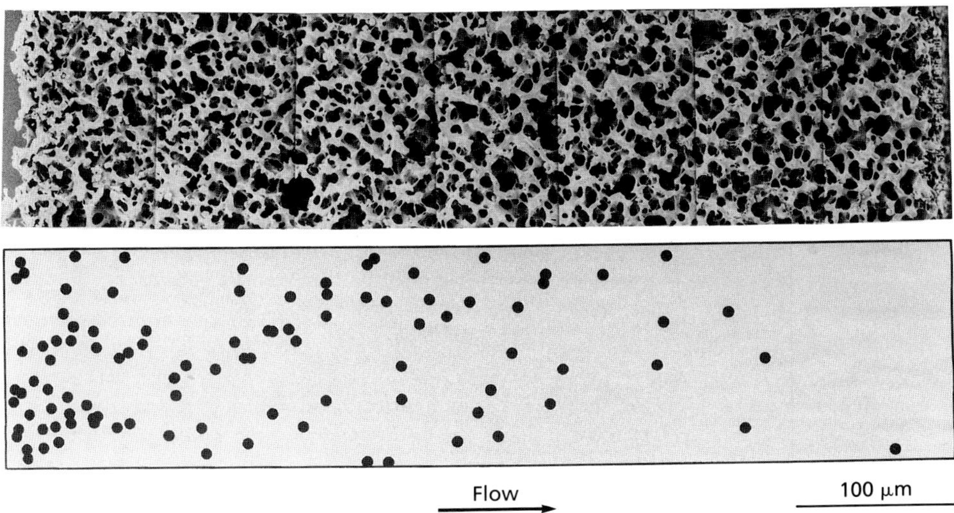

Fig. 10.3 A longitudinal section of a porous polyurethane sheet after filtration. After filtration, the porous polyurethane sheet was treated as described in Figure 10.2. Photographs were taken in longitudinal section from the blood-entering side (left) to the blood-leaving side (right) and pasted on to each other to form a complete longitudinal-section view (top). Black dots (bottom) indicate the location of trapped leukocytes.

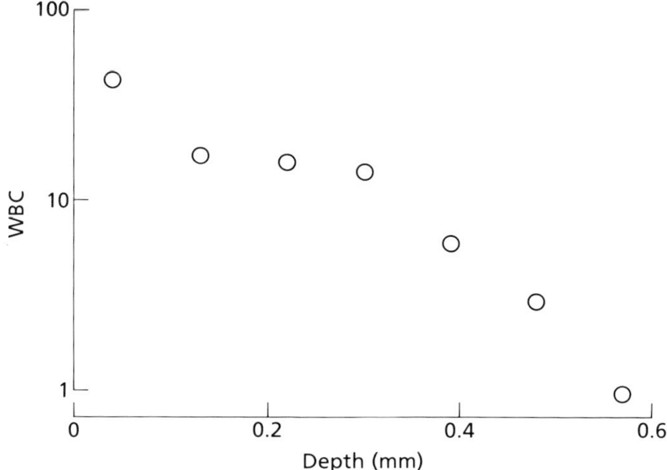

Fig. 10.4 Relationship between the number of trapped leukocytes (WBC, white blood cells) and the depth from the blood-entering surface of a filter. The bottom part of Figure 10.3 was divided into seven sections and the logarithm of the number of leukocytes in each section was plotted against the distance from the blood-entering surface to each section.

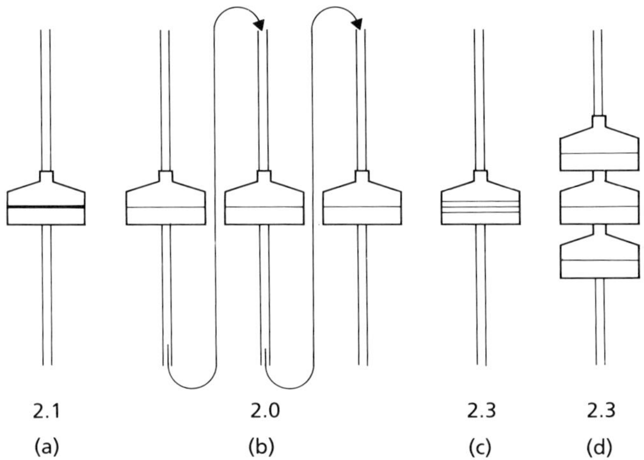

Fig. 10.5 Log_{10} reduction rates of one 0.9 mm thick porous sheet and three 0.3 mm thick sheets. Log_{10} reduction rates of (a) one 0.9 mm thick sheet; (b) three 0.3 mm thick sheets in separate holders; (c) three 0.3 mm thick sheets stacked in one holder; and (d) three 0.3 mm thick sheets in separate holders connected serially were compared.

summarized in Figure 10.6, clearly presented a linear relationship between the thickness of porous material and the log_{10} reduction rate for leukocytes.

Next, we tried to find out why leukocytes were selectively trapped in the porous material; in other words, why erythrocytes were not trapped in it. The results shown in Figure 10.7 revealed that leukocyte removal rates were lowered when

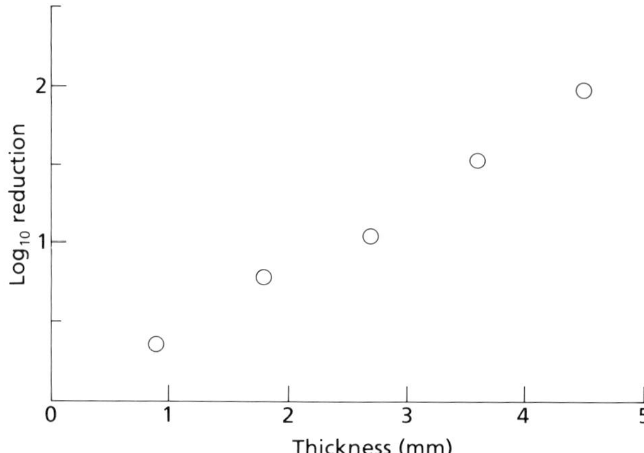

Fig. 10.6 The relationship between the thickness of a porous sheet and the $\log_{10}$ removal rate for leukocytes. Porous polyurethane sheets 0.9 mm thick were stacked up to five pieces. Leukocyte removal rates, expressed as $\log_{10}$ removal rates, were plotted against the thickness of the polyurethane material.

hematocrit of applied blood became higher, suggesting competition between leukocytes and erythrocytes for the capture sites. However, considering the large difference between the number of erythrocytes and that of leukocytes in a CRC unit, the affinity of erythrocytes for the sites must be far lower than those of leukocytes.

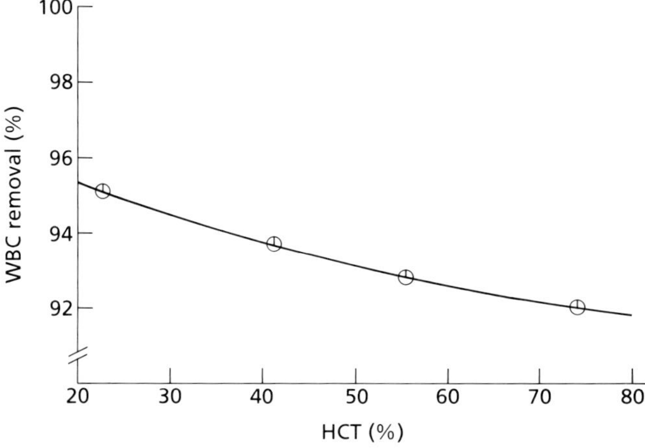

Fig. 10.7 Relationship between hematocrits (HCT) of concentrated red cells (CRCs) and leukocyte (WBC, white blood cell) removal rates. Freshly prepared CRCs were further concentrated by centrifugation and their hematocrits were adjusted by dilution with autologous plasma. After adjustment, each CRC was filtered and the leukocyte removal rate was measured.

Table 10.1 Effect of preservation on leukocyte removal rate. Concentrated red cells (CRCs) were prepared and stored at 4 ± 2°C. On the day of preparation, on day 8, and on day 14, 40 ml aliquots were sampled from each CRC unit and applied to two types of porous sheet (identified as A and B). Results from four independent CRC units were expressed as mean ± s.d.

| | Leukocyte removal rate (%) | | |
| | | Preserved blood | |
Porous sheet	Fresh blood	Day 8	Day 14
A	15 ± 4	41 ± 15	59 ± 11
B	68 ± 9	90 ± 12	89 ± 15

In a preliminary experiment, we found that nondeformable erythrocytes, which were fixed with glutaraldehyde, were almost completely captured in the porous filter material (data not shown). Therefore a large difference in affinity for filter material between erythrocytes and leukocytes was suggested to be based on the difference in deformability.

If this is the case, highly deformable leukocytes can also break away from the sites. This must be the reason for relatively lower reduction rates for leukocytes in fresh CRCs than those in stored CRCs, as shown in Table 10.1.

Table 10.2 demonstrates that leukocytes kept at low temperature for longer than 1 h had a tendency to be trapped in the porous material more efficiently than those kept at room temperature. As granulocytes are reported to lose their deformability by low temperature treatment [2], these results also support the idea.

Additionally, we investigated the effect of some inhibitors on leukocyte removal from fresh CRCs by porous material. Results are shown in Figure 10.8. A metabolic inhibitor, sodium azide, and a cytoskeleton-decomposer, colchicine, increased the leukocyte removal rate (Fig. 10.8a and b), although a Ca^{2+}-chelator, ethyleneglycol-bis-(β-aminoethyl ether)-N,N,N′,N′-tetroacetic acid (EGTA) which has an ability to reduce the adhesiveness of leukocytes to foreign surface, had no effect (Fig. 10.8c).

Table 10.2 Effect of low temperature treatment on leukocyte removal rate. Freshly prepared concentrated red cell (CRC) units were divided into two aliquots. Each fraction was held at room temperature or 8°C for up to 5 h and submitted to filtration experiment. Refrigerated samples were warmed to room temperature before filtration. Results from three independent CRC units were expressed as mean ± s.d.

| | Leukocyte removal rate (%) | | | |
Temperature	Initial	1 h	3 h	5 h
23°C	70 ± 10	78 ± 6	88 ± 8	88 ± 6
8°C		91 ± 8	93 ± 5	91 ± 5

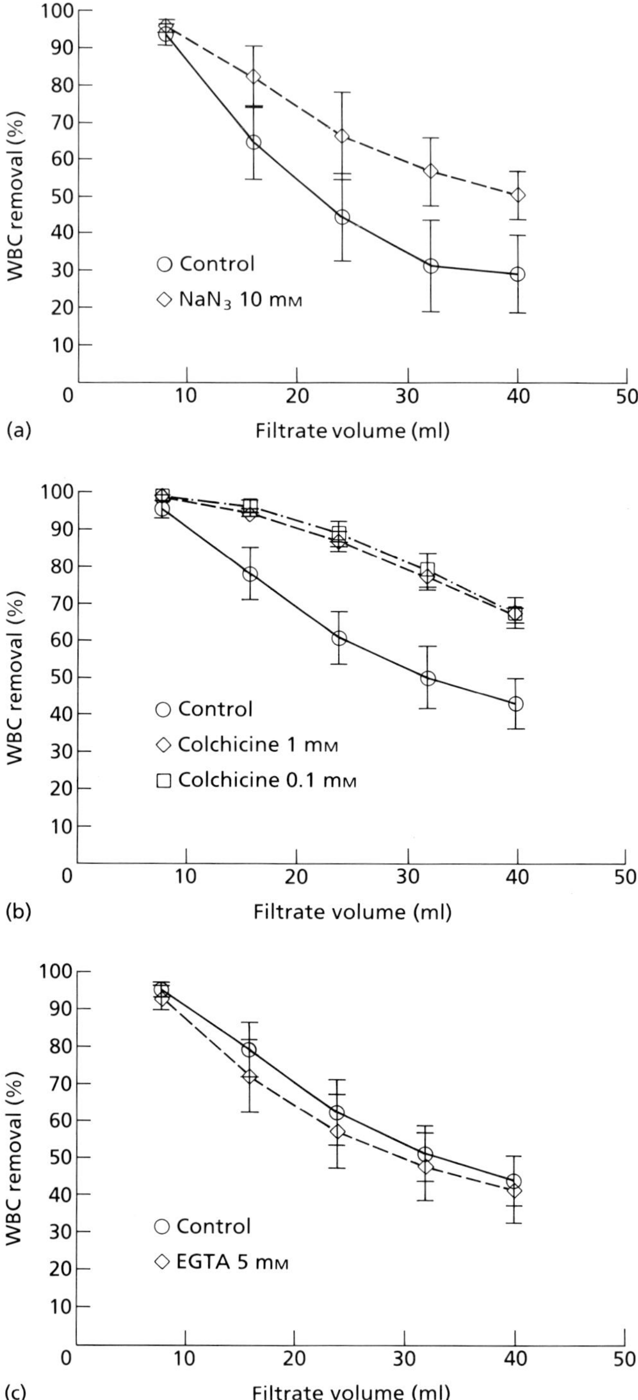

100
90
80
70
60
50
40
30
20
10
0
WBC removal (%)
Control
NaN$_3$ 10 mM
0 10 20 30 40 50
Filtrate volume (ml)
(a)

100
90
80
70
60
50
40
30
20
10
0
WBC removal (%)
Control
Colchicine 1 mM
Colchicine 0.1 mM
0 10 20 30 40 50
Filtrate volume (ml)
(b)

100
90
80
70
60
50
40
30
20
10
0
WBC removal (%)
Control
EGTA 5 mM
0 10 20 30 40 50
Filtrate volume (ml)
(c)

These findings are extra evidence for the significance of deformability of cells in withdrawal action from the capture sites.

Summary

Leukocytes trapped in the porous polyurethane material did not show an indication of energy-dependent morphologic change such as phagocytic action. Besides, when the metabolic activity of leukocytes was diminished by preservation or by addition of sodium azide, the removal rate was augmented. These findings strongly suggest that leukocytes behaved as nonbiologic particles in the filter.

We found a linear relationship between the thickness of the filter material and $\log_{10}$ reduction rate for leukocytes. This finding suggests that the probability of capture when a leukocyte passes through a unit thickness of filter material is equal everywhere in the porous element. If we denote the probability as a constant α, the number of trapped leukocytes ($-dN$) when N cells were entered to a thin portion of the porous sheet of area S, and the thickness dt should be:

$$-dN = N\alpha S\, dt$$

This can be solved as:

$$-\ln (N/N_0) = \alpha St$$

where N_0 is the total number of leukocytes applied to the filter. Now we can surmise the relationship between the $\log_{10}$ reduction rate and filter thickness as follows.

$$\log_{10} \text{ reduction} = -\log_{10}(N/N_0) = (\alpha S/\ln 10)t$$

As αS is a constant, this equation means that the $\log_{10}$ reduction rate is proportional to the thickness of the filter material. When the leukocyte removal filter is made of porous material, we believe that this log–linear relationship stands for up to at least four $\log_{10}$ reductions because Chianese *et al.* [3] reported that a series of two 2-$\log_{10}$ filters exhibited the $\log_{10}$ reduction value of 4. This log–linear relationship, as discussed above, is based on the homogeneity of distribution of the capture sites and it implies neither cell–cell interaction nor allosteric effect between capture sites involved in the trap mechanism.

The relationship depicted here is not unique to leukocyte removal filters. On the contrary, it is well known as a common feature of any depth filters intended to trap

---

Fig. 10.8 Effect of some inhibitors on removal rate for fresh leukocytes (WBC, white blood cells). Inhibitor, (a) sodium azide (NaN$_3$, 10 mM); (b) colchicine (0.1 and 1 mM); or (c) EGTA (5 mM), was added to freshly prepared concentrated red cells (CRCs). After incubation at room temperature for 10 min, 40 ml of each CRC was filtered. Filtered CRC was collected into five 8 ml fractions and leukocyte removal rates of each of them were measured. Data are expressed as mean ± s.d. of five independent experiments.

nonbiologic particles. Therefore, no particular biologic interaction seems necessary to account for the trap mechanism of leukocytes.

Furthermore, we also found that deformability of cells plays a substantial role in their capability of evacuation from the capture sites. Difference in deformability between leukocytes and erythrocytes must be a major reason for the selective removal of leukocytes by porous filter material.

Acknowledgments

The authors thank Mr Yoshitaka Omura and Mr Osamu Kaneko for their technical assistance.

References

1 Takahashi T, Hosoda M, Mogi Y *et al.* A new porous polyurethane filter to remove leukocytes from platelet concentrates. *Jpn J Transfus Med* 1991;37:24–31.
2 Miyamoto M, Sasakawa S. Studies on granulocyte preservation: I. Changes of granulocyte functions during liquid storage and the influence of storage temperature and pH. *Jpn J Transfus Med* 1984;29:612–617.
3 Chianese D, Nardone D, Miripol J. The effect of filter configuration on leukocyte removal from AS-5 red cells. *The 1990 ISBT/AABB Book of Abstracts* S42:11. ISBT & AABB Joint Congress, Los Angeles, 1990. American Association of Blood Banks: Arlington, USA.

Discussion

Ito (Kyoto University Medical School): You used the expression that "the leukocytes are caught into a labyrinth." If this phenomenon is the same as in gel filtration, it is considered more difficult for molecules with lower molecular weight to come out of the filter than for those with higher molecular weight. How do cell membrane deformability and cell adhesion, contribute to the leukocyte removal?

Kora: I think the problem of how these different factors work is one of degree. If a differently sized latex particles having a small range of diameters is used, bigger particles cannot pass through, but if we use smaller particles, there is a point at which they abruptly begin to go through. I think there is a relationship between this phenomenon and the mechanisms of leukocyte depletion.

Okumura: Lymphocytes, leukocytes or polymorphonuclear leukocytes, any blood cells will do. As you know, cell membrane is actively flowing, just like the ocean, and it is possible to measure the fluidity. Membrane fluidity is greatly affected by temperature, colchicine, and sodium azide. So what is the meaning of deformability of cell membrane? Do you mean the membrane fluidity or the changing of its shape?

Kora: As with granulocytes, I'm thinking of energy-dependent conformational change.

OKUMURA: We can measure the rapidity of the movement of surface molecules. Has it any relation to the adhesion?

KORA: I'm sorry but we have as yet been unable to examine it.

TAKAHASHI: Do you think that the mechanism of filtration is due to sifting? The microporous Imgard filter has different specificity according to the properties of the cells, as mentioned in the first presentation. That is to say, adhesion is one of the mechanisms for filtration and the tendency is well observed in Imgard microporous materials. As for the experiment with colchicine, the colchicine-treated cells seemed to swell. I suppose it depends not on the theory of membrane fluidity but on the sifting effect that the cells treated with colchicine were removed effectively by filtration. Do you look at the cells through a microscope? In my view, colchicine-treated cells seem to be larger in size.

KORA: I have no microscopic data. However, no difference was observed even if a very high concentration of colchicine was used. As we carried out the experiments in the presence of red cells, I suppose the red cells absorbed large amounts of the reagents. Red cells, especially, have many adhesion sites for cytochalasin. Regarding the depletion depending on the difference in subset, I agree with you, although we don't have enough data.

11 · Development of polymeric adsorbents for separation of lymphocyte subpopulations

K. Kataoka

Department of Material Science, and Research Institute for Biosciences, Science University of Tokyo, Yamazaki 2641, Noda, Chiba 278, Japan

Abstract

There is widespread consensus that the separation of lymphocyte subpopulations is important in assessing immunologic status in human diseases as well as in the therapy of immunologic disorders. The purpose of this work is to develop novel polymeric adsorbents for the separation of lymphocyte subpopulations. Based on our strategy of separating lymphocyte subpopulations through their differential ionic affinity toward polymer matrices, a series of graft copolymers with polyamine side chains was prepared. These polyamine adsorbents were found to show selective retention of B cells, which lend these adsorbents practical usage as a separating column for lymphocytes. Further, quaternization of amino groups in these graft copolymers even allows the efficient separation of T-cell subsets by this copolymer column, suggesting the promising feature of synthetic adsorbent as a major tool for separating a wide spectrum of cell populations.

Introduction

With recent progress in the biomedical sciences, the development of cell separation systems becomes especially important [1–3]. Among the great many cell populations of interest, lymphocyte subpopulations are the ones whose separation has received the most practical interest because their successful separation is the critical process in precise assays and effective therapy of serious diseases, especially those related to immune responses.

Important goals of our research include the development of new synthetic polymers with specific affinity toward a particular subpopulation of lymphocytes, and the application of these polymers as an adsorbent used for separation of lymphocyte subpopulations. Worthy of mention is that even morphologically indistinguishable cell populations often have distinctive surface properties due to differences in their plasma membrane composition. This may lead to differential cellular adsorption on to materials with distinctive chemical structures. We gave special attention to the differential ionic character of surfaces of lymphocyte subpopulations arising from differences in the number and species of acidic functional groups expressed on their plasma membranes [4]. Thus, basic amino groups were chosen as the main component for the design of polymeric materials expected to have specific ionic interactions with lymphocyte subpopulations.

Polyamine graft copolymers as novel polymeric adsorbent for separation of lymphocyte subpopulations

Our systematic study on the interaction of lymphocyte with synthetic polymeric materials having amino groups led to the finding that polyamine graft copolymers with poly(2-hydroxyethylmethacrylate) backbone (HA copolymer; Fig. 11.1) selectively adsorb B cells out of a lymphocyte suspension prepared from rat lymph nodes [5]. Further, these graft copolymers showed excellent performance as a column adsorbent for the separation of B and T cells. By passing a lymphocyte suspension derived from rat lymph node through the column packed with HA-coated glass beads, T-cell suspension with more than 95% purity was obtained as column effluent in a yield of nearly 100% [6]. Worthy of further mention is the simple operational condition of the HA column system. Passage of lymphocytes through the column takes less than 5 min, insuring a low incidence of cellular damage due to a prolonged handling process. HA columns worked successfully even at temperatures as low as 4°C, indicating that the resolution of B and T cells by these graft copolymer columns is based on the differential physicochemical affinity of B and T cells on graft copolymer surfaces and not on the differential energy-dependent activation of these cells triggered by the contact with these surfaces [7].

Lymphocytes attached on graft copolymer surfaces maintain their original spherical shape. This feature offers the great advantage of high recovery of attached B cells from the column [8]. Indeed, as can be seen from Table 11.1, a B-cell population with more than 90% purity and 90% yield was successfully recovered from an HA copolymer column by a gentle pipetting procedure. Recently, the HA copolymer column was found to be useful for the separation of spleen lymphocytes as well as lymph node lymphocytes [9]. However, efficacy of separation was somewhat lower for spleen lymphocytes compared with lymph node lymphocysts. This is probably due to the competitive retention of null cells as well as to the considerably heterogeneous

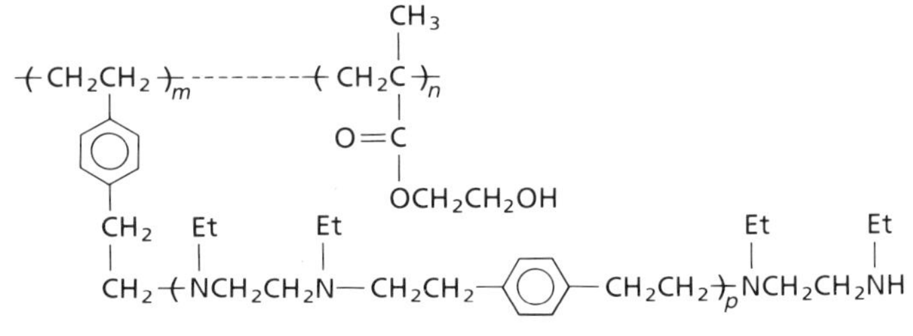

Fig. 11.1 Structural formula of poly(2-hydroxyethylmethacrylate) (HA copolymer).

Table 11.1 Purity and recovery of B and T cells separated by poly(2-hydroethylmethacrylate) (HA copolymer) column

pH of cell suspension	T cells		B cells*	
	Purity (%)	Recovery (%)	Purity (%)	Recovery (%)
7.0	92.4 ± 3.1	69.4 ± 3.2	60.6 ± 3.8	94.7 ± 4.0
7.2	93.1 ± 3.5	95.7 ± 2.9	90.1 ± 3.7	93.1 ± 2.1
7.3	96.3 ± 2.7	99.2 ± 0.8	97.3 ± 1.0	92.4 ± 2.3

* B cells are recovered from the column by gentle pipetting with addition of 1% bovine serum albumin.

features of spleen lymphocytes in their electrostatic properties of plasma membrane surfaces.

Separation mechanisms of polyamine graft copolymer columns

It is important to gain insight into the mechanisms involved in the separation of B and T cells by graft copolymer columns. Because lymphocyte adsorption on these copolymers was significantly affected by pH and the ionic strength of the medium, ionic interaction is suggested to have a principal role [10]. Most likely is the ionic interaction of protonated amino groups in the copolymer with acidic groups on the cellular plasma membrane surface. Diamine units in polyamine grafts were found to undergo two-step protonation, as illustrated in Figure 11.2. Protonation degree (α) of these amino groups was drastically changed in the physiologic pH range. Further, it was found that the transition in conformation of polyamine grafts took place around the protonation degree of 0.5, as schematically shown in Figure 11.3: a change from hydrophilic extended state to hydrophobic compact state due to deprotonation of amino groups.

This conformational change of the polyamine chain has a striking effect on the retention of lymphocytes on the HA copolymer column, as shown in Figure 11.4 [11]. The sudden increase in T-cell retention in the range of $\alpha > 0.5$ is well correlated with the conformational change of the polyamine chain from the aggregated compact state to the extended state. That is, the T cell interacts negligibly with polyamine in the

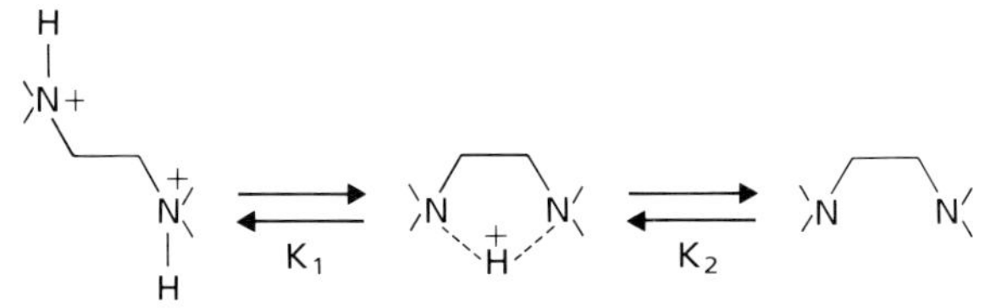

Fig. 11.2 Two-step protonation of diamine unit in copolymer.

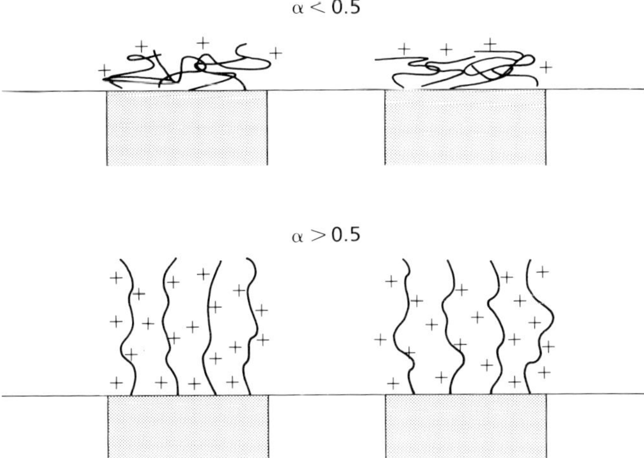

Fig. 11.3 Morphologic change of polyamine grafts with protonation of amino groups.

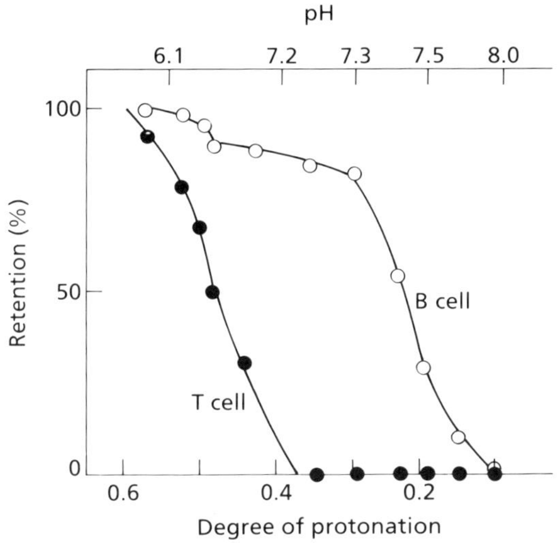

Fig. 11.4 Effect of protonation degree on retention of B and T cells on HA13 column.

compact state. This is in sharp contrast with the B cell which interacts considerably with polyamine in the compact state as well as in the extended state. Consequently, in the range of $\alpha = 0.3$–0.4, which approximately corresponds to the physiologic pH range of 7.0–7.4, the HA column adsorbed more than 90% of loaded B cells with negligible retention of T cells, resulting in a T-cell-enriched population with more than 95% purity in nearly 100% yield as the column effluent.

Recently, our group and the group of Giddings, University of Utah, have collaborated to develop a new cell separation method named hybrid field-flow fractionation

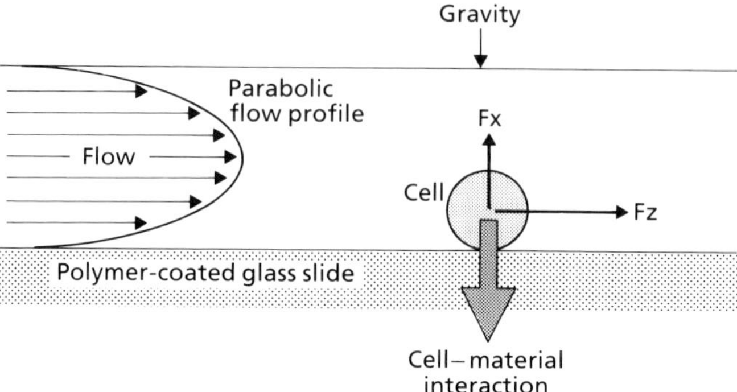

Fig. 11.5 Schematic view of field-flow fractionation/adsorption chromatography apparatus. Fx, perpendicular lift force; Fz, viscous drag force.

(FFF)/adsorption chromatography [12]. A thin ribbon-like chamber with an open-flow channel was used in this method (Fig. 11.5). The inner-bottom surface of the chamber was coated with HA13. Lymphocytes were introduced into the chamber, settled for a given time period and subsequently recovered from the chamber by stepwise increases in flow. By regulating the mode of stepwise flow increase, complete separation of B and T cells was achieved by this new method.

Column separation of T-cell subsets using a partially quaternized HA copolymer as adsorbent

Our most recent interest focused on the design of synthetic adsorbents for T-cell subsets, including helper, suppressor, and killer T cells. Although the monoclonal antibody-based method for separating lymphocyte subsets has become a powerful tool, there still exist many disadvantages including unfavorable biologic responses, low storage stability, and high cost for the preparative process. These disadvantages can be alleviated through the development of synthetic cellular adsorbents with an adequate affinity toward particular T-cell subsets. Recently, we have found that the partially quaternized HA copolymer (HQA, Fig. 11.6) can be used for resolving helper and suppressor T cells.

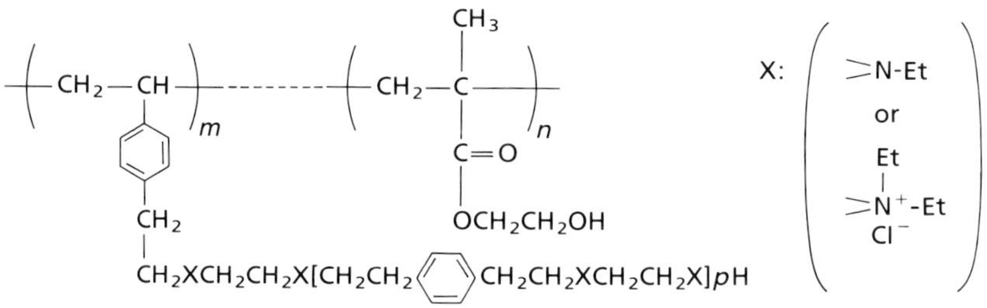

Fig. 11.6 Structural formula of quaternized HA copolymer.

Immunofluorescence assay using fluorescein isothiocyanate-labeled monoclonal antibody revealed that at pH 7.4, HQA preferentially adsorbed suppressor T cells as well as B cells (derived from the lymph node of a Wistar rat). No such resolution was observed with the HA column, indicating a crucial role of the quaternary ammonium groups for this resolution. The degree of quaternization of amino groups also has an important effect. The sample with the highest degree of quaternization, 28.9% (HQA 13 (28.9)) yielded the most enriched helper T-cell population, with more than 60% purity as column effluent (Fig. 11.7).

In conclusion, our results demonstrated a successful separation of lymphocyte subpopulations through differential ionic affinity to synthetic adsorbents, indicating a promising feature of cellular adsorption chromatography as a major tool for separating a wide spectrum of cell populations.

Acknowledgments

Our work cited in this paper was performed in collaboration with the research groups of Prof. Teiji Tsuruta, Science University of Tokyo, and Prof. Yasuhisa Sakurai, Tokyo Women's Medical College. Funding for most of this work was provided by the Ministry of Education, Science, and Culture, Japan through Grant-in-Aid for Scientific Research (Priority Area Research Program: New Functionality Materials — Design, Preparation, and Control), and by the TEPCO Research Foundation.

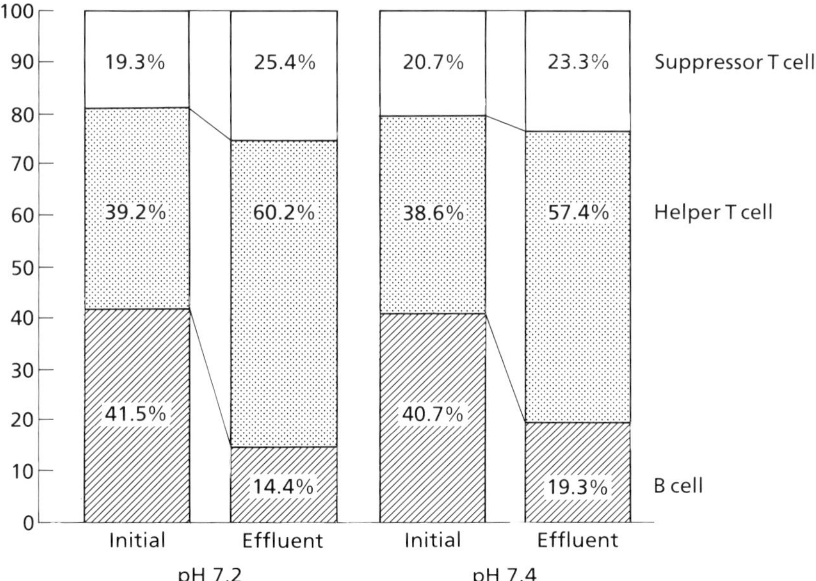

Fig. 11.7 Change in the ratio of lymphocyte subpopulations due to quaternized HA copolymer column treatment.

References

1 Kataoka K, Sakurai Y, Tsuruta T. Microphase separated polymer surfaces for separation of B and T lymphocytes. *Makromol Chem* 1985; (suppl. 9):53–67.
2 Kataoka K, Sakurai Y, Tsuruta T. Affinity selection of cells on solid-phase matrices with immobilized proteins. In: Brash JL, Horbett TA, eds. *Proteins at Interfaces, Physicochemical and Biochemical Studies.* Washington, DC: American Chemical Society, 1987:603–614.
3 Kataoka K. Polymers for cell separation. *CRC Crit Rev Biocompatibility* 1988;4:341–369.
4 Marchalonis JJ, Wang A-C, Galbraith RM, Baker WC. Lymphocyte membrane glycoproteins: molecular and functional properties. In: Marchalonis JJ, ed. *The Lymphocyte, Structure and Function.* New York: Dekker, 1988:307–390.
5 Maruyama A, Tsuruta T, Kataoka K, Sakurai Y. Separation of B- and T-lymphocytes by cellular adsorption chromatography using poly(2-hydroxyethylmethacrylate)/polyamine graft copolymer as column adsorbent. *J. Biomed Mater Res* 1988;22:555–571.
6 Kataoka K, Nabeshima Y, Tsuruta T. Molecular design of cellular specific polymers and their application to separation of lymphocyte subpopulations. In: Okamura S, Tsuruta T, Imanishi Y, Sunamoto J, eds. *Fundamental Investigations on the Creation of Biofunctional Materials.* Kyoto: Kagaku Dojin, 1991:151–159.
7 Maruyama A, Tsuruta T, Kataoka K, Sakurai Y. Elimination of cellular active adhesion on microdomain-structured surface of graft-polyamine copolymers. *Biomaterials* 1989;10:291–298.
8 Maruyama A, Tsuruta T, Kataoka K, Sakurai Y. Separation of B and T lymphocytes by cellular adsorption chromatography with polyamine graft copolymers as column matrices. II. Recovery of adsorbed B cell enriched populations from the column. *Biomaterials* 1989;10:393–399.
9 Kikuchi A, Mizutani S, Kataoka K, Tsuruta T. Resolution of lymphocyte subpopulations derived from rat spleen by polyamine-graft-PHEMA copolymer. *Polymers Adv Technol* 1991;2:245–251.
10 Maruyama A, Tsuruta T, Kataoka K, Sakurai Y. Polyamine graft copolymer for separation of rat B and T lymphocytes. Role of ionic interaction between polymer matrix and lymphocytes. *Makromol Chem Rapid Commun* 1987;8:27–30.
11 Kataoka K, Okano T, Sakurai Y, Maruyama A, Tsuruta T. Controlled interactions of cells with multiphase-structured surfaces of block and graft copolymers. In: Tsuruta T, Nakajima A, eds. *Multiphase Biomedical Materials.* Utrecht: VSP, 1989:1–19.
12 Bigelow JC, Giddings JC, Nabeshima Y *et al.* Separation of B and T lymphocytes by a hybrid field-flow fractionation/adhesion chromatography technique. *J Immunol Methods* 1989;117:289–293.

Discussion

YUASA (Juntendo University): Now the conformation of filter membranes is becoming complicated and we can select their specificities for cells according to the chemical and physical characteristics of the membrane surface. It is said that the polymer does not activate cells. How about such improved filters like these? Is there any possibility of activation of complement, alternation of cell membrane or changing in conformation of antigen molecules?

KATAOKA: This is an important problem. Although we do not examine all functions of the separated cells, at least for the T cells which passed through the column, one physical method, cell electrophoresis, can be applied. This method is very sensitive and if the membrane proteins are removed or changed, the isoelectric point shifts immediately. We could not find any changes on T cells analyzed with this method. As for B cells, which adhere to the column and are eluted from it, we observed no alternation on viability, but a slight shift in the isoelectric point was found. However, I have no idea whether it affects the function of the B cells, and whether complete recovery will occur during cultivation *in vitro*. We are going to analyze this in detail in the future.

OKUMURA: We separate T and B cells by use of the Leukopack, which is a classical but still very popular method. I can say that the responses of the cells separated by this method are reversible as far as we could determine with available immunochemical methods. There may be some functional effects, but the cells recover as far as I know.

HANDA: You showed us the photograph of the filter with platelets. In my view adsorption is generally nonspecific. What do you think of the relation between specific binding and nonspecific binding? When platelets adhere to the surface of macromolecules, extracellular adhesive glycoproteins, for example fibrinogen, stick to the surface and then the platelets adhere to them via their adhesive molecules. Did you perform the adhesion test in the presence of proper serum glycoproteins or serum factors? Is there any possibility of binding via a certain receptor on platelets?

KATAOKA: We used cell suspension in our study.

HANDA: The cells were washed and there were no proteins in the medium.

KATAOKA: As you said, various proteins adhere to the surface of the polymer and I think we should consider such effects when we filter whole blood and platelet-rich plasma.

HANDA: How about whole blood?

KATAOKA: Although it is not yet demonstrated completely, modification of the functional groups on the polymer may affect the kinds of proteins that will be absorbed on it, or the conformation of absorbed protein. Perhaps the structure of the functional groups may affect the potentials of the cells, whereas some proteins may act as amplifiers to transport information to the cell. But how to control this is currently unknown.

OKUMURA: About the last question, a slight change in oxygen pressure or other factors may occur in such a situation and they can induce down- or upregulation of adhesion molecules on the cells. This phenomenon has become an important subject of discussion when we think of immunological response and graft-versus-host disease. I think this is a very interesting model to explain this phenomenon *in vitro*.

12 · Leukocyte depletion of HTLV-I carrier red cell concentrates by filters

M. Kobayashi, M. Yano, K.-W. Kwon, T.A. Takahashi, H. Ikeda, and S. Sekiguchi

Hokkaido Red Cross Blood Center, Yamanote 2-2, Nishi-ku, Sapporo 063, Japan

Abstract

To determine whether leukocyte depletion by filters could reduce or prevent the transmission of viruses carried in leukocytes, we filtered human T lymphotropic virus type I (HTLV-I)-positive red cell concentrate (RCC) with a Sepacell R-500 filter and examined the HTLV-I proviral DNA and infectivity of the residual leukocytes in the filtrates. We used the polymerase chain reaction (PCR) to detect proviral DNA with the primer for the pX region of HTLV-I. HTLV-I-specific DNA was confirmed in two cases out of five filtered samples. To investigate the HTLV-I infectivity *in vitro* of these residual leukocytes, we used the syncytium induction assay in which HTLV-I-infected leukocytes from carrier donors were cocultivated with the human epidermoid cancer cells (ME-180). We filtered 7 HTLV-I positive RCCs. In only one case of seven filter-passed leukocytes did we detect HTLV-I proviral DNA, but no significant increased syncytium formation was observed in any case. Morphologic damage to the cellular organelle in the residual leukocytes was observed. These findings indicate that, although leukocyte depletion is insufficient for complete removal of HTLV-I from seropositive blood, the filtration may contribute to the prevention of HTLV-I transmission by cell damage during filtration and subsequent reduction of cell-to-cell contact.

Introduction

There are many kinds of viruses transmitted by blood transfusion, such as hepatitis B (HBV) and C virus (HCV), HTLV-I, and cytomegalovirus (CMV). These viral transmissions can be classified mainly into two types in transfusion medicine. One is viral transmission mediated by leukocytes, and the other is that mediated by cell-free plasma. Some viruses are carried in specific types of leukocytes: CMV is largely carried in granulocytes; human immunodeficiency virus (HIV) and HTLV-I by T lymphocytes; Epstein–Barr virus (EBV) in B lymphocytes, and HIV also in monocytes. Alloimmunization and viral transmission are two major adverse effects of blood transfusion, and they are caused by the leukocytes in blood products. Clinical studies indicate that alloimmunization could be prevented by reducing the number of leukocytes in blood components. Viruses in fresh frozen plasma can be removed directly by a virus removal filter, the Bemberg microporous membrane (BMM), which has been developed recently in our blood center in collaboration with Asahi Chemical Industry (Tokyo, Japan) [1,2]. Viruses in blood components could be removed in several ways. From RCCs, viruses can be removed by washing the cells, and removal of leukocytes by means of filters should be effective in preventing leukocyte-mediated viral transmission. However, the possibility of avoiding viral transmission by depleting leukocytes in blood products has not as yet been confirmed.

To determine if leukocyte depletion by a filter could prevent leukocyte-mediated infection, we selected HTLV-I as a model virus. HTLV-I is a causative agent of adult T-cell leukemia and is usually found in T lymphocytes. Japan is one of the endemic areas of HTLV-I infection. About 1% of Japanese blood donors are considered to be healthy carriers of this virus, which is apparently transmitted by cell-to-cell contact. Since the virus is found in T lymphocytes, we tried to remove leukocytes from HTLV-I-positive blood in order to prepare HTLV-I-free blood. In order to test whether leaked leukocytes contained HTLV-I, we tried to detect proviral DNA by the PCR [3,4] method using primer pairs for the constant HTLV-I pX region. We also studied the *in vitro* HTLV-I infectivity by the syncytium induction assay [5].

Materials and methods

Filtration of HTLV-I seropositive blood

We filtered HTLV-I seropositive RCC using a Sepacell R-500 filter (Asahi Medical, Tokyo, Japan) and prepared mononuclear cells from the filtrate by Ficoll gradient. HTLV-I antibody was evaluated by particle agglutination assay using Serodia-HTLV-I (Fujirebio, Tokyo, Japan) and indirect immunofluorescence.

Polymerase chain reaction method

We prepared template DNA from pre- and postfiltration samples using proteinase K and phenol/chloroform extraction. We performed 35 cycles of amplification with a primer set of HTLV-I pX [6] and analyzed samples by dot blotting using a γ-^{32}P-adenosine triphosphate-labeled 20mer probe that was complementary to internal sequences of the amplified fragment.

In vitro HTLV-I infectivity

We evaluated *in vitro* HTLV-I infectivity by the syncytium induction assay. We cocultivated HTLV-I-permissive (ME-180) cells and lymphocytes separated from pre- and postfiltration samples. After subcultivation, syncytia (multinucleated giant cells) were detected by microscopy. The infectivity of HTLV-I was expressed as the ratio of the number of syncytia formed by the addition of lymphocytes to the number of syncytia formed spontaneously in ME-180 cells without addition of lymphocytes (syncytium formation ratio).

Electron microscopic observation

We prepared leukocytes from pre- and postfiltration RCC. After fixation with glutaraldehyde and osmic acid, they were dehydrated and mounted in epoxy resin. Then they were observed by electron microscopy (JEM-1200 EX, Japan Electron, Tokyo, Japan).

Leukocyte viability

Leukocytes of pre- and postfiltration samples were cultivated overnight and stained by fluorescein diacetate (FDA, Sigma, St Louis, MO, USA) and ethidium bromide (EB). Viable cells were stained green and dead cells were stained red. We evaluated leukocyte viability by counting each cell number by microscopy.

Leukocyte subset ratio

We filtered a pool of buffy coat (derived from 200 ml of whole normal blood) at room temperature and collected 20 ml fractions of filtrate. In the filtrate that contained 2×10^6 leaked leukocytes, lymphocytes were analyzed for leukocyte surface antigen markers with a monoclonal antibody by FACS-Analyzer (Beckton Dickinson, Rutherford, NJ, USA). Leu2 (CD8) and Leu3 (CD4) were used as helper/inducer and suppressor/cytotoxic T-cell markers, respectively. Leu4 (CD3) was treated as a pan T cell and surface immunoglobulin (sIg) as a B-cell marker.

Induction of HTLV-I antigen in filtrated leukocytes

The lymphocytes from pre- and postfiltration samples were cultured for 2–3 weeks and tested for the expression of HTLV-I core protein with anti-HTLV-I p19 monoclonal antibody by the indirect immunofluorescence method.

Results

Sensitivity of proviral DNA detection by the polymerase chain reaction method

We analyzed a serial 10-fold dilution of HTLV-I complementary DNA (PHT-M[3.9]), a kind gift from Dr K. Shimotohno (National Cancer Center Research Institute, Tokyo, Japan).

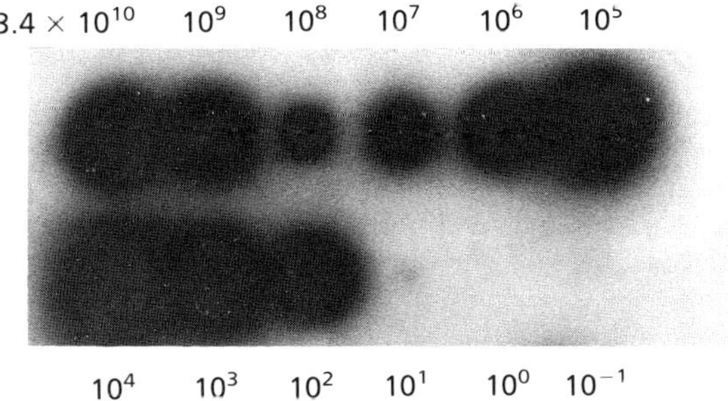

Fig. 12.1 Sensitivity of the polymerase chain reaction method by amplification of human T lymphotropic virus type I complementary DNA.

We could detect about 30 copies (3.4×10 copies) by dot blotting analysis (Fig. 12.1).

Leukocyte removal percent and proviral DNA detection

We examined whether HTLV-I proviral DNA (the pX region) could be detected in the residual leukocytes after Sepacell filtration (Table 12.1). The total number of leukocytes in the prefiltration blood was 1.60×10^8–2.74×10^9 cells and that at post-filtration was 6.96×10^5–5.16×10^7 cells. The leukocyte removal percentage was 98.12–99.97%.

HTLV-I proviral DNA was detected in all samples before filtration and also in two of the five filtered samples (Table 12.1, no. 1 and no. 2). Figure 12.2 shows the autoradiography of the PCR experiments.

There was no significant correlation between PCR results and the number of leukocytes leaked.

Table 12.1 Detection of human T lymphotropic virus type I (HTLV-I) proviral DNA in Sepacell R-500 filtrate

	Experiment no.				
	1	2	3	4	5
Total WBC	2.32×10^9	1.60×10^8	1.61×10^8	1.57×10^9	2.74×10^9
Pre-PCR	+	+	+	+	+
HTLV-I Ag*	+	−	+	+	−
Total WBC	6.96×10^5	2.47×10^7	2.40×10^6	8.28×10^5	5.16×10^7
Post-PCR	+	+	−	−	−
Leukocyte removal (%)	99.97	98.44	99.85	99.95	98.12

* Induction of human T lymphotropic virus I (HTLV-I) antigen p19 in PBL.
PCR, polymerase chain reaction; WBC, white blood cells.

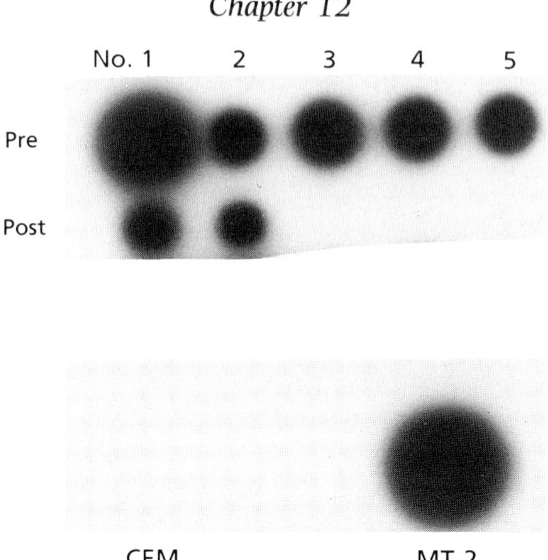

Fig. 12.2 Dot blot analysis of polymerase chain reaction products of the human T lymphotropic virus I pX gene in pre- and postfiltration samples. MT-2, positive control; CEM, negative control.

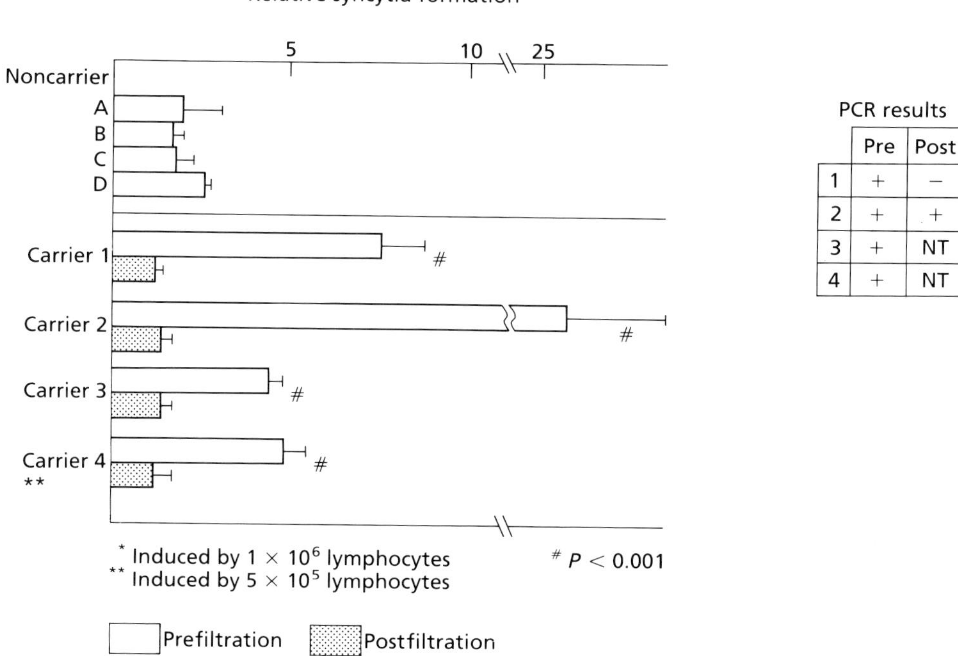

Fig. 12.3 Syncytium formation and polymerase chain reaction (PCR) in pre- and postfiltration samples. NT, not tested.

Evaluation of *in vitro* HTLV-I infectivity in filtrated leukocytes

We studied proviral DNA and the ability of syncytium formation of seven of pre- and postfiltrated RCC samples. Proviral DNA was detected in all prefiltration samples and among the filtrated samples, it was still detected in carrier 2. The syncytium formation ratios at prefiltration (Fig. 12.3, carrier 1 and carrier 2) were 7.5 and 27.5, respectively. But those at postfiltration were reduced to 1.1 and 1.2. The other samples also showed similar results.

Consequently, the syncytium formation ratio at postfiltration was significantly lower than that at prefiltration ($P < 0.001$).

Lymphocyte subset ratios of pre- and postfiltration samples

There was no significant change in the ratio of $CD8^+:CD3^+$ and $CD4^+:CD3^+$ between pre- and postfiltration (Fig. 12.4). The $CD4^+:CD8^+$ ratio at postfiltration was higher than that before filtration. $CD8^+$ cells were likely to be better removed than other cell markers. B lymphocytes were also likely to be better removed than T lymphocytes. However, all results showed no significant change.

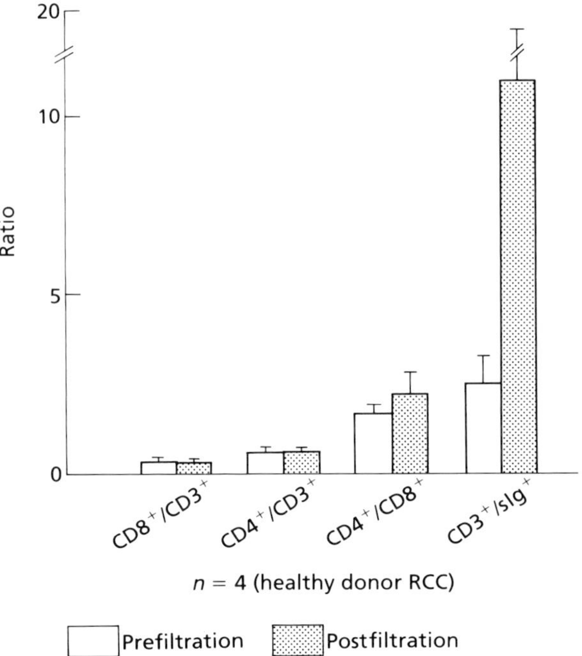

Fig. 12.4 Lymphocyte subset ratios of pre- and postfiltration samples.

Leukocyte viability in pre- and postfiltration samples

Figure 12.5 shows the viability of leukocytes from healthy donors (HTLV-I-negative) at overnight culture and immediately after filtration. There were significant changes of viability in Sepacell-filtered leukocytes in both cases.

Induction of HTLV-I antigen in pre- and postfiltration samples

In prefiltration lymphocytes, 0.3–5.2% of cells were HTLV-I antigen-positive (Table 12.2). But the filtrated lymphocytes did not survive more than 24 h in culture, regardless of the HTLV-I carrier state. Thus we could not confirm whether HTLV-I-positive cells were present or not in the filtrated lymphocytes.

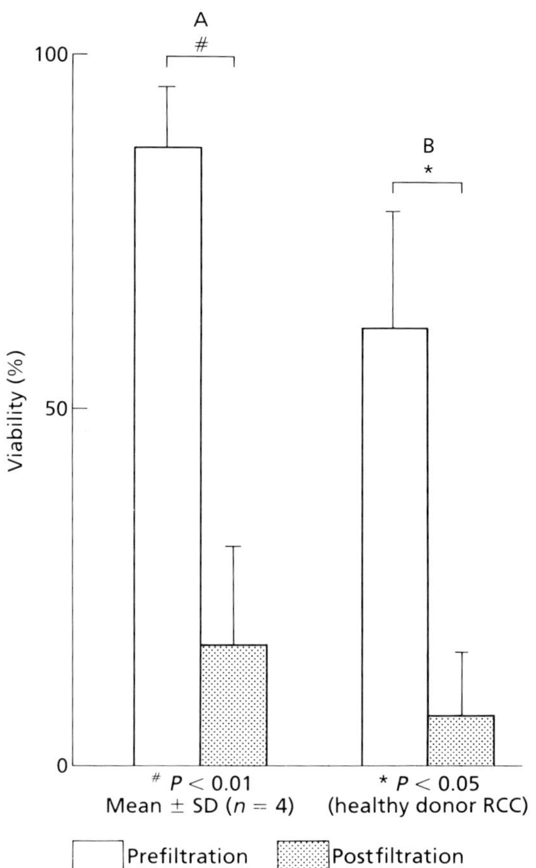

Fig. 12.5 Leukocyte viability in pre- and postfiltration samples. (A) Within 1 h of filtration; (B) overnight culture after filtration.

Table 12.2 Induction of human T lymphotropic virus I (HTLV-I) p19-positive cells in filtered leukocytes

	%HTLV-I-positive cells	
Experiment no.	Prefiltration	Postfiltration
1	0.3	—*
2	5.0	—
3	5.2	—
4	3.6	—

* Lymphocytes did not survive in culture beyond 24 h.

Morphology of leukocytes in pre- and postfiltration

Filtered and unfiltered leukocytes from HTLV-I-negative blood were examined by electron microscopy. As shown in Figure 12.6, most of the filtered leukocytes appeared to be injured.

Summary

One of our major purposes was to find effective ways to reduce the possibility of leukocyte-mediated virus infection [7].

HTLV-I is usually found in $CD4^+$ lymphocytes and is transmitted by cell-to-cell contact. In this study, however, there was no significant change of T-cell subpopulations in the filtrates (Fig. 12.4). The Sepacell filter did not appear to remove $CD4^+$ cells selectively, but removed B cells rather than T cells.

To determine if Sepacell-passed leukocytes can transmit HTLV-I to other cells, we employed the syncytium induction assay, in which HTLV-I-infected leukocytes from carrier donors were cocultivated with human epidermoid cancer cells (ME-180). Although there were PCR-positive samples among the Sepacell-passed leukocytes, they lost syncytium induction activity (Fig. 12.3).

In order to clarify the reason for this, we evaluated leukocyte viability (Fig. 12.5) and induction of HTLV-I antigen (Table 12.2), as well as carrying out observations by electron microscopy (Fig. 12.6). As with any assay, it is possible to assume that the filtered lymphocytes were injured during the filtration so that they could no longer survive *in vitro*. When observed by electron microscopy, most of the filtered leukocytes appeared to be injured.

Bruisten *et al.* [8] performed research similar to ours. They studied how to diminish the risk of blood transmission of HIV by the reduction of HIV-I-infected white blood cells. Their results indicate that complete removal of infected white blood cells cannot be achieved by current filters. However, as shown in their paper, the development of filters with an enhanced ability to remove (possibly infected) white blood cells may have the additional benefit of improving the safety of donor blood.

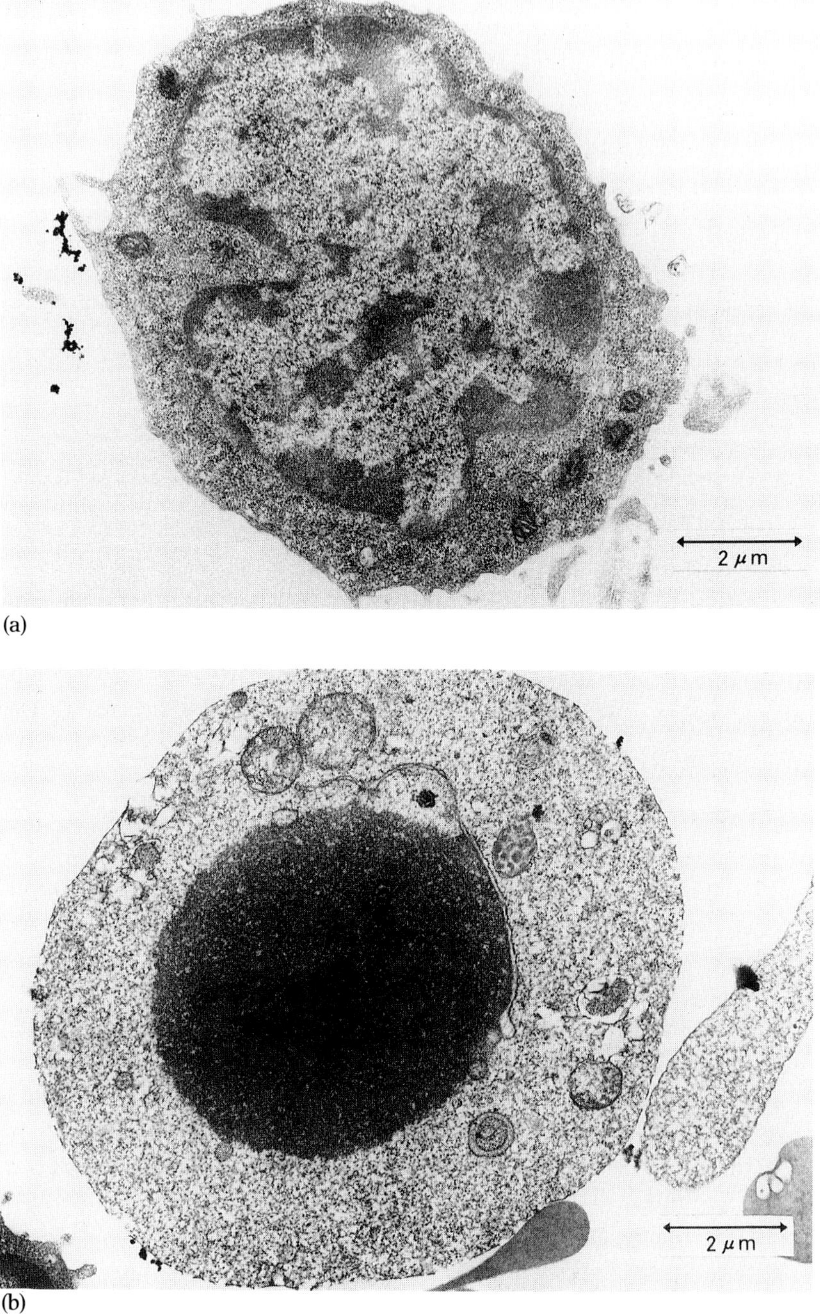

Fig. 12.6 Morphologic changes observed in the lymphocytes passed through the Sepacell R-500. (a) Control lymphocytes; (b) filtered lymphocytes.

In addition to our current study, we must also carry out more detailed evaluations of filter-passed leukocyte *in vivo* viral infectivity. In the future we expect that leukocyte depletion will be applied to prevent HTLV-I infection from donor blood.

References

1 Sekiguchi S, Ito K, Kobayashi M *et al*. Possibility of hepatitis B virus (HBV) removal from human plasma using regenerated cellulose hollow fiber (BMM). *Membrane* 1989;14:253–261.
2 Sekiguchi S, Ito K, Kobayashi M *et al*. An attempt to prepare hepatitis B virus (HBV)-free plasma by ultra-filtration using microporus regenerated cellulose hollow fiber. *Transfus Sci* 1990;11:211–216.
3 Saiki RK, Gelfand DH, Stoffel S *et al*. Primer-directed enzymatic amplification of DNA with a thermostable DNA polymerase. *Science* 1988;239:487–491.
4 Duggan DB, Ehrlich GD, Davey FP *et al*. HTLV-I induced lymphoma mimicking Hodgkin's disease diagnosis by polymerase chain reaction of specific HTLV-I sequences in tumor DNA. *Blood* 1988;71:1027–1032.
5 Yano M, Kwon KW, Ikeda H, Sekiguchi S. Syncytium induction assay for HTLV-I infected cells using ME180-syncytia formation by peripheral blood lymphocytes from healthy HTLV-I carriers. *Jpn J Transfus Med* 1992;38:34–39.
6 Kwok S, Ehrlich G, Poiesz B, Kalisch R, Sninsky JJ. Enzymatic amplification of HTLV-I viral sequences from peripheral blood mononuclear cells and infected tissues. *Blood* 1988;72:1117–1123.
7 Sekiguchi S, Takahashi TA. Leukocyte-depleted blood products and their clinical usefulness. In: Brozović B, ed. *The Role of Leukocyte Depletion in Blood Transfusion Practice*, Oxford: Blackwell Scientific Publications, 1989:26–34.
8 Bruisten SM, Tersmette M, Wester MR, Vos AHV, Koppelman MHGM, Huisman JG. Efficiency of white cell filtration and a freeze-thaw procedure for removal of HIV-infected cells from blood. *Transfusion* 1990;30:833–837.

Discussion

OHTO (Fukushima Medical College): Is there any possibility that the DNA of the HTLV-I virus is integrated into blood cells other than T4 lymphocytes, especially erythroblast strains? Are the immature erythroblast-strain cells removed by leukocyte-depletion filters or do they come out of them?

KOBAYASHI: HTLV-I is a retrovirus and is thought to infect T4 lymphocytes. Therefore, we examined the leukocyte reduction by filtration.

OHTO: One recent report said that rabbits existed that do not produce antibody against HTLV-I and that the HTLV-I DNAs were inserted into the white cells of half of them. If this fact can be applied to human cases, the screening method now in use may lose its validity.

KOBAYASHI: Are you asking whether there are any samples that are serologically negative but are PCR positive?

IKEDA: HTLV-I DNA, at least, could not be observed in any peripheral blood lymphocytes from seronegative donors when analyzed by the PCR method.

SHIMIZU: How many negative samples did you analyze?

IKEDA: Not so many. There were samples that were positive for only particle agglutination assay but these samples are PCR-negative. If we include these samples in the seronegative group, we examined about 40 samples. The samples that were positive for immunofluorescence were almost all PCR-positive. Thus, we consider immunofluorescence-positive donors to be carriers because they were PCR-positive.

ITO (Kyoto University): Your working hypothesis is that filtration with the Sepacell can prevent infection because it can remove all CD4 cells, isn't it? If this is so, you must examine the presence of CD4 cells, but PCR is not suitable because such a highly sensitive detection method may exaggerate the presence of infected cells.

KOBAYASHI: But techniques such as the immunoabsorbant method are the only way to remove T4 lymphocytes specifically. If a leukocyte-removal filter is used the infectiousness of the leaked leukocytes is a problem. I have reported that some morphological damage might occur in such leukocytes, as confirmed by electron micrographs.

ITO: If you would like to investigate it thoroughly, I suppose inactivation of white cells by UV irradiation or by some other way would be appropriate.

KOBAYASHI: We think that the use of leukocyte-depletion filters is one of the simplest methods.

SHIMIZU: Are viruses killed by radiation?

ITO: No, viruses are not killed. CMV or HTLV-I are thought to infect by contact between live cells. Thus, I suppose killing of live cells can prevent infection.

SHIMIZU: Is there any evidence?

ITO: Well, there is no evidence but this hypothesis is thought to be right, and some previous experimental results seem to support it.

13 · Mechanisms of immune responses to allo-MHC Class I

M. Minami

Department of Transfusion Medicine and Immunohematology, Faculty of Medicine, Yokohama City University, Fukuura 3–9, Kanazawa-ku, Yokohama 236, Japan

Abstract

To examine the role of Ia molecules in T-cell responses to allo-class I major histocompatibility antigens, a series of allo-Class I-reactive T-cell hybridomas was established. Of 134 T-cell hybridomas obtained from the fusion of C3H/HeJm or B10.HTT T cells stimulated with C57BL/6 splenocytes, nine T-cell hybridomas were reactive to Class I antigens and 126 T-cell hybridomas were reactive to Class II antigens. Six of nine interleukin-2 (IL-2) producing T-cell hybridomas were further analyzed: five mapped to H-$2K^b$ and the other mapped to H-$2D^b$. Three of these T-cell hybridomas, HTB-157.7, HTB-176.10, and HTB-177.2, could react to the EL-4 cell line that expresses H-$2K^b$ and H-$2D^b$ Class I antigens but lack Class II I-A^b molecules. Furthermore, the activation of these three T-cell hybridomas with C57BL/6-derived asplenocytes was not blocked by anti-I-A. In contrast, the other three T-cell hybridomas, CB-127.6, CB-221.7, and HTB-102.7, failed to react with EL-4 but reacted with the LB cell line which expresses class I (H-$2K^b$, H-$2D^b$) and class II (I-A^b) molecules. Although Class II molecules were required for activation of the latter clones there was no apparent I-A allele specificity, suggesting that a relatively nonpolymorphic Ia determinant was involved. The activation of the three latter T-cell hybridoma clones with C57BL/6 splenocytes could be blocked completely by anti-I-A. The data are interpreted in terms of possible T-cell receptor models for recognition of Class I with nonpolymorphic Class II determinants.

Introduction

It is not surprising that leukocytes contaminating red cells and platelets for transfusions preparations were initially accepted by blood bankers and transfusionists as normal and noncontroversial passengers. Alloimmunization is a matter for serious concern in multiple transfusions. In 1971 Terasaki *et al.* and Patel *et al.* had published data showing that kidney transplants could be compromised by preexisting immunization against human leukocyte antigens (HLAs).

Immune responses to HLA, especially antibody responses to HLA Class I, induce an adverse reaction after transfusion. Thus, it is important to elucidate the mechanisms of immune responses to HLA and especially Class I.

The immune system consists of the humoral and the cellular immune systems. The humoral system is responsible for the production of antibody by B cells. The cellular immune system comprises a rich tapestry of antigen-presenting cells (APCs), monocytes, macrophages, and T cells, stimulation of which results in the secretion of a variety of lymphokines and the development of both cytotoxic and superior activities.

With a few exceptions, an immune response to an antigen starts with APCs. These are bone marrow-derived cells capable of presenting antigen in a form recognizable by T lymphocytes.

All APCs express both Class I and Class II MHC molecules on their surface. In humans these are, respectively, HLA A, B, and C, and HLA DR, DP, and DQ. Class II molecules are normally expressed only by certain cells of bone marrow origin, specifically macrophages, B cells, Langerhans cells of the skin, endothelial cells, and dendritic cells. Class I antigens, HLA A, B, and C, are expressed by all nucleated cells and also by platelets.

Proliferation in the mixed leukocyte reaction (MLR) is generally stimulated by Class II alloantigens. However, strong proliferative responses to Class I alloantigens have been reported [1–5]. This finding raises the important question of whether the proliferating T cell recognizes allo-H-2K/H-2D antigens in the same manner as allo-Ia antigens. A requirement for an Ia-bearing cell in Class I MLR has been described [3,6,7]. Furthermore, a primary MLR to Class I alloantigens is blocked by the addition of anti-Ia antibody, suggesting that Ia molecules are involved in the activation of Class I-reactive T cells [1]. In contrast, we have previously demonstrated that proliferation of a secondary Class I MLR can be stimulated with Ia-accessory cells [7]. This is an apparent disparity between the requirement for Ia molecules in primary and secondary Class I MLR. In this chapter, we describe several IL-2-producing T-cell hybridoma clones that react to allo-Class I molecules. Analysis of the requirements for Ia molecules in the activation of these T-cell hybridomas revealed that there are at least two types of IL-2 producing Class I-reactive T-cell hybridoma clones. One type of Class I-specific T-cell hybridoma clone required concomitant recognition of Ia molecules for activation.

The present data suggest that this type of T-cell hybridoma clone may recognize determinants on Ia molecules which are of limited polymorphism. In contrast, the second type of T-cell hybridoma clones do not require recognition of Ia molecules for activation, and may represent an Ia-independent inducer (IL-2-producing) clone or may be related to cytotoxic T lymphocytes.

Materials and methods

Mice

C57BL/6, C3H/He Jms, and BALB/c mice were supplied by the animal breeding unit of the Institute of Medical Science, Tokyo, or were obtained from The Jackson

Laboratory, Bar Harbor, ME, USA. Breeding pairs of B10HTT, B10MBR, B10A(3R), B10A(4R), bm12, B10GD, B10HTG, and B10.WB strains were bred and were maintained in our own animal colony. Mice were used at 6–10 weeks of age for experiments.

Monoclonal antibodies

Antibody-producing hybridoma culture supernatants were centrifuged and were filtered before use as a source of monoclonal antibodies. The monoclonal antibodies, their specificities, and their sources are as follows: 28.16.8S [8], anti-I-A^{b,d} was made available by Dr V. Oi [9]; and Ho13.4, anti-Thy-1.2 was obtained from the Cell Distribution Center of the Salk Institute (La Jolla, CA).

T-cell hybridomas

T-cell blasts for construction of alloreactive T-cell hybridomas were derived from bulk MLR cultures after 4 days of stimulation, as described elsewhere [10]. In brief, nylon wool-nonadherent C3H/HeJms (CB series) or B10.Htt (HTB series) T cells $(1-2 \times 10^7)$ were cultured in 10% CO_2 (Napco Incubator, National Instruments, Portland, OR) with an equal number of 800 rad-irradiated (^{137}Cs source, γ-cell 40; Atomic Energy of Canada, Ottawa, Ontario, Canada), erythrocyte-free splenocytes from C57BL/6 mice in a 25 ml flask. Four days later, responding T-cell blasts were recovered and were fused at a 1 : 1 ratio to the hypoxanthine guanine phosphoribosyltransferase-negative T-cell lymphoma line BW5147. Hybridomas were selected by culture in the medium with hypoxanthine, aminopterine, and thymidine. They were tested for their IL-2 production when cultured with C57BL/6-derived, 800 rad-irradiated spleen cells, as described below. All hybridomas described in this report were further cloned by limiting dilution after the initial screening. HTB-9.3 hybridoma is an HTB series of hybridoma and was characterized previously to be reactive to I-A^b molecules [10].

Cell culture

Hybridomas were tested for their alloreactivity *in vitro* as described elsewhere [10]. In brief, $1-5 \times 10^4$ T-cell hybridomas were cultured with or without various numbers of irradiated mitomycin C-treated stimulator cells. Cultures were incubated at 37°C for 18–24 h, at which time 100 µl of culture supernatant was harvested and the IL-2 content of the culture supernatant was measured with an IL-2 addicted T-cell line, CTLL. CTLL cells (4×10^3) were added to test supernatants and were incubated at 37°C for 20–24 h with 0.25 µCi[^{3}H] thymidine ([^{3}H]TdR) added over the final 6 h. Cells were harvested on to glass fiber filter strips with a semiautomated harvesting device. Incorporation of [^{3}H]TdR was determined by liquid scintillation counting.

Background counts per minute (cpm) of unstimulated CTLL cells

CTLL + supernatant of stimulator cells alone, or CTLL + supernatant of T-cell hybridoma alone (with or without antibody) was between 100 and 500 cpm.

Cell preparation

T-cell-depleted spleen cells were used as stimulator cells. They were prepared by treating spleen cells with monoclonal anti-Thy-1.2 antibody plus complement and were irradiated at 800 rad.

Cell lines

EL-4 cells and LB.15.13 (LB) cells, Ia + B cell hybridomas [11] were treated with 50 µg/ml of mitomycin C (Sigma Chemical, St. Louis, MO) for 45 min at 37 °C before being used as stimulator cells.

Results

H-2 specificity of alloreactive T-cell hybridomas used in these studies

A series of T-cell hybridomas was derived from C3H/HeJ or B10.HTT T cell blasts which had been stimulated with allogenic C57BL/6-irradiated splenocytes. The T cells were fused to the BW5147 lymphoma cell line. In total, 629 hybridomas were examined, from which 186 IL-2-producing, alloreactive T-cell hybridomas were identified. The reactivity of these 134 alloreactive T-cell hybridomas was examined for their intra-H-2 specificity. Nine hybridomas were reactive to Class I antigens, and 126 hybridomas were reactive to Class II antigens [10]. Of these nine Class I antigen-reactive hybridomas, six clones were analyzed further for this report. As shown in Table 13.1, only one hybridoma, HTB-102.7, was stimulated by C57BL/6-, B10.A(4R)-, B10.GD-, B10.HTG-, or B1.0WB-derived stimulator cells and was not stimulated by B10.MBR, B10.A(3R), or C3H/HeJ splenocytes, indicating that the HTB-102.7 hybridoma detected an antigen which mapped to the H-2D^b region. The other five hybridoma clones were stimulated by C57BL/6, B10.MBR, B10.A(3R), and bm 12 splenocytes but were not stimulated by B10.GD, B10.HTG, and C3H/HeJ splenocytes, indicating that these five hybridomas were reactive to H-2K^b molecules.

Reactivity of Class I-reactive T-cell hybridomas to the EL-4 and LB cell lines

The reactivity of the Class I-reactive T-cell hybridomas was tested with both the EL-4 cell line (which expresses Class I antigens, but not Class II antigens) and the LB cell line (which expresses both Class I and Class II antigens). As shown in Table 13.2,

Table 13.1 Specificity of alloreactive T-cell hybridomas used in this study

Responder T-cell hybridomas	Stimulator cells*					
	C57BL/6 (b,b,b,b)†	C3H/HeJ (k,k,k,k)	BALB/c (d,d,d,d)	B10.MBR (b,k,k,q)	B10.A(4R) (b,b,k,d)	B10.A(3R) (k,k,b,b)
Experiment 1						
HTB-102.7	15.0	1.1	0.0	0.1	0.0	10.7
CB-127.6	27.3	0.1	0.0	22.4	20.5	0.0
CB-221.7	19.9	0.0	0.0	18.3	18.3	0.0
HTB-157.7	19.2	0.0	0.0	16.3	12.2	0.0
HTB-176.10	19.9	0.0	0.0	21.2	17.0	0.1
HTB-177.2	19.4	0.0	0.0	19.6	11.8	0.1

* See materials and methods for protocol and preparation of stimulator cells and assay of interleukin-2 (IL-2) production. Data are given as net cpm $\times 10^{-3}$ (Δ cpm) of IL-2 activity, calculated as mean cpm in responder and stimulator cell cultures minus mean cpm in responder cell cultures and mean cpm in stimulator cell cultures. Standard deviation is within 15% of mean Δcpm.
† Parentheses indicate H_2 allele formula: (K, I-A, I-E, D).

Table 13.2 Reaction of Class I-reactive T-cell hybridomas to EL-4 and LB stimulator cells*

Responder T-cell hybridomas	Stimulator cells†		
	C57BL/6 spleen cells	EL-4	LB
HTB-102.7	7.8 ± 1.1	0.0 ± 0.0	6.7 ± 0.4
CB-127.6	6.3 ± 0.7	0.0 ± 0.0	10.1 ± 1.1
CB-221.7	11.1 ± 1.5	0.0 ± 0.0	8.7 ± 0.5
HTB-157.7	11.4 ± 0.9	13.0 ± 1.0	13.3 ± 1.2
HTB-176.10	14.9 ± 1.1	16.7 ± 0.5	16.7 ± 0.8
HTB-177.2	9.4 ± 0.9	7.4 ± 0.4	8.7 ± 1.1

*See footnotes to Table 13.1 for protocol. Data are expressed as net cpm $\times 10^{-3}$ of interleukin-2 activity. Mean cpm in stimulator spleen cell culture was 199 ± 2; mean cpm in EL-4 culture was 126 ± 21; and mean cpm in LB culture was 114 ± 15.
† Stimulator cells included 5×10^5 irradiated spleen cells from C57BL/6 mice, 1×10^5 mitomycin C-treated LB cells.

three of five T-cell hybridomas which were reactive to H-2K^b molecules reacted with mitomycin C-treated EL-4 cells to produce IL-2. In contrast, clones CB-127.6 and CB-221.7, which were also reactive to H-2K^b molecules, and the HTB-102.7 cells, which were reactive to H-2D^b molecules, could not be stimulated by EL-4. It is unlikely that the failure of these clones (CB-127.6, CB-221.7, and HTB-102.7) to respond to EL-4 is due to the weak stimulation of EL-4 as compared to whole spleen cells, because the EL-4 nonreactive CB-221.7 hybridoma consistently showed stronger responses to splenic stimulator cells than the EL-4-reactive HTB-177.2

clone. These T-cell hybridomas also failed to respond to various numbers of EL-4 (1×10^3 to 5×10^5), whereas the HTB-157.7, HTB-176.10, and HTB-177.2 hybridomas were able to respond to this range of EL-4 stimulator cells by producing IL-2 (data not shown). In contrast, all Class I-reactive hybridomas could react to the LB cell line, which expresses both Class I and Class II products [11]. Preliminary experiments suggest that the inability of selected T-cell hybridomas to respond to EL-4 is not attributable to the IL-1 dependence of the latter hybrids.

CB-127.6, CB-221.7, and HTB-102.7T cell hybridomas require corecognition of Class I and Class II antigens for activation

Several reports have shown that the primary MLR response to Class L antigens requires Ia$^+$ stimulator cells [1–5]. Thus, we tested whether some Class I-reactive T-cell hybridomas reactive to whole spleen cells but not to EL-4 require recognition of Class L antigens and Ia for activation.

To test whether Ia molecules are involved in the stimulation of these six hybridoma clones, blocking experiments were performed with monoclonal anti-IA antibodies. Hybridoma cells (2×10^4) were cultured with 5×10^5 irradiated splenocytes from C57BL/6 or B10.MBR mice. Monoclonal anti-I-A^k antibody was added at the initiation of the culture as the blocking reagent. Controls, including stimulation of the I-A^b or anti-I-A^k antibody, were added at the initiation of the culture as the blocking reagent. Controls included stimulation of the I-A^b-reactive HTB-9.3 clone with C57BL/6-derived spleen cells which could be blocked by anti-I-A^b antibody. As shown in Table 13.3, stimulation of the HTB-157.7, HTB-176.10, and HTB-177.2 clones was not blocked with monoclonal anti-Ia antibodies. In contrast, stimulation of the CB127.6, CB-221.7, and HTB-102.2 clones was completely blocked with monoclonal anti-Ia antibody of the relevant specificity. Nonspecific blocking by monoclonal antibodies of irrelevant specificity was not observed.

These results indicate that there are two distinct types of Class I-reactive clones in terms of the requirements for recognition of Ia molecules. The first type is activated by stimulation with Class I molecules alone. The other type of clone requires recognition of both Class I and Class II antigens for activation. Furthermore, it should be noted that the responses of the CB-127.6 and CB-221.7 T-cell hybridomas to stimulator spleen cells from CB57BL/6(H-2^b) mice were blocked by anti-I-A^b antibody (28-16-8S), and the responses of these hybridomas to spleen cells from B10.MBR (b,k,k,q) mice were blocked by anti-I-A^k antibody [10]. These results suggest that the CB-127.6 and CB-221.7 T-cell hybridomas recognize Ia determinants which display little or no polymorphism.

Summary

The role of Class II antigens on stimulator cells in allo-Class I-mediated MLR has been poorly understood. Previously, we reported that in a primary MLR to allo-Class I MHC

Table 13.3 Effect of monoclonal anti-Ia antibody on the response of allo-active T-cell hybridomas[*]

Responder T-cell hybridomas	Stimulator spleen cells[†]	Antibody added[‡]		
		Medium	Anti-I-A^b	Anti-I-A^k
Experiment 1				
HTB-102.7	C57BL/6	8.9 ± 0.7	0.0 ± 0.1	NT[‡]
CB-127.6		9.8 ± 1.0	0.0 ± 0.0	NT
CB-221.7		11.6 ± 1.7	0.0 ± 0.0	NT
HTB-157.7		17.2 ± 0.8	16.9 ± 0.8	NT
HTB-176.10		8.8 ± 1.7	8.7 ± 0.5	NT
HTB-177.2		13.7 ± 0.8	13.5 ± 0.2	NT
HTB-9.3[§]		14.7 ± 1.8	0.0 ± 0.0	NT
Experiment 2				
CB-127.6	B10.MBR	10.9 ± 1.3	10.2 ± 2.0	0.0 ± 0.1
CB-221.7		13.9 ± 0.8	13.9 ± 1.3	0.0 ± 0.0
HTB-157.7		23.6 ± 0.4	23.9 ± 2.1	22.8 ± 0.8
HTB-176.10		11.8 ± 0.8	11.8 ± 0.3	11.6 ± 1.2
HTB-177.2		15.8 ± 1.1	15.5 ± 2.3	15.3 ± 1.7

*See footnotes to Table 13.1 for protocol.
† Irradiated spleen cells (5×10^5) were used as stimulator cells.
‡ Each anti-Ia antibody was added at the beginning of culture at a final concentration of 2%.
§ See materials and methods.
NT, not tested.

antigens, Ia-bearing stimulator cells were required [3]. Furthermore, the primary MLR to allo-Class I antigens is blocked by the addition of anti-Ia antibody, indicating that in a primary MLR to allo-Class I, antigen recognition of Class II MHC antigens is required [1,2]. In contrast, we reported previously that in a secondary MLR to allo-Class I antigens, Ia$^-$ stimulator cells can induce a T-cell proliferative response [7]. The present study describes several T-cell hybridomas reactive to allo-Class I antigens, and examines the role of Class II antigens in the response to Class I antigens. The data demonstrate two types of allo-Class I reactive T-cell hybridomas; one requires the recognition of Class II antigens, and the other does not.

We characterized six allo-Class I-reactive T-cell hybridomas in the current study. The specificity of five clones mapped to the H-2K^b region and one mapped the H-2D^b region. There have been few reports of Class I-reactive, IL-2-producing T-cell hybridomas [12]. Endres *et al.* [12] described a T-cell hybridoma which was reactive to self-Class I (H-2D region) antigens and which produced IL-2.

The self-Class I-reactive, IL-producing T-cell hybridomas reported by Endres *et al.* [12] also possessed cytolytic activity. Hybridoma clones which mediated delayed-type hypersensitivity reactions to hapten-modified Class I products have also been identified [13]. Other investigators described T-cell hybridomas with cytolytic activity specific for Class I molecules plus viral antigens [14–17]. All of these examples involve

T-cell hybridomas which are restricted to self-Class I determinants, whereas the present report characterizes allo-Class I-restricted T-cell hybridomas.

Swain *et al.* [18] initially reported that the frequency of allo-helper T cells generated by primary stimulation across H-2K differences between the mutant B6.C-H-2^{ba} and wild-type B6 was approximately one-half of the frequency of allo-helper T cells to whole H-2 differences. In one experiment, the ratio of T-cell hybridoma reactive to Class I antigens compared to Class II antigens was 9:125 (7%). The lower frequency of Class I-specific cells in the present studies may be due to the different strain combination used or to the preference of BW5147 cells to hybridize with Class II antigen-reactive T cells, and/or the differences in the assay systems.

Three of six I-reactive T-cell hybridomas were reactive to EL-4 cells which express Class I antigens but lack Class II antigens (Table 13.2). Thus, some T cells could respond to Class I antigens without obligate recognition of Class II antigens. The presence of some T-cell hybridoma clones which react to Class I antigens independently of Class II antigens and others which see Class I in the context of Ia is consistent with our previous reports [3–7]. The three Ia-dependent hybridomas, CB-127.6, CB-221.7, and HTB-102.7, were nonreactive with Ia$^-$ EL-4 cells, although they were reactive to Ia$^+$ LB cells (Table 13.2). Furthermore, the requirements of corecognition of Class II MHC antigens for activation of CB-127.6, CB-221.7, and HTB-102.7 T-cell hybridoma clones was also shown by blocking experiments with relevant monoclonal anti-I-A antibodies (Table 13.3). However, there is no evidence for allele specificity in Ia recognition. HTB-102.7 cells could recognize H-2D^b determinant in the context of the I-A^b, I-A^k, I-A^{bm12}, I-A^d, or I-A^j alleles, whereas the CB-127.6 and CB-221.7 clones recognized H-2K^b with I-A^b, I-A^{bm12}, or I-A^k (Table 13.1). Therefore, these T-cell hybridomas seem to recognize specific Class I determinant and Class II MHC antigens which express limited polymorphism.

Although T cells that recognize allogenic Class I MHC antigen and express helper function have been described [18,19,20], in general, helper T cells are restricted to Class II antigen recognition. T cells that are reactive to Class I antigens are generally cytotoxic T cells. Our preliminary results show that at least one of these clones (HTB-157.7) shows weak cytotoxic activity for EL-4 target cells in 20-h ^{51}CR-release assays. In contrast, CB-127.6, CB-221.7, and HTB-102.7 cells were not cytotoxic under the same experimental conditions (data not shown). Recognition of Class I determinants in the absence of Class II molecules has been characteristic of cytotoxic T cells, and some cytotoxic clones produce IL-2 [21]. Thus the HTB-157.7, HTB-176.10, and HTB-177.2 clones may be of cytotoxic T-cell lineage; alternatively, they may represent Class I-specific IL-2-producing helper cells, which were previously noted in the secondary MLR.

It was reported that anti-Lyt-2 antibody can block function of cytotoxic T cells restricted by Class I MHC antigens [22–25]. However, the activation of the allo-Class I-reactive T-cell hybridomas used in these studies was not blocked with either of two batches of monoclonal anti-Lyt-2 antibody, and none of the clones appear to express

Lyt-2 antigens on their membranes (data not shown). Because Lyt-2 molecules are presumably involved in auxiliary functions for cytolytic ability of the T-cell hybridoma (HTB-157.7) may correlate with the absence of Lyt-2 molecules.

In conclusion, the results reported here resolve an apparent disparity in the activation requirement of primary and secondary MLR. The data demonstrate that there are two types of allo-Class I MHC antigen-reactive T cell hybridomas. One recognizes Class I molecules and Class II MHC antigens; the other type recognizes Class I antigens alone. The former clones resemble proliferative and helper T cells which are stimulated by normal antigen in the context of self-Ia determinants. However, in this system, the reactions are dependent on Ia but are not restricted by self-Ia. This resembles the reactive patterns noted for Mls-reactive clone [26]. The exact role of Ia antigens in allo-Class I reactions remains an issue for investigation.

We can interpret the specificity of these reactions as recognition of Class I molecules in the context of Class II MHC antigens, implying that the receptor on these T cells recognizes Class I plus a nonpolymorphic portion of a Class II molecule. An alternative interpretation is that these T cells recognize Class I antigens with their receptors in a normal fashion, but that successful interaction between T cells and the targets requires the recognition of a nonpolymorphic determinant on Class II molecules by CD4. Finally, the Class II-requiring hybridomas may recognize a nonpolymorphic Ia determinant in the context of Class I molecules — a case similar to the recognition of viral antigens by Class I-restricted cells.

References

1 Rock KL, Barnes MC, German RN, Benacerraf B. The role of Ia molecules in the activation of T lymphocytes. II. Ia-restricted recognition of allo K/D antigens is required for class I MHC-stimulated mixed lymphocyte reactions. *J Immunol* 1983;130:457.

2 Weinberger O, German RN, Burakoff SJ. Responses to the H-2K^{ba} mutant proceed via recognition of syngeneic Ia. *Nature* 1983;302:429.

3 Minami M, Shreffler DC, Cowing C. Characterization of the stimulator cells in the murine primary mixed leukocyte response. *J Immunol* 1980;124:1314.

4 Bach FH, Alter BJ. Alternative pathway of T lymphocyte activation. *J Exp Med* 1978;148:829.

5 Wettstein PJ, Bailley DW, Mobraaten LE, Klein J, Frelinger JA. T lymphocyte response to H-2 mutants. I. Proliferation is dependent on Ly 1$^+$2$^+$ cells. *J Exp Med* 1978;147:1395.

6 Ahmann GB, Nadher PI, Brinkrant A, Hodes RJ. T cell recognition in the mixed lymphocyte response. II. Ia-Positive splenic adherent cells are for non-I-region-induced stimulation. *J Immunol* 1981;127:2308.

7 Minami M, Shreffler DC. Ia-positive stimulator cells are required in primary, but not in secondary, mixed leukocyte reactions against H-K and H-D differents. *J Immunol* 1981;126:1774.

8 Ozato K, Mayor N, Saches DH. Hybridoma cell lines secreting monoclonal antibodies to mouse H-2 and Ia antigens. *J Immunol* 1980;124:533.

9 Oi VT, Johnse PP, Goding JW, Herzenberg LA. Properties of monoclonal antibodies to mouse Ig allotypes, H-2, and Ia antigens. *Curr Op. Microbiol Immunol* 1978;81:115.

10 Minami M, Kawasaki H, Taira S, Nariuchi H. Alloantigen presentation by B cells: two types of alloreactive T cell hybridomas, B cell-reactive and B cell-nonreactive. *J Immunol* 1985;135:111.

11 Kappler J, White J, Wegmann D, Marrack P. Antigen presentation by Ia + B cell hybridomas to H-2 restricted T cell hybridomas. *Proc Natl Acad Sci USA* 1982;79:3604.

12 Endres R, Marrack P, Kappler JW. An IL 2-secreting T cell hybridoma that responds to a self class I histocompatibility antigen in the H-2D region. *J Immunol* 1983;131:1656.

13 Minami M, Okuda K, Sunday ME, Dolf ME. H-2K, H-2I and H-2D restricted hybridoma contact sensitivity effectors cells. *Nature* 1982;297:231.

14 Kaufman Y, Berker G, Eashhar Z. Cytotoxic T lymphocyte hybridomas that mediate specific tumor-cell lysis *in vitro*. *Proc Natl Acad Sci USA* 1981;78:2502.

15 Whitaker BR, Kauffman RS, Che M, Finberg R. CT hybridomas: tumor cells capable of lysing virally infected target cells. *J Immunol* 1982;129:900.

16 Nabholz M, Cianfriglia M, Acuto O, Conzelmann A, Haas W, Boehmer HV, McDonald HR, Pohlit H, Johnson JP. Cytolytically active murine T cell hybrids. *Nature* 1980;287:437.

17 Conzelmann A, Silva A, Cinfriglia M, Tougne C, Sekaly RP, Nabholz M. Correlated expression of T cell growth factor dependence, sensitivity to *Vicia villosa* lectin and cytolytic activity in hybrids between cytolytic T cells and T lymphomas. *J Exp Med* 1982;156:1335.

18 Swain SL, Panfili PR, Dutton RW, Lefkovits I. Frequency of allogeneic helper T cells responding to whole H-2 differences and to an H-2K differences alone. *J Immunol* 1979;123:1062.

19 Panfili PR, Dutton RW. Alloantigen-induced T helper activity. I. Minimal genetic differences necessary to induce a positive allogenic effect. *J Immunol* 1978;120:1897.

20 Swain SL, Panfili PR. Helper cells activated by allogenic H-2K or H-2D differences have Ly phenotype distinct from those responsive to I differences. *J Immunol* 1979;122:583.

21 Andrus L, Granelli-Piperno A, Reich E. Cytotoxic T cells both produce and respond to Interleukin-2. *J Exp Med* 1984;159:647.

22 Swian SL. Significance of Lyt phenotypes: Lyt 2 antibodies block activities of T cells that recognize class I MHC antigens regardless of their function. *Proc Natl Sci USA* 1981;78:7101.

23 Shinohara N, Hammerling U, Sachs D. Mouse allo antibodies capable of blocking cytotoxic T cell function. II. Further study on the relationship between the blocking antibodies and the products of the Lyt-2 locus. *Eur J Immunol* 1980;1:589.

24 Hollander N, Pillemer N, Weissman L. Blocking effect on Lyt-2 antibodies of T cell function. *J Exp Med* 1980;152:674.

25 McDonald HR, Glasebrook AL, Bron C, Kelso A, Cerottini JC. Clonal heterogeneity in the functional requirement for Lyt-2,3 molecules on cytotoxic T lymphocytes (CTL): possible implications for the affinity of CTL antigen receptors. *Immunol Rev* 1982;68:69.

26 Lynch DH, Gress RE, Needleman BW, Rosenberg SA, Hodes RJ. T cell responses to Mis determinations are restricted by cross-reactive MHC determinants. *J Immunol* 1985;134:2071.

Discussion

Oнто(Fukushima Medical School): It is said that alloimmunization cannot be observed for about 2 months after birth. Have you measured the MLR response in newborn babies?

Minami: Immediately after birth?

Oнто: With cord blood.

Minami: I haven't investigated it and so I don't know much about it. Several reports have suggested it to be low.

Oнто: Does that mean there was no response, or that it was positive but impossible to detect?

MINAMI: I suppose there is some positive reaction. But I did not examine it, so I am not sure.

KANO (Olympus BRC): What is your conclusive answer to the question that you first proposed, 'Is it possible that the helper T cells are activated only by platelet transfusion?'

MINAMI: Though I have no definitive answer, one group demonstrated that host's APC can deal with soluble allo-HLA Class I antigen in an *in vitro* CTL response. However, the efficiency of immunization by this system is likely to be very low in comparison with the case immunized by intact cells.

KIYOKAWA(Fukuoka Red Cross Blood Center): If UV-irradiated platelet concentrates are infused into allosensitized patients, the number of circulating platelets does not increase due to the antigen–antibody reaction. But we must consider the side-effects, and the cell populations responsible for such side-effects. Do you have any comments on this point?

MINAMI: Concerning UV-irradiated cells? I'm not sure if irradiated white cells or granulocytes cause the febrile reaction or not.

IKEDA: In relation to the question by Dr Kano, we have tried to inject UV-irradiated platelets intravenously, not subcutaneously. In this case, it seems that alloimmunization may occur through such a system as the platelets are captured into APC and presented on the APC, after which antigens are recognized. We have not arrived at a conclusion yet, but we have data suggesting that allosensitization likely occurs even with UV-irradiated platelets through this system.

TAKAHASHI: I suppose, there is something that absorbs UV rays when blood components are irradiated. Is it possible that some molecules, such as proteins and amino acids, are especially sensitive to UV irradiation?

MINAMI: That is a very difficult question. Actually, UV-irradiation causes various phenomena but I have no idea what exactly happens in detail. I myself would like to explore the mechanisms.

14 · UV-B irradiation to platelet concentrates and its effects *in vivo* and *in vitro*

H. Ikeda, T. Kobata, S. Nakata, T. Mitani, and S. Sekiguchi

Hokkaido Red Cross Blood Center, Yamanate 2-2, Nishi-ku, Sapporo 063, Japan

Abstract

Platelet transfusions are indispensable for aplastic anemia or hematologic malignancies in order to reduce the risk of thrombocytopenic hemorrhage during intensive chemotherapy and bone marrow transplantation. However, a considerable number of thrombocytopenic multitransfused patients become refractory [1]. Allosensitization is mainly responsible for the refractoriness and is mostly caused by contaminating lymphocytes in platelet concentrates [2,3]. The use of single donor platelets [4] or lymphocyte-depleted platelet concentrates is effective in preventing allosensitization [5,6], but they are not 100% effective.

It has been known that ultraviolet (UV) irradiation abolishes both responder and stimulator functions of lymphocytes in mixed lymphocyte reaction (MLR) [7,8]. Platelets appear to be relatively insensitive to UV irradiation. UV-irradiated platelets function normally *in vitro* [8] and their survival *in vivo* is comparable with that of unirradiated platelets [9,10]. Also, UV-B irradiated platelets are effective to prevent allosensitization in dogs [11]. However, the mechanism of its suppressive effect is largely unknown.

We have been studying various effects of UV-B irradiation on rat platelets and its mechanism of prevention of allosensitization. We have found that lack of allosensitization with UV-B-irradiated cells is not due to the reduction of viability or disappearance of cell surface antigens on irradiated cells. Alloantigens of UV-B-irradiated cells were well recognized by allosensitized rats *in vivo*. Inhibitory effects of UV-B irradiation on cell surface capping may be relevant to the failure of recognition of alloantigens on UV-irradiated cells by T cells. Effects of UV-B irradiation on cell surface appear to have little influence on platelet functions. UV-B-irradiated platelets are functionally comparable to nonirradiated platelets *in vivo* as well as *in vitro*.

Allosensitization followed by multiple platelet transfusions is caused by contaminating lymphocytes. Transfusion-associated (TA) allosensitization in rats is dependent on the number of transfused lymphocytes (Fig. 14.1). The number of transfused platelets appears to be irrelevant, as reported elsewhere [2,3]. Accordingly, prevention of TA allosensitization can be achieved either by depletion or inactivation of contaminating lymphocytes. We carried out the study of inactivation of the lymphocytes by UV-B irradiation mainly with rats.

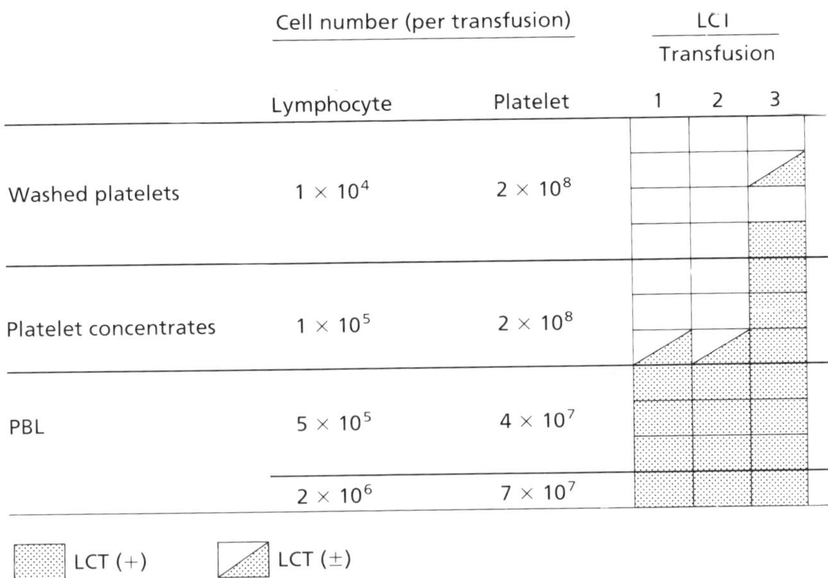

Fig. 14.1 Transfusion-associated allosensitization in rats. LCT, lymphocyte cytotoxicity test; PBL, peripheral blood lymphocyte.

Peripheral blood lymphocytes (PBLs) of inbred WKA strain rats were subjected to 500–1000 J/m UV-B irradiation and transfused to allogeneic inbred ACI strain rats. The recipients' sera were monitored for allosensitization by microcytotoxicity test. Antidonor antibody was not detected after several transfusions of UV-B-irradiated cells (Fig. 14.2). MLR was also abrogated by UV-B irradiation to stimulator cells (Fig. 14.3). Mitomycin (MMC) treatment of lymphocytes did not affect TA allosensitization or MLR. Frozen-thawed lymphocytes were ineffective for allosensitization, indicating that viable cells were mostly efficient at provoking allosensitization, although alloantigens could be presented by host antigen-presenting cells (APCs) [12]. The viability of rat lymphocytes at 2 h after UV-B irradiation was comparable to untreated or MMC-treated cells (Table 14.1). The results indicate that absence of allosensitization with UV-B-irradiated cells is not due to low viability of irradiated cells.

Results on expression of MHC molecules of UV-B-irradiated cells are variable among studies [13–17]. Reduction or even disappearance of MHC antigens [13] was reported. Binding of antirat Class I monoclonal antibody to lymphocytes at saturation was examined by flow cytometry after cells were UV-irradiated or MMC-treated. No significant difference was observed between UV-B and MMC treatments in Class I antigen expression at 2 h after treatments (Table 14.1 and Fig. 14.4). At 48 h after UV-B irradiation to lymphocytes, a minor peak of weaker fluorescence appeared with a concomitant reduction of the major peak (data not shown). With MMC treatment, 90% of the cells were dead after 24 h. No significant difference in MHC Class II

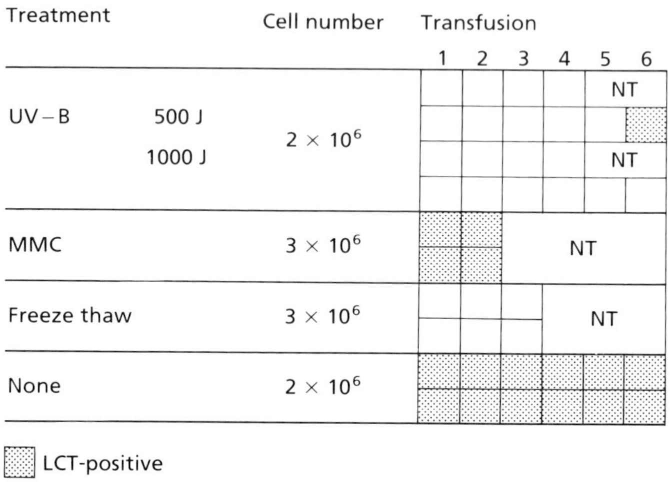

Fig. 14.2 Treatment of PBL and its effect on allosensitization. LCT, lymphocyte cytotoxicity test; MMC, mitomycin; NT, not tested; UV-B, ultraviolet B.

expression at 2 h after UV-B or MMC treatment was observed. Since expression of MHC molecules and viability of UV-irradiated cells are comparable to those of MMC-treated cells at 2 h after treatment, the absence of allosensitization with UV-irradiated cells is not assumed to mean the reduction of viability or disappearance of irradiated cells.

As mentioned above, UV-B irradiation does not induce an immediate influence on alloantigen expression in the irradiated cells. The results were also confirmed *in vivo*.

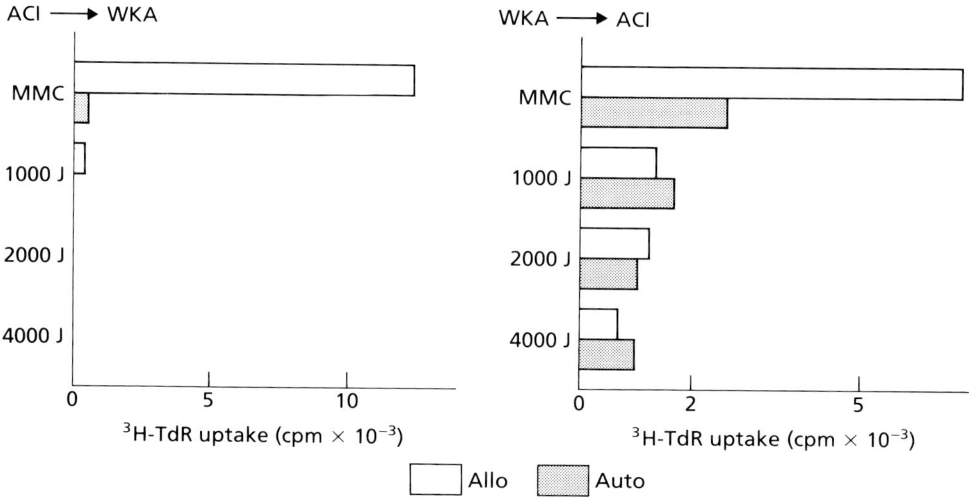

Fig. 14.3 Ultraviolet B irradiation on mixed lymphocyte reaction stimulators. MMC, mitomycin; ³HTdR, ³H thymidine.

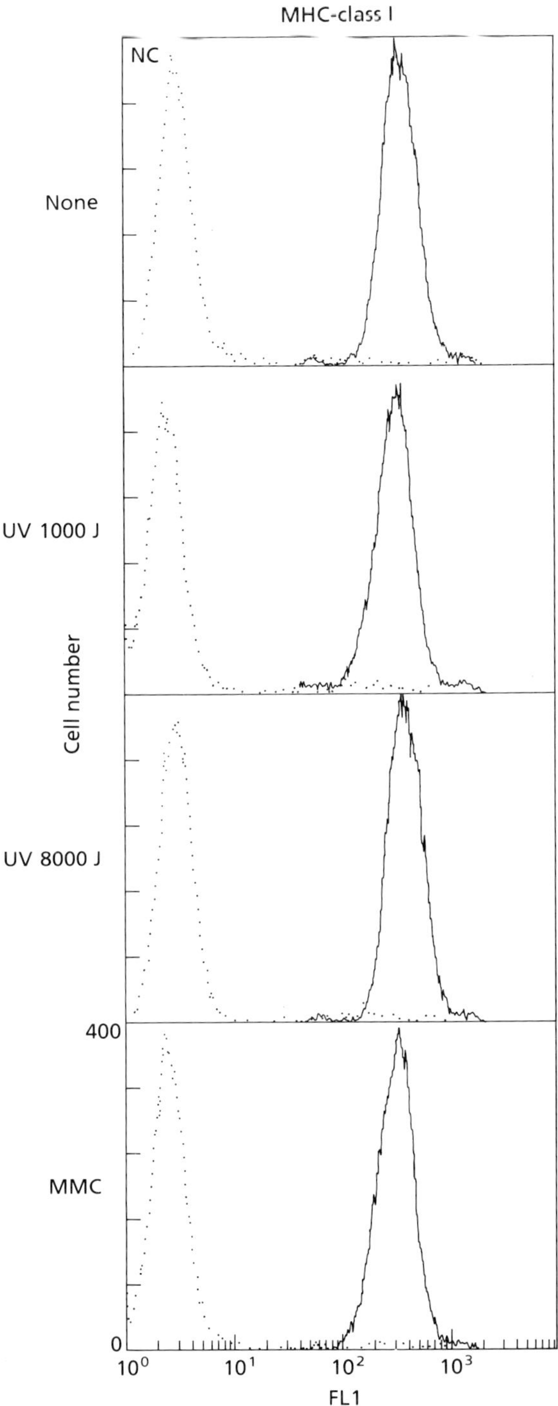

Fig. 14.4 Major histocompatibility complex (MHC), Class I antigens of ultraviolet (UV)-irradiated rat lymphocytes. MMC, mitomycin; NC, normal control.

Table 14.1 Viability and major histocompatibility complex (MHC) antigens of lymphocytes after treatment

	Viability (%)		MHC Class I		MHC Class II	
Treatment	2 h	24 h	2 h	18 h	2 h	18 h
Ultraviolet B 500 J	95.3	92.6	100	100	100	100
Co^{60} 20 Gy	100	20.8	100	NT	100	NT
Mitomycin	100	10.0	100	NT	100	NT
None	100	100	100	100	100	100

NT, not tested.

Rats were lethally irradiated and received platelet transfusion. Transfusion of UV-B-irradiated platelets from allogeneic rats was effective if the animals were not yet sensitized but ineffective if the rats were already allosensitized (Fig. 14.5). Also, a rapid rise in antidonor antibody was observed when UV-B-irradiated PBLs were transfused to allogeneic rats that had been previously immunized with the same donor cells (Fig. 14.6). *In vitro*, UV-B-irradiated cultured B cells functioned as effective target cells for cytotoxic T cells which had been generated with the same cultured B cells (Fig. 14.7). The cytotoxic lymphocytes (CTLs) were cytotoxic to other B cells (KT-3) which share HLA-B7 and Cw-7.

The results indicate that alloantigens on the UV-B-irradiated platelets are responsive and efficient at the effector phase of immune reaction and that transfused platelets were destroyed in alloimmunized rats.

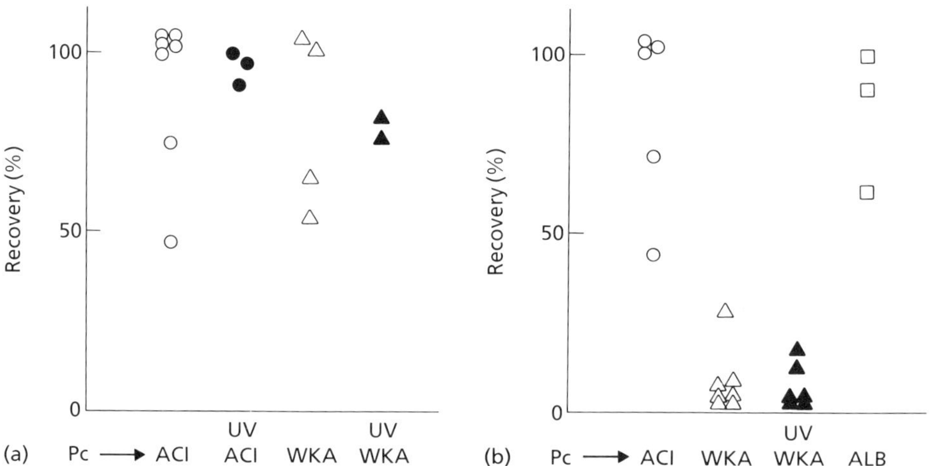

Fig. 14.5. Recovery of transfused platelets. (a) Nonsensitized (ACI); (b) sensitized ACI (anti-WKA). UV, ultraviolet.

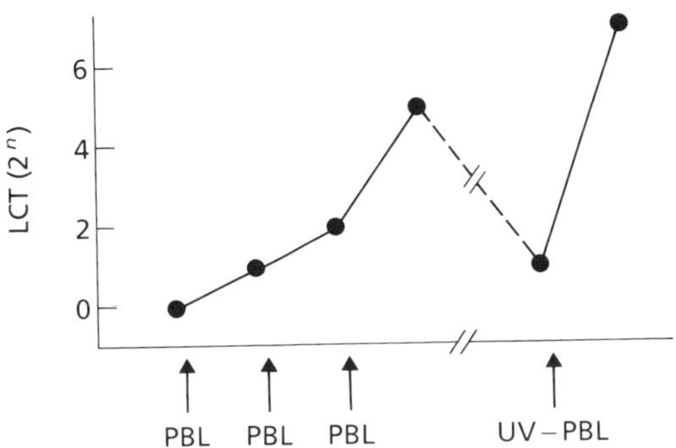

Fig. 14.6 Booster effect of UV-B irradiated PBL (UV-PBL).

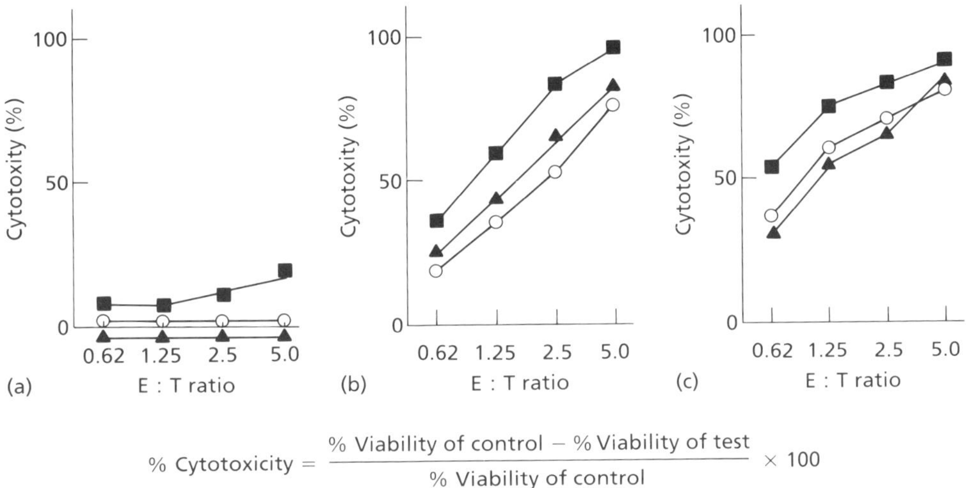

$$\% \text{ Cytotoxicity} = \frac{\% \text{ Viability of control} - \% \text{ Viability of test}}{\% \text{ Viability of control}} \times 100$$

Fig. 14.7 CTL-activity of ultraviolet-irradiated cells. (a) Target : Wa; (b) target : KT-13; (c) target : So. O–O, 0 J; ▲–▲, 1000 J; ■–■, 8000 J.

For alloantigen recognition and subsequent T-cell activation to occur, the alloantigen must have interactions with T-cell receptor (TCRs). However, stimulation of TCRs only may not be sufficient to induce a proliferative response of resting T cells. Other ligand–receptor interactions that form clustering between T cells and APCs will provide additional signals for T-cell activation [18–20]. It is possible that UV irradiation induces certain damages in APCs so that clustering between T cells and damaged APCs is hampered [21–23].

We found that the capping formation of UV-B-irradiated cells is markedly inhibited. After UV-B irradiation, cells were incubated with antibodies for 30 min at

Table 14.2 Capping formation (percentage) of cell surface molecules after ultraviolet B or mitomycin treatment of ER cells

	HLA Class I		HLA Class II		ICAM I	
	4°C	37°C	4°C	37°C	4°C	37°C
Ultraviolet B 0 J	0	77.4	0	90.7	0	75.3
Mitomycin	0	78.3	0	83.0	0	81.0
Ultraviolet B 10 000 J	0	10.4	0	3.0	0	8.0
NaN$_3$	0	0	0	0	0	0

HLA, human leukocyte antigen; ICAM-I, intercellular adhesion molecule 1 (CD54).

37°C, followed by incubation with fluorescein isothiocyanate (FITC)-anti-Ig for 30 min at 37°C. Capping of Class I, Class II, or ICAM-1 was markedly inhibited (Table 14.2). Treatment of cells with MMC did not have any effect on capping. Capping formation represents movements of cell surface molecules that may be required for the clustering between T cells and APCs.

Functions of UV-irradiated platelets were examined next. It was possible that UV-B irradiation induced some damage on the platelet surface which would affect platelet functions. Rat platelets were UV-B-irradiated and tested for their functions *in vitro*. Collagen- and adenosine diphosphate-induced aggregation or %HSR were unchanged up to 8000 J/m^2, compared to unirradiated platelets (Table 14.3). UV-B-irradiated platelets are effective *in vivo*. UV-B-irradiated platelets were transfused to lethally irradiated syngeneic rats and peripheral blood was sampled at 1 and 24 h after transfusion. Transfusions of UV-B platelets and normal platelets equally improved extended bleeding time after lethal irradiation (Fig. 14.8). Adenosine diphosphate-induced aggregation of platelets from the rats reconstituted with UV-B-irradiated platelets was comparable to that from the rats reconstituted with unirradiated

Table 14.3 Function of ultraviolet B (UV-B)-irradiated rat platelets

	Maximum aggregation (%)			
UV (J/m^2)	ADP (5 µmol/l)	ADP (25 µmol/l)	Collagen (20 µmol/l)	%HSR
0	46	53	67	95.6
1000	48	56	78	52.2
2000	40	54	72	90.5
4000	44	52	74	69.9
8000	49	56	75	NT

ADP, adenosine diphosphate; NT, not tested.

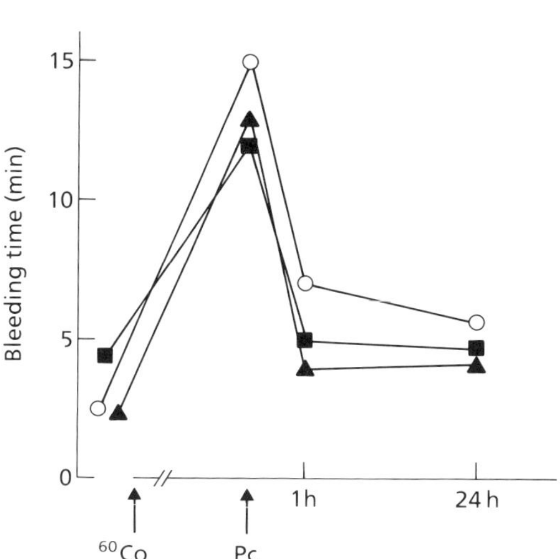

Fig. 14.8 Function of ultraviolet B-irradiated platelets *in vivo*. ○, 0 J; ▲, 4000 J; ■, 4000 J. Pc, platelet concentrate.

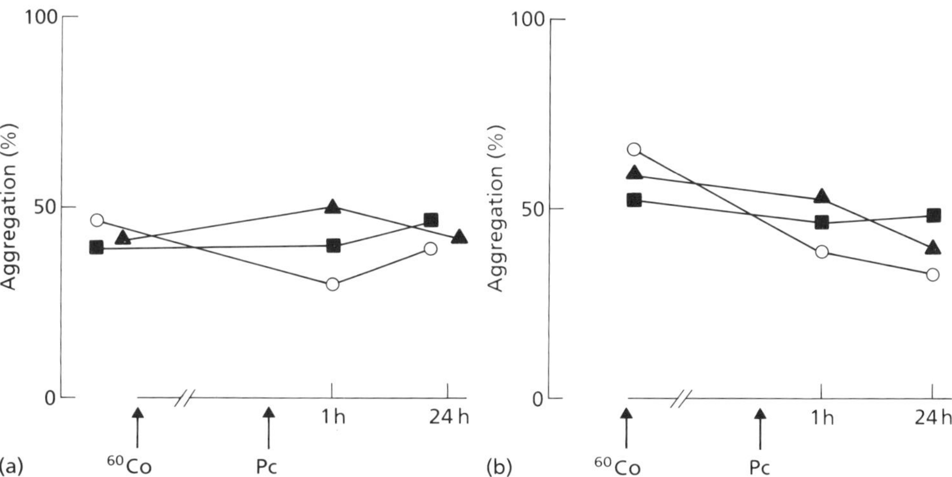

Fig. 14.9 Function of ultraviolet B-irradiated platelets *in vivo*. ○, 0 J; ▲, 4000 J; ■, 4000 J.
(a) Adenosine diphosphate 4 µm/l; (b) adenosine diphosphate 25 µm/l. ^{60}Co, 60-cobalt; Pc, platelet concentrate.

platelets (Fig. 14.9). The results are in accord with the reports that UV-B irradiation does not impair platelet function *in vivo*.

In conclusion, UV-B-irradiated platelets are functionally comparable to non-irradiated platelets *in vivo* as well as *in vitro*.

References

1 Slichter SJ. Transfusion and bone marrow transplantation. *Transfus Med Rev* 1988;2:1–17.
2 Welsh KI, Burgos H, Batchelor JR. The immune response to allogeneic rat platelets: Ag-B antigens in matrix form lacking Ia. *Eur J Immunol* 1977;7:267–272.
3 Claas FHJ, Smeenk RJT, Schmidt R, van Steenbrugge GJ, Eernisse JG. Alloimmunisation against the MHC antigens after platelet transfusions is due to contaminating leucocytes in the platelet suspension. *Exp Hematol* 1981;9:84–89.
4 Sintnicolaas K, Sizoo W, Haije WG *et al*. Delayed alloimmunisation by random single donor platelet transfusions. A randomized study to compare single donor and multiple donor platelet transfusions in cancer patients with severe thrombocytopenia. *Lancet* 1981;1:750–754.
5 Murphy MF, Metcalfe P, Thomas H *et al*. Use of leukocyte-poor blood components and HLA-matched platelet donors to prevent HLA alloimmunisation. *Br J Hematol* 1986;62:529–534.
6 Sniecinski I, O'Donnell MR, Nowicki B, Hill LR. Prevention of refractoriness and HLA alloimmunization using filtered blood products. *Blood* 1988;71:1402–1407.
7 Kahn RA, Duffy BF, Rodey GG. Ultraviolet irradiation of platelet concentrate ablogates lymphocyte activation without affecting platelet function *in vitro*. Transfusion 1985;25:547–550.
8 Pamphilon DH, Corbin S, Saunders J, Tandy N. Application of ultraviolet light in the preparation of platelet concentrates. *Transfusion* 1989;29:378–383.
9 Bucholz DH, Mitipol J, Aster RH *et al*. Ultraviolet irradiation of platelets to prevent recipient alloimmunization. *Transfusion* 1988;28:26S.
10 Pamphilon DH, Potter M, Cutts M *et al*. Platelet concentrates irradiated with ultraviolet light retain satisfactory *in vitro* storage characteristics and *in vivo* survival. *Br J Hematol* 1990;75:240–244.
11 Slichter SJ, Deeg HJ, Kennedy MS. Prevention of platelet alloimmunization in dogs with systemic cyclosporine and by UV-irradiation or cyclosporine-loading of donor platelets. *Blood* 1987;69:414–418.
12 Lechler RI, Batchelor JR. Restoration of immunogenicity to passenger cell-depleted kidney allografts by the addition of donor strain dendritic cells. *J Exp Med* 1982;155:31–41.
13 Gruner S, Volk HD, Noark F *et al*. Inhibition of HLA-DR antigen expression and of the allogeneic mixed leukocyte reaction by photochemical treatment. *Tissue Antigens* 1986;27:147–154.
14 Slater IM, Murray S, Liu J *et al*. Dissimilar effects of ultraviolet light on HLA-D and HLA-DR antigens. *Tissue Antigens* 1980;15:431.
15 Pretell JO, Cone RE. Comparison of altered expression of histocompatibility antigens with altered immune function in murine spleen cells treated with ultraviolet radiation and/or TPA. *Transplantation* 1985;39:175–181.
16 Aprile JA, Deeg HJ, Castner T. *et al*. Impaired expression of class-II antigens on canine dendritic cells following ultraviolet irradiation. *Exp Hematol* 1987;15:452–456.
17 Deeg HJ, Aprile J, Sevens E *et al*. Phenotypic and functional alternations of recipient lymphocytes after transfusion of UV-irradiated and normal blood: implication for marrow transplantation. *Transplant Prod* 1987;19:2709–2714.
18 Dougherty GJ, Murdock S, Hogg N. The function of human intercellular adhesion molecule-1 (ICAM-1) in the generation of an immune response. *Eur J Immunol* 1988;18:35–39.
19 Springer TA, Dustin ML, Kishimoto TK, Marlin SD. The lymphocyte function-associated LFA-1, CD-2 and LFA-3 molecules: cell adhesion receptors of the immune system. *Annu Rev Immunol* 1987;5:223–252.
20 Altmann DM, Hogg N, Trowsdale J, Wilkinson D. Cotransfection of ICAM-1 and HLA-DR reconstitutes human antigen presenting cell function in mouse L cells. *Nature (Lond)* 1989;338:512–514.
21 Pamphilon DH, Alnaqdy AA, Wallington TB. Immunomodulation by ultraviolet light: clinical studies and biological effects. *Immunol Today* 1991;12:119–123.

22 Deeg HJ. Ultraviolet irradiation in transplantation biology. *Transplantation* 1988;45:845–851.
23 Krutmann J, Khan IU, Wallis RS *et al.* Cell membrane is a major locus for ultraviolet B-induced alteration in accessory cells. *J Clin Invest* 1990;85:1529–1536.

Discussion

MINAMI: Was it a secondary response you got when you transfused intact allolymphocytes after immunization with irradiated leukocytes?

IKEDA: I suppose the response was the first sensitization judging from the rising titers of the antibodies produced after the change in antigenic cells from UV-irradiated cells.

MINAMI: Were there any booster effects observed when you transfused UV-irradiated leukocytes into rats immunized with intact leukocytes?

IKEDA: A booster effect was observed with UV-irradiated PBL.

TSUKUI (The Central Blood Center): The conformation of surface antigen molecules seems to be altered owing to UV irradiation. What is your opinion on this?

IKEDA: I'm not sure that there are conformational changes in the whole molecular structure of surface antigens after UV irradiation, as we did not investigate this. But at least I think we can say that the epitopes are intact.

TSUKUI: It is not surprising that the conformation was changed because such a high dose of UV irradiation was used.

IKEDA: I think that it is quite possible.

SHIMIZU: Are there any practical problems in the UV-irradiation system?

TAKAHASHI: A UV-irradiation machine has already been completed and is being used for platelet products at Hotel Dieu Hospital in Paris, France. Moreover, in the USA, some groups investigated a UV-irradiation system in a cooperative study comprising many institutions and they are now asking for permission from the FDA to use an irradiation machine. We are planning to evaluate this system here at the Hokkaido Red Cross Blood Center in the near future.

JUJI (Tokyo University): I think that the possibility of mutagenesis after UV irradiation will become a subject of discussion when the Ministry of Health and Welfare considers whether to permit the use of this system. We should examine this point and confirm its safety.

IKEDA: That's true. But I think it may not be so serious because transfused blood cells would be metabolized and disappear within a few days. Some people still worry about the safety of UV irradiation. It may be the same as for ^{60}Co irradiation. We should confirm the safety of the system before its clinical application.

SHIMIZU: How do they deal with the problem in France or in the USA?

TOHYAMA: Oliphat and other people performed UV irradiation of plasma and blood to inactivate hepatitis virus between 1957 and 1959. I have heard that they did not succeed in inactivation of the virus, but I have not heard of any side-effects caused by UV-irradiated blood products.

Part 4
Clinical Aspects

15 · The effects of leukocyte depletion on alloimmunization by platelet transfusions

H.T. Meryman, H. Braine,* K. Holland,* and
T. A. Takahashi

*Transplantation Laboratory, American Red Cross, Jerome H. Holland
Laboratory 15601 Crabbs Branch Way, Rockville MD 20855, USA and
The Johns Hopkins Oncology Center, 550 N. Broadway, Baltimore, MD 21205, USA

Abstract

A particular hazard for thrombocytopenic patients is refractoriness to platelet transfusion, a problem which should be substantially alleviated by the prevention of alloimmunization against the Class I antigen expressed by platelets and white cells but not by red cells. A number of studies have shown that alloimmunization from red cell transfusions can be prevented by reducing the residual leukocyte count and available data suggest that leukocyte depletion to about 5×10^6 or less is sufficient for red cells. However, the effectiveness of leukocyte depletion in preventing alloimmunization by platelet transfusions is less clear. This chapter discusses the immunology of alloimmunization and describes a clinical study currently in progress.

Introduction

Although an increasing number of reports over the last few years have provided evidence that leukocyte depletion of red cells, and more recently of platelets, does decrease the incidence of alloimmunization, the mechanism by which alloimmunization occurs is unfamiliar to many clinicians and it may be useful to review the current understanding of the process in order better to interpret the clinical data now being accumulated.

The recognition of foreign antigen by T cells is generally preceded by the processing of antigen by antigen presenting cells (APCs), which are most commonly dendritic cells, macrophages, or Langerhans cells in the skin. Extracellular protein is internalized by the APC, degraded to peptide in its acid compartments, and coupled to the Class II major histocompatibility complex (MHC) which is synthesized within the APC. The MHC–peptide complex is then expressed on the surface of the APC (Fig. 15.1). This process appears to be unselective, with the APC processing any and all protein, self or foreign.

The Class II MHC–peptide complex is recognized by the CD4 or helper T cell, which contacts the MHC–peptide complex with its receptor. If the MHC is occupied by peptide derived from self protein, the clones of T cells capable of recognizing that

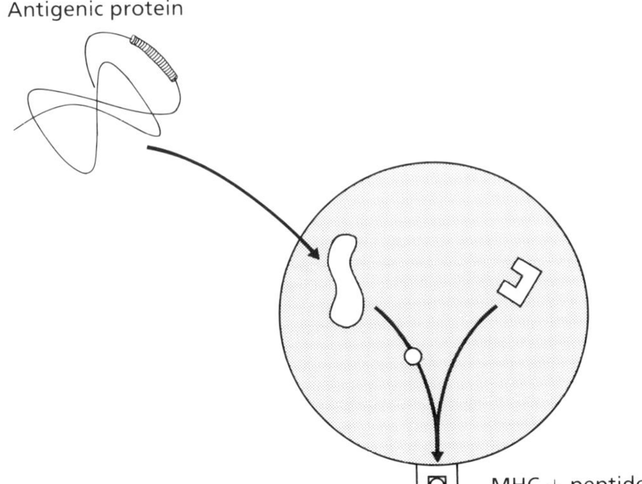

Fig. 15.1 Extracellular protein is internalized and degraded in the acid compartments of the antigen presenting cell (APC). Class II major histocompatibility complex (MHC) is synthesized in the APC, conjugated with the peptide products of antigen degradation, and the MHC–peptide is expressed at the APC surface.

specific complex will have been deleted in the thymus during fetal development. If the peptide is derived from foreign protein it will be recognized but only by a T cell whose receptor is capable of recognizing that particular MHC–peptide complex. Any other T cell will separate without further response.

When the T cell recognizes a foreign peptide on the Class II MHC this induces in the T cell a response which includes increases in calcium and inositol triphosphate, the secretion of diacylglycerol (DAG), activation of protein kinase C, and expression of the interleukin-2 (IL-2) receptor on the T- cell surface (Fig. 15.2). However, the CD4 cell requires IL-2 for proliferation and the MHC–peptide signal alone does not induce IL-2 secretion [1].

Recognition of its Class II complex on the APC by the CD4 cell results in a clustering of other surface molecules around the MHC and these are contacted by counterparts on the CD4 cell (Fig. 15.3). This cluster of molecules constitutes a costimulating signal, also known as the accessory or second signal. It is believed to include such molecules as ICAM-1 and ICAM-2, CD2 and LFA-3, as well as lymphokines, including IL-1 and IL-6 [2]. The complete nature of the costimulatory signal is not yet known. The presence of this second signal causes the secretion of IL-2 by the CD4 cell which not only leads to proliferation of the CD4 cell itself but also provides the stimulus (help) for the proliferation of CD8 (cytotoxic) T cells and B cells.

The foregoing sequence of events occurs in the normal function of the immune system with host APCs presenting antigen-derived peptide to host CD4 cells for potential recognition. The introduction of foreign, or donor, leukocytes is quite a different matter and it is not immediately obvious how immunization against the

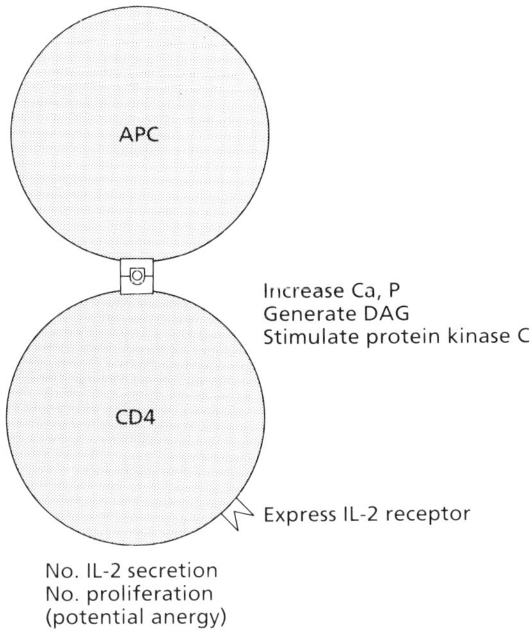

Fig. 15.2 Attachment to the major histocompatibility complex (MHC)–peptide by the T-cell receptor on a CD4 cell capable of recognizing that particular complex as foreign results in a number of intercellular events and expression of the interleukin-2 (IL-2) receptor on the T-cell surface. IL-2 is not secreted. APC, antigen presenting cell; Ca, calcium; DAG, diacylglycerol; P, phosphorus.

foreign MHC will occur. Two alternatives can be proposed (Fig. 15.4). First, recipient APCs may process and present to recipient T cells soluble MHC shed from donor cells. Alternatively, recipient T cells may recognize MHC–peptide on the surface of donor APCs. In an experiment reported by us, donor APCs were lysed by freezing and thawing, a procedure that has been shown to result in the shedding of surface molecules [3]. When cell-free lysate was added to recipent APCs and T cells, no T-cell proliferation resulted, implying that soluble antigen was not processed or, more likely, that peptide fragments of the donor MHC were not recognized as foreign by CD4 cells.

On the contrary, when viable donor APCs were incubated with recipient T cells, T-cell proliferation occurred, leading to the conclusion that allograft recognition by CD4 cells requires the presence of intact, viable donor APCs [4]. This is an important conclusion since it implies that, in general, allograft responses may require the presence of viable donor APCs for their initiation.

The foregoing discussion has focused only on presentation of the Class II MHC and its recognition by CD4 T cells. Both the cytotoxic and the humoral elements of alloimmunization are generally directed against the Class I molecules present on all nucleated cells; however, without CD4 activation and proliferation, support for CD8 and B-cell function, primarily by IL-2, will not be available.

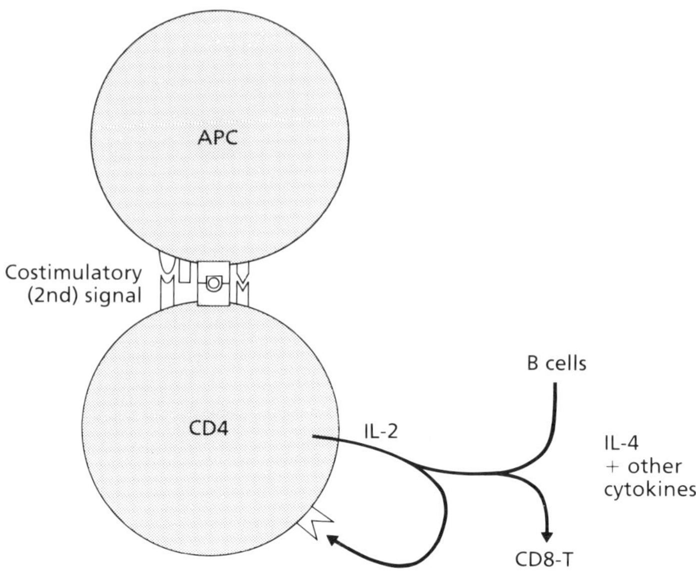

Fig. 15.3 Recognition of the major histocompatibility complex (MHC)–peptide by an appropriate CD4 cell results in a clustering of other surface molecules around the MHC–T-cell attachment as well as the secretion of cytokines. This accessory signal stimulates the secretion of interleukin-2 (IL-2) by the CD4 cell. APC, antigen presenting cell.

- When is the MHC foreign?
- Do T cells recognize alloMHC fragments or only intact alloMHC on cells?

Presentation of alloMHC fragment *AlloMHC on allo cells*

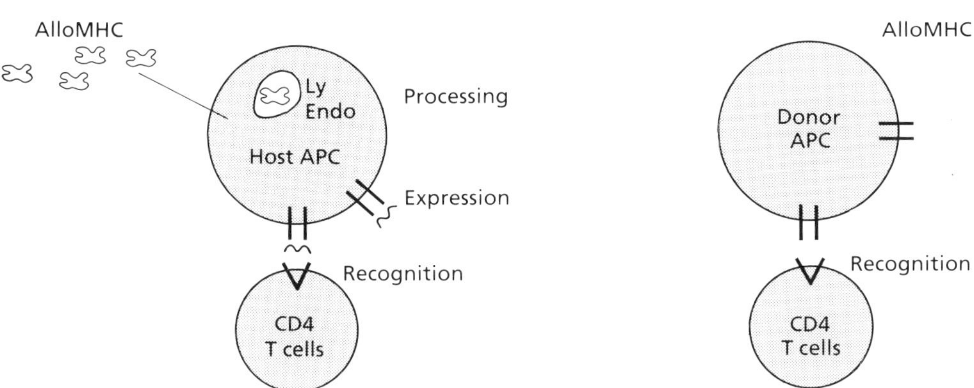

Fig. 15.4 When the antigen presenting cell (APC) is foreign (donor) there are two possible ways by which recipient T cells could be activated: processing by recipient T cells of donor major histocompatibility complex (MHC) shed by donor APCs, or recognition of donor MHC–peptide on intact donor APCs.

The Class I MHC molecule is also present on the APC but, unlike the Class II molecule, it presents only endogenous peptide from the cell interior. The presumed function of the Class I system is to present peptide derived from abnormal cell contents such as viruses and malignancies and thereby lead to destruction of such cells. The Class I MHC–peptide complex can be recognized by the CD8 cytotoxic T cell and by the B cell. Figure 15.5 shows a proposed model of an alloimmune response. The donor APC presents peptide of exogeneous origin to be recognized by the CD4 cell. It is irrelevant whether the peptide is of donor or recipient origin. Since the MHC is foreign, even recipient peptide will appear foreign to recipient T cells, CD8 cells will be activated, and IL-2 will be secreted. The endogenous peptide presented on the donor Class I MHC is presumably similar to that presented on Class I MHC molecules on other donor cells and the Class I cellular and humoral responses initiated by the APC will be directed against them.

It the case of red cell transfusions, since human red cells do not express Class I antigen, prior immunization by foreign leukocytes will have no effect on them but will be directed against contaminating leukocytes and platelets. The resulting lysis of donor leukocytes, particularly of granulocytes, is responsible for nonhemolytic febrile reactions. Relatively large numbers of leukocytes are required for a clinically

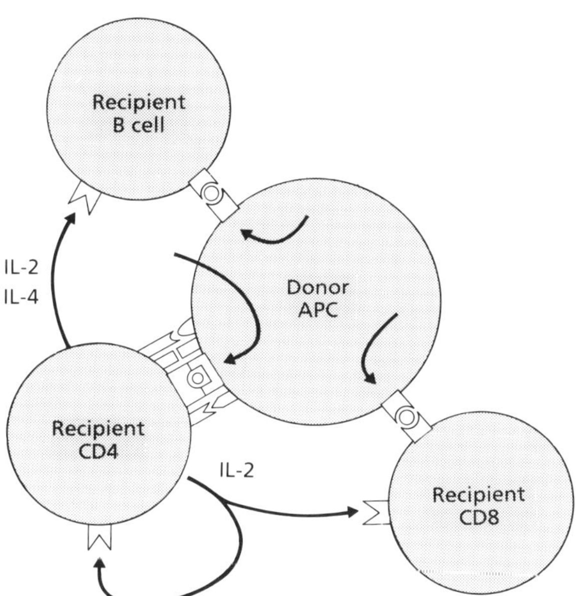

Fig 15.5 A proposed model of alloimmunization. Donor (foreign) major histocompatibility complex (MHC) on donor antigen presenting cells (APCs) presents peptides to recipient CD4 cells. The combination appears foreign regardless of the source of peptide. Class I MHC on the APC presents donor peptide of intracellular origin to recipient CD8 cells and B cells. The activated CD4 cells provide the lymphokine support necessary for CD8 and B-cell proliferation. I-2, interleukin-2.

significant reaction so that modest leukocyte depletion, such as that achieved by red cell washing or by microaggregate filtration, can prevent the febrile response.

Platelets, on the other hand, express Class I antigen, and, when transfused into a patient previously immunized against any of the Class I alleles carried by the platelets, will be destroyed. Platelet destruction appears to be primarily through a humoral (antibody) response rather than a cellular-mediated process. It should be noted that alloimmunization can often be directed against portions of the MHC molecule that are common to many human leukocyte antigen (HLA) phenotypes so that immunization induced by one donor can result in the development of antibodies with broad specificity that may be effective against the cells from other donors of different phenotypes. Viral infections or other events triggering a Class I response can also induce an antibody response to HLA molecules through the same mechanism.

In addition, there is the possibility that Class I MHC shed by donor cells and present as soluble antigen can be processed and presented in conventional fashion by recipient APCs. Alloimmunization by cell-free blood components has been reported [5,6] but this route of immunization may be relatively uncommon since leukocyte depletion alone does appear to be quite effective in preventing alloimmunization and several days of storage may be necessary to release sufficient antigen to induce an immune response [7].

A number of clinical studies of patient response to leukocyte-depleted red cells have been reported and are summarized in [8]. The data from these reports suggest that more than 5×10^6 contaminating leukocytes are necessary to induce alloimmunization from red cell transfusions. One cannot predict from these data, however, whether a comparable leukocyte depletion would prevent alloimmunization from platelet transfusions since the platelets will present a very large amount of Class I antigen in addition to that on the contaminating leukocytes. To answer this question clinical trials are essential.

Several studies of alloimmunization by leukocyte-depleted platelets have already been reported [8,9,10]. We also have a clinical study in progress and a multi-institutional study being conducted in Japan (by Handa *et al.*) is reported in these proceedings (see Chapter 19). Our study is designed to answer two questions: first, does leukocyte depletion by filtration reduce the incidence of alloimmunization against HLA antigen in bone marrow transplant patients and, second, if some immunization is seen using filtered platelets, is this because the leukocyte depletion is insufficient or is there a source of immunization other than that induced by donor white cells?

The study is being conducted with bone marrow transplant patients. To the extent possible, patients never transfused and never pregnant are randomized into the study but the difficulty of finding such patients led us also to include a subgroup of patients previously pregnant or having received fewer than 5 transfusions but seronegative for HLA at the time of admisson into the study.

In order to avoid the possibility of immunization from red cell transfusions, red cells are filtered twice, once shortly following collection using the Pall RC-100 filter, and again at the time of transfusion using a second Pall RC-100 filter in line at the bedside. In a series of six test units, the mean residual leukocyte count was $3.38 \times 10^5 \pm 5 \times 10^5$ cells as measured by the method of Sadoff *et al.* [11].

Platelets are collected as single donor units by hemapheresis using either the Haemonetics V50 or the Fenwal CS-3000. Cytomegalovirus-negative donors are selected for cytomegalovirus-negative patients. In the filtered group, platelets are filtered through the Pall PL-100, which achieves a mean residual leukocyte count of $3.8 \times 10^5 \pm 3 \times 10^5$, as determined in a series of three hemapheresis units sacrificed for this purpose.

A second study group receives platelets depleted of leukocytes by elutriation. This centrifugal procedure separates cells on the basis of sedimentation velocity rather than by density difference and was shown by one of us (TT) to be ideal for the separation of leukocytes from the much smaller platelets. Elutriated platelets have a mean residual leukocyte count of $1.29 \times 10^4 \pm 1.08 \times 10^4$ based on samples from 269 transfusions.

Based on published data, leukocyte depletion of platelets does appear significantly to reduce the incidence of alloimmunization. However, some patients receiving leukocyte-depleted platelets do alloimmunize despite leukocyte depletion comparable to that which prevents immunization from red cell transfusions. This suggests that there may be a source of immunization other than contaminating leukocytes—possibly soluble Class I antigen shed by platelets. As data from our study permit us to compare the immunization rate from filtered platelets with that from elutriated platelets containing only contaminating leukocytes, a better understanding of alloimmunization by platelet transfusion may become possible.

References

1 Mueller DL, Jenkins MK, Schwartz RH. An accessory cell-derived costimulatory signal acts independently of protein kinase C activation to allow T-cell proliferation and prevent the induction of unresponsiveness. *J Immunol* 1989;142:2617.

2 Mincheff MS, Meryman HT, Costimulatory signals necessary for induction of T cell proliferation. *Transplantation* 1990;49:768–772.

3 Takahashi T, Inada S, O'Shea JJ, Brown EJ. Osmotic stress and the freeze-thaw cycle cause shedding of Fc and C3b receptors by human polymorphonuclear leukocytes. *J Immunol* 1985;134: 4062–4068.

4 Mincheff Ms, Meryman HT. Induction of primary mixed leukocyte reactions with ultraviolet B or chemically modified stimulator cells. *Transplantation* 1989;48;1052–1056.

5 Diepenhorst P, Engelfriet C. Removal of leukocytes from whole blood and erythrocyte suspensions by filtration through cotton wool. V. Results after transfusion of 1,820 units of filtered erythrocytes. *Vox Sang* 1975;29:15–22.

6 Pellegrino MA, Indiveri F, Fagiola U, Antonello A, Ferrone S. Immunogenicity of serum HLA antigens in allogeneic combinations. *Transplantation* 1982;33:530–533.

7 Engelfriet CP, Diepenhorst P, Giessen MVD, von Riesz E. Removal of leukocytes from whole blood and erythrocyte suspensions by filtration through cotton wool. IV. Immunization studies in rabbits. *Vox Sang* 1975;29:15–22.

8 Meryman HT. Transfusion-induced alloimmunization and immunosuppression and the effect of leukocyte depletion. *Transfus Med Rev* 1989;3:180–193.

9 Schiffer CA. Prevention of alloimmunization against platelets. *Blood* 1991;77:1–4.

10 Kooy M van M, van Prooijen HV, Moes M, Bosma-stants I, Akkerman JWN. Use of leukocyte-depleted platelet concentrate for the prevention of refractoriness and primary HLA alloimmunization: a prospective, randomized trial. *Blood* 1991;77:201–205.

11 Sadoff BJ, Dooley DC, Kapoor V, Law P, Friedman LI, Stromberg RR. Methods for measuring a 6 $\log_{10}$ white cell depletion in red cells. *Transfusion* 1991;31:150–155.

Discussion

Whyte: The situation in the bone marrow transplant, as distinct from the leukemia situation, is that you have in fact three donors interacting. You have the recipient, the transplant donor, and the transfused donor. The source therefore for the APCs can come from either of those three and you've only really dealt with one of them by the elutriational filtration mechanism. The antigen which can be presented by the isologous APC may also come from three different sources and unless you have (and given your selection criteria, it's very unlikely) identical twin donors for each of these transplant recipients, you have a rather more complex situation in which I'm surprised that residual alloimmunization is in fact present, as you've shown. But you're really measuring an epiphenomenon about that, above a baseline of immunization.

Meryman: But it is encouraging that in fact the reduction in alloimmunization from the transfusion, which I presume is what we're seeing, *is* significant and in the light of your comments one would really have expected more alloimmunization in the depleted group than we saw because of the interaction between the donor and recipient. So what you're telling us is that there is yet another explanation for the residual alloimmunization and of course you're quite correct.

White: And one is impressed at the reduction, in the complexity of the situation.

Meryman: Yes.

Ikeda: Sometimes in transfused patients we find alloimmunization against platelet-specific antigens. Is it possible that this can occur in response to antigens picked up by host APC?

Meryman: We were looking only at HLA. But your point is well taken. If you can develop antibodies against the platelet antigen in the absence of any other source, then that implies that other antigens on the platelets such as HLA could also be recognized and immunization against them could be possible. This is certainly one possible explanation for the residual alloimmunization that we see. But again the fact that we and others do see a substantial reduction in immunization by removing the white cells tells us that the dominant source of antibody is from the leukocytes in the transfusion.

Ikeda: How did you confirm that the bone marrow transplant patients were not in a sensitized state before transfusion?

MERYMAN: We simply used the standard complement-aided cytolysis assay that I guess most hospitals use in their panels as our primary assay. We are now in the process of going back through the serum samples using more sensitive assays to see whether the antibody level persisted longer than it appears from the conventional panel assay or not.

IKEDA: So, with a more sensitive method you might discover that some of these patients had been sensitized?

MERYMAN: No. In the patients that we have looked at so far — and this is not yet all of them, even by a more sensitive assay — we do not find antibodies prior to the appearance of a panel-reactive assay.

WOODFIELD (Auckland Regional Blood Services, New Zealand): I think that we need to know a bit more about the specificity of those particular antibodies appearing so early. Are they truly HLA antibodies? If so, they should be able to be identified. One possible cause might be that antibodies appearing so early in nonpregnant, nontransfused patients may easily be immunoglobulin M antibodies, which are being quite commonly recognized now and can be identified, or at least removed, by DDT treatment or heat treatment. The other possibility is that they could be immunoglobulin A antibodies that the test that you are using identifies.

MERYMAN: Unfortunately, this project is being funded as a clinical study and not an academic study and it may be difficult for us to launch a project to analyze what is going on. [If there is] anybody here who would like to receive some *very small* aliquots from our serum samples and who *guarantees* to produce useful results, we would be delighted to share them.

SNIECINSKI: Are these early antibodies associated with clinical refractoriness related to transfusion?

MERYMAN: I wish I could answer the question, but these bone marrow transplant patients present such a complex picture as far as refractoriness, which is simply defined as the failure of the platelet increment to be what you think it should be. There is some degree of refractoriness in most of these patients whether they are alloimmunized or not. With this small number of patients we can't really draw any conclusions as to whether this is important or not. Some of the patients have a dramatic response to alloimmunization and at least two of the deaths were associated with the appearance of antibodies and almost total refractoriness, but in others there was really little change in their response to the platelet transfusions before, during, and after the immunization. But they were all responding badly and requiring a lot of platelets.

OTO (Fukushima Medical College): Can we expect a decrease of alloimmunization against red cell antigens by depleting APCs?

MERYMAN: I don't see why. I can't answer categorically but it seems to me that that's probably an immune response that's launched by the recipient and not necessarily involving donor APCs. But that's just a guess.

OTO: My opinion is that red cells are destroyed by APCs and presented by APCs and that alloimmunization is caused by soluble antigens. MHC may be destroyed and alloimmunization may occur by the second process.

MERYMAN: But not necessarily donor APCs. It could be the recipient system. I can't answer the question.

16 · Leukocyte depletion of red cell and platelet concentrates: clinical importance to patients awaiting organ transplantation

E. Richter, D. Barz,‡ O. Blauärmel,‡ G. Staffa,* T. Manger,*
H. Goldschmidt,§ W. Schultze,† and G. Matthes

*Institute of Transfusion Medicine, *Clinic of Surgery and †Clinic of Internal Medicine, Humboldt
University of Berlin, Medical Faculty (Charité) and ‡Blood Transfusion Center, German Red Cross,
Berlin 1040, and §University of Heidelberg, Schumannstrasse 20, Germany*

Abstract

Alloimmunization against human leukocyte antigens (HLAs) is an undesirable result
of contaminating leukocytes transmitted to the patient during transfusion of red cells
and platelets. Leukocyte depletion therefore is needed to prevent alloimmunization or
to perform effective transfusions to patients with alloantibodies.

Before 1990 cryopreservation of red cell concentrates was used to eliminate the
white cells. This method reduced the application of leukocyte-depleted red cell
concentrates to patients after kidney and bone marrow transplantation. Buffy coat-
free resuspended red cell concentrates have been in general use since 1978. In 1990
filter systems were brought into use for the leukocyte depletion of red cells and
platelets.

This retrospective analysis includes 116 patients awaiting liver transplantation
and five after bone marrow transplantation. Among this group there were 27 patients
with red cell antibodies and five patients with HLA antibodies.

The study was completed by 219 leukemic patients (179 with acute lymphoblastic
leukemia (ALL), 29 with acute myeloblastic leukemia (AML), 11 with aplastic anemia)
who were transfused within the prefiltration period. Thirty-four HLA antibodies were
detected. From the 11 aplastic anemia patients, four became alloimmunized (34%). In
contrast 16 leukemic children, mostly suffering from aplastic anemia, were treated
with filtered red cell and platelet concentrates. No antibodies have been detected in
this group so far.

Introduction

There are different reasons for eliminating leukocytes from red cell and platelet
concentrates before transfusion. Two major tasks of leukocyte depletion are the
prevention or even reduction of the recipient alloimmunization against HLAs and the

prevention of cytomegalovirus (CMV) transmission or reactivation from CMV-positive blood [1,2].

Various methods are known to be more or less effective in reducing the amount of residual leukocytes in red cell concentrates, such as buffy coat removal, washing with saline, cryopreservation, filtration and, the latest innovation, ultraviolet (UV) irradiation.

From 1978 buffy coat-free red cell concentrates were generally used in the former East Germany. Together with the buffy coat, about 70% of the containing white cells were removed [3]. To prevent alloimmunization, washed red cell concentrates or cryopreserved red cells were prepared as leukocyte-depleted blood. Washed red cells are known to be insufficiently leukocyte-depleted as the white cells are reduced by only 80–85% [4]. Cryopreservation is effective but cost- and work-intensive [2].

Methods

Cryopreserved red cell concentrates

We studied the transfusion efficiency of cryopreserved red cell concentrates in patients suffering from hematologic disorders in one trial and on transplantation patients in the other. The data were compared with the posttransfusion efficiency of buffy coat-free resuspended red cells. The mean white blood cell (WBC) count obtained from 137 routinely frozen red cell concentrates was 0.38×10^7 by manual counting. The transfusion efficiency was calculated from the patient's hemoglobin (Hb) concentration before transfusion, the volume and the Hb of the transfused unit, and the patient's total blood volume together with the Hb concentration after transfusion [5]. The maximum Hb increase was observed 40 h after transfusion of saline-adenine-glucose-mannitol resuspended red cell concentrates. We found the highest transfusion efficiency after transfusion of cryopreserved red cell concentrates, because of the selection of the red cell population during the freezing and washing procedure. Figure 16.1 also indicates that $-25°C$ storage using a high concentration of glycerol is less effective; it is the same as citrate-dextrose-sucrose–adenine-guanosine (CDS-AG)-preserved red cell concentrates. The reason for this could be the saccharose content of that preservative, which makes the erythrocyte membrane rigid and therefore detectable by the spleen, as demonstrated by rheologic studies [6].

Patients awaiting kidney transplantation or after transplantation were treated with cryopreserved red cell concentrates to prevent alloimmunization. Opelz and Terasaki [7] demonstrated the effect of the development of immune tolerance after transfusion of red cell concentrates containing white cells to patients before kidney transplantation, but this immune tolerance-inducing effect was only present if the patients received no more than five transfusions. Otherwise the situation became completely inverse and complicated, and in some cases prevented the transplantation by becoming alloimmunized.

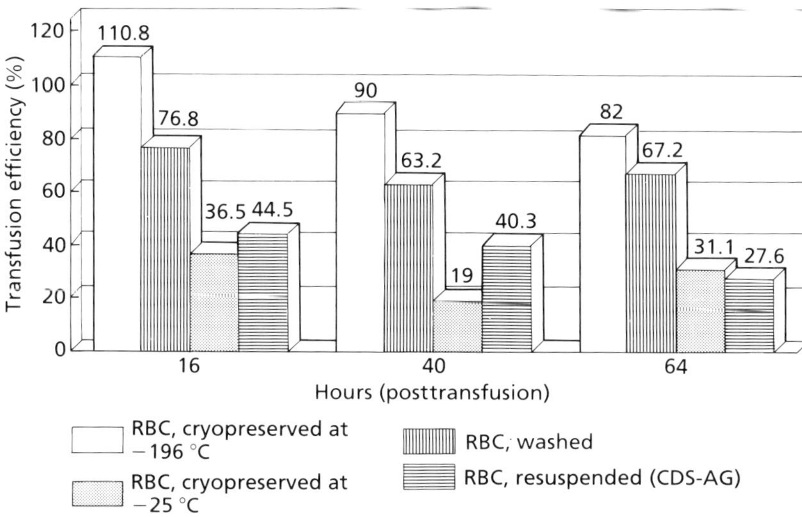

Fig. 16.1 Comparison of the transfusion efficiency of different red blood cell (RBC) preparations.

As patients on dialysis treatment need red cell transfusions continuously, the limit of five is difficult to achieve and will be reached within 2 months of initiation of the treatment. On the other hand most patients are on a waiting list for kidney transplantation for longer than a year. Leukocyte depletion therefore seems necessary for their blood supply.

A comparable situation is found in leukemic patients, especially those with aplastic anemia. These patients have no immunosupppression, need blood products chronically and therefore often develop alloantibodies. Some of 210 leukemic patients (179 with ALL, 20 with AML, and 11 with aplastic anemia) received transfusions within the prefiltraton period. At least 34 were alloimmunized, forming HLA antibodies with a ratio of 16%. This is less than published data—20–50% [8,9].

All these patients received transfusions not only of red cell concentrates but also of platelets [10]. Table 16.1 shows the transfusion frequency of AML patients. Even if red

Table 16.1 Transfusions of red blood cells and platelet concentrates to patients with acute myeloblastic leukemia in the prefiltration period

	Red blood cells		Platelet concentrates	
	Buffy coat-free	Cryopreserved	Multiple donor	Single donor
Adults (*n* = 11)	34	88	48 (7–23)	97 (6–23)
Children (*n* = 9)	4	10	0	20 (1–7)

Table 16.2 Frequency of alloimmunization of patients suffering from aplastic anemia after red cell and platelet concentrate transfusion within the prefiltration period

Patients (*n*)	Red blood cell	Platelet concentrate	Antibody
6	Cryopreserved	Single donor, random	3
1	Cryopreserved	Single donor, human leukocyte antigen-matched	0
1	Cryopreserved	Multiple donor	0
3	Buffy coat-free	Multiple donor	1
Total			4/11 (36%)

cell concentrates were leukocyte-depleted by cryopreservation, platelet concentrates were not. Mostly single donor preparations were used, containing at least $1{-}2 \times 10^8$ leukocytes. As there was a relatively low antibody incidence overall, 36% allosensitization was found among the 11 patients suffering from aplastic anemia shown in Table 16.2. The seroconversion we found was transient in most cases. A typical picture is given in Figure 16.2 [11].

Filtered red cell concentrates

Since leukocyte removal filters were introduced in 1990 we have processed more than 650 red cell concentrates routinely. The residual WBC count of less than 0.2×10^7 reached the limits of routine counting and needs special counting techniques to be detected [12,13].

We followed 135 patients awaiting organ transplantation from 1989 to 1991. The patients are characterized as shown in Table 16.3 and Figure 16.3. The majority were

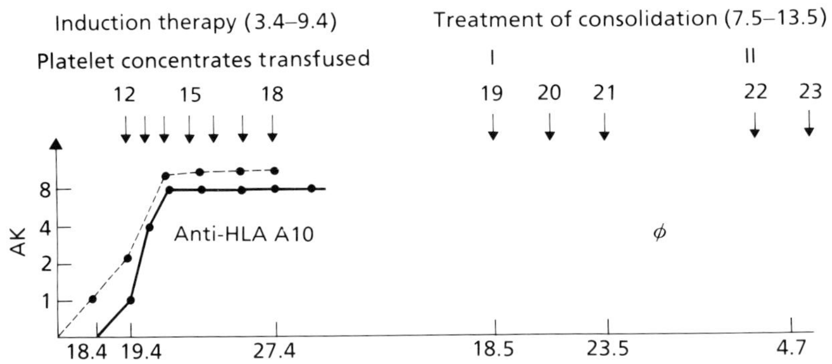

Fig. 16.2 Antibody titer of human leukocyte antigen (HLA) antibody of a patient with acute myeloblastic leukemia (AML).

Table 16.3 Patients on the waiting list for organ transplantation

Organ to be transplanted	n
Liver	116
Grafted	45*
Died after transplantation	8
Died on waiting list	16
Still waiting	35
Rejected from waiting list	12
Heart	8/1†
Pancreatic islets	3/2†
Liver and kidney	2/1†
Kidney and pancreas	1
Bone marrow	5/5†

*Plus one retransplantation.
†The second number refers to organs grafted.

awaiting liver transplantation. Beside HLA antibodies, which developed in four out of 116 patients (3.5%), antibodies against red cell antigens were also observed. Table 16.4 summarizes our findings. The overall percentage of 24% of the patients with red

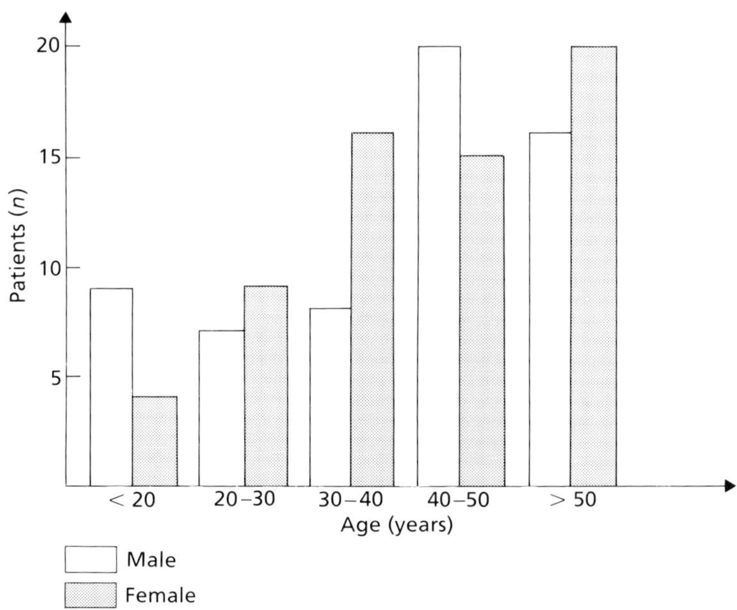

Fig. 16.3 Age distribution of patients awaiting liver transplantation.

Table 16.4 Frequency of occurrence of human leukocyte antigen and ABO antibodies in patients awaiting liver transplantation ($n = 116$)

Human leukocyte antigen system	4 (3.5%)		
Red cell antigens	27 (24%)		
Anti-I	5	Anti-e, C	1
Anti-D	2	Anti-A_1	2
Anti-D, E	2	Anti-Le^a	1
Anti-E	2	Anti-W^a	1
Anti-E, c	1	Anti-W^a, I	1
Anti-c	2	Anti-K	2
Anti-c, C^w	1	Anti-K, E	1
Anti-C^w, P, I	1	Anti-e, H	1
Anti-e	1		

cell antibodies seems high but corresponds well with the findings of Ramsey *et al.* [14] who analyzed 496 adults in this special patient group: 22% of their patients were alloimmunized against ABO antigens. One of our patients with the anti-e/anti-H combination could only be substituted with cryopreserved red cell concentrates. Of course, additional HLA antibodies would complicate the blood supply of these patients. Therefore methods to prevent allosensitization must be used.

Table 16.5 documents the blood supply to our patients. All four patients with HLA antibodies — which had already been detected before transplantation — received significantly ($P < 0.05$) more transfusions than the others. Two of them were treated with washed red cell concentrates and single donor platelets during the prefiltration period. The other two received filtered blood products. None of them showed complications with regard to the blood supply as they were immunosuppressed, including with cyclosporin A.

Another reason to transfuse patients awaiting organ transplantation with leukocyte-depleted blood is the high risk of virus transmission, which complicates or

Table 16.5 Average blood supply (mean ± s.d.) to patients awaiting liver transplantation before and after the transplantation, in comparison with the four patients who were alloimmunized (HLA antibody)

	Whole blood	Red cell concentrate	Platelet concentrate
Before transplantation ($n = 35$)	0.4 ± 1.1	2.7 ±4.5	0
After transplantation ($n = 45$)	6.2 ± 5.4	15.8 ± 5.1	3.0 ± 1.6
Patients with HLA antibodies ($n = 4$)	9.3 ± 14.5	41.7 ± 27.5	6.7 ±6.1

Table 16.6 Frequency of alloimmunization of bone marrow transplantation patients after transfusions of leukocyte-depleted red cell and platelet concentrates

	Red blood cells	Platelet concentrate	Antibody
Without leukocyte depletion ($n = 1$)	6	25	–
With leukocyte depletion ($n = 3$)	5.8 ± 0.2	13.5 ± 0.5	
With HLA antibody ($n = 1$)	7	30	+

prevents organ transplantation. Is CMV predominant; not only is it transmitted to CMV-negative patients by blood transfusions but also the disease can be reactivated in CMV-positive patients. It is now accepted that filtered red cells and platelet concentrates could be safely transfused instead of CMV-negative blood products [15,16]. This is important because of the limitations of the blood supply to patients with red cell antibodies. The effective removal is based on the strong association of the CMV to the leukocytes [17]. Therefore Rawal *et al.* [18] proposed early filtration; otherwise virus transmission could be caused by viruses released from lysed white cells during storage.

A severe complication of patients who undergo bone marrow transplantation is interstitial pneumonia, for which CMV is responsible. As we have only just started the program only five patients are involved (Table 16.6). One patient was already alloimmunized before transplantation. There was no influence of filtered red cell or platelet concentrates on the antibody titer.

Filtered platelet concentrates

Although platelets express HLA Class I antigens, it was demonstrated that the contaminating leukocytes in platelet concentrates are responsible for alloimmunization [19].

Following this, leukocyte depletion is needed for platelet transfusions, even in patients who are not immunosuppressed and who need a blood supply chronically, such as in aplastic anemia. We followed 16 children suffering from aplastic anemia, who were treated with filtered platelet concentrates. A total of 137 single donor platelet concentrates (Haemonetics V-50) were routinely prepared and filtered using PL-10N (Table 16.7). The white blood cell contamination was reduced from 2.3×10^8 to 0.2×10^7. None of our patients were allosensitized, or developed refractoriness (Table 16.8).

In contrast to Fisher *et al.* [20], who reported alloimmunization after two transfusions of platelet concentrates, Carr *et al.* [21] found the first sign of alloimmunization, refractoriness, after seven platelet transfusions. This number was reached in only seven of our 16 patients, showing that a longer observation period is needed in our study.

Table 16.7 Results of leukocyte depletion of routinely prepared platelet concentrates (n = 137) using the PL-10N filter

Parameter	Content
Platelets	$3.0 \pm 1.3 \times 10^{11}$
White blood cells	$0.18 \pm 0.21 \times 10^{7}$
Red blood cells	$1.3 \pm 0.39 \times 10^{10}$
Volume	200–300 ml

Table 16.8 Transfusions of leukocyte-depleted platelet concentrates to patients suffering from aplastic anemia (n = 16)

Patients	Filtered platelet concentrate* n = 75
Unit/patient	4.7 (1–11)
Antibody	0

*Pall PL-100 filter.

Conclusions

Patients awaiting organ transplantation need transfusions of leukocyte-depleted blood products. From the clinical point of view there is no question as to how to remove residual leukocytes from red cell or platelet concentrates, but the process should be effective to diminish all risks complicating or preventing organ transplantation. However, even if leukocyte depletion is carefully done to less than 10^{6} residual leukocytes, below the so-called critical immunogenic leukocyte loud (2×10^{6}) dose, allosensitization is possible, as Meryman *et al.* [23] have reported recently.

References

1 Earnisse JG, Brand A. Prevention of platelet refractoriness due to HLA antibodies by administration of leucocyte-poor blood components. *Exp Hematol* 1981;9:77–83.

2 Brady M, Anderson D, Milan J. Prevention of posttransfusion cytomegalovirus infection in neonates by the use of frozen-washed red blood cells. *Clin Res* 1982;30:895.

3 Strauss D, Seidel B, Meurer W, Markova NA. Das buffy-coat-arme Erythrozytenkonzentrat: Herstellung, Konservierung und Qualitätsbewertung. *Folia Haematol (Lpzg)* 1980;107:104–124.

4 Luban NC, Williams AE, McDonald M. Low incidence of cytomegalovirus infection in neonates transfused with washed red blood cells. *Am J Dis Child* 1987;141:416–419.

5 Zschoch S, Matthes G, Ihle R. Bewertung des Transfusionserfolges unterschiedlich konservierter Erythrozytenkonzentrate. *Folia Haematol (Lpzg)* 1988;115:629–640.

6 Kucera W, Wegner G, Lerche D. Investigations on the deformability of human red blood cells stored in different preservative solutions. *Biomed Biochim Acta* 1985;44:1459–1467.

7 Opelz G, Terasaki PI. Poor kidney-transplant survival in recipients with frozen-blood transfusions or no transfusions. *Lancet* 1974;2:696–698.

8 Perkins HA. HLA antigens and blood transfusions effect on renal transplants. *Transplant Proc* 1977;9:229–232.

9 Kickler TS. The challenge of platelet alloimmunization: management and prevention. *Transfus Med Rev* 1990;4:8–18.

10 Reuter G, Barz D, Dörffel W, Selle B, Leverenz S. Thrombozyten substitution bei Kindern—Indikation, Effektivität, immunologische Aspekte: Ergebnisse einer prospektiven Studie. 15. Tagung der Gesell Hämatol Bluttransf Schwerin, 6-9. März 1990

11 Leverenz S, Ihle R, Dörffel W, Reuter G, Richter E, Fünfhausen G. Results of platelet transfusions in pediatric and in adult leucemic patients. Symp. Trilaterale on Transfusion Medicine, Zakopane, 6-7. November 1984

12 Takahashi TA, Hosoda M, Sekiguchi S. A flow cytometric method to detect residual leucocytes in platelet and red cell concentrates. *Jpn J Transfus Med* 1990;36:429–437.

13 Friedman LI, Sadoff BJ, Stromberg R. White cell counting in red cells and platelets: how few can we count? *Transfusion* 1990;30:387–389.

14 Ramsey G, Cornell FW, Hahn LF, Larson P, Issitt LB, Starzl TE. Red cell antibody problems in 1000 liver transplants. *Transfusion* 1989;29:396–400.

15 Murphy MF, Grint PCA, Hardiman AE, Lister TA, Waters AH. The use of leucocyte-poor blood components to prevent primary cytomegalovirus (CMV) in patients with acute leukaemia. *Br J Haematol* 1988;79:253–255.

16 Gilbert GL, Hayes K, Hudson IL, James J. Prevention of transfusion-acquired cytomegalovirus infection in infants by blood filtration to remove leucocytes. *Lancet* 1989;1:1228–1231.

17 Wagner SJ, Friedman LI, Dodd RY. Approaches to the reduction of viral infectivity in cellular blood components and single donor plasma. Proc. 2nd Hokkaido Symp. on Transfusion Medicine Sapporo, pp 99–128, 1991

18 Rawal B, Yen TSB, Vyas GN, Bush M. Leucocyte filtration remove infectious particulate debris but not free virus derived from experimentally lysed HIV-infected cells. *Vox Sang* 1991;60:214–218.

19 Class FHJ, Smeek RJT, Schmidt R, van Steenbrugge GJ, Earnisse JG. Alloimmunization against the MHC antigens after platelet transfusions is due to contaminating leucocytes in platelet suspension. *Exp Hematol* 1981;9:84–89.

20 Fisher M, Chapman JR, Ting A, Morris PJ. Alloimmunization to HLA antigens following transfusion with leucocyte-poor and purified platelet suspensions. *Vox Sang* 1985;49:331–335.

21 Carr R, Hutton JL, Jenkins JA. Transfusion of ABO-mismatched platelets leads to early platelet refractoriness. *Br J Haematol* 1990;75:408–413.

22 Meryman HT, Braine H, Holland K, Kickler T, Takahashi TA. Alloimmunization in bone marrow transplant patients receiving leucocyte-depleted platelets and red cells. First German–Japanese Symp. on Transfusion Medicine, Berlin, 8. May 1991

23 Meryman HT, Mincheff M. Immunomodulation by blood transfusion. In: Smit Sibinga CTh, Das PC and The TH, eds. *Immunology and Blood Transfusion*. Dordrecht: Kluwer Academic Publishers, 1992 (in press).

Discussion

YUASA (Juntendo University): You just mentioned the number of transfused blood units for the liver transplantation before and after transplantation. Does the number of units transfused after transplantation include the units of blood transfused during the surgery?

RICHTER: Yes, it does.

YUASA: And you also showed that the cryopreserved red blood cell is very effective for hematologic patients. Do you still use that kind of blood?

RICHTER: No, now we use filter-depleted blood. The reason is that before 1990 filter systems were not available.

SNIECINSKI: We have also studied the efficacy of filtration by various filters and evaluated the efficacy of the freshly collected units in comparison to the stored units and I'd just like to confirm your results that the efficacy of the white cell removal from the freshly collected units is somewhat decreased as compared to the efficacy of the white cell removal from stored units. Also one question: could you perhaps postulate the mechanism, explaining your observation that in the freshly collected units that have been filtered the only remaining cells are the granulocytes?

RICHTER: No, we still have no idea about that; except that in fresh blood, of course, the amount of granulocytes is much higher than in 1-day stored blood, as the granulocytes *fall down* during the 4°C storage. So you couldn't find such amounts in stored blood. And perhaps the filter material has an effect, as we only used the Sepacell in this study.

SEKIGUCHI: Dr Takahashi, do you have any comment on this question?

TAKAHASHI: Yes, we also observed granulocyte leakage when we filtered fresh, not cooled, whole blood or red cell concentrates using filters made of nonwoven polyester fibers. So it is true that granulocytes come out when we filter fresh blood. But I'm not sure how it affects the clinical results.

SNIECINSKI: If we postulate that the granulocytes disintegrate during storage, and that is true, and that's why we do not see them in the filtered blood, then we would propose that the filters don't remove granulocytes at all.

RICHTER: Yes, maybe, but only partly.

MAEDA: Do you perform liver transplantations for patients with anti-HLA antibodies in your country?

RICHTER: No, we don't. The liver, of course has a very high amount of antigen. So sometimes even the blood type is not considered for the liver transplantation. In the case of HLA antibodies a lymphocytotoxic cross-match was done to find a compatible organ for the liver transplantation.

SEKIGUCHI: Do you think that patients awaiting transplants need leukocyte-depleted blood?

RICHTER: Yes, I think so, in general, as you could diminish the complications. In-line filtration may be the choice in future.

17 · Use of leukocyte-depleting filters for prevention of HLA alloimmunization and refractoriness to platelet transfusion

H. Maeda, Y. Hitomi, R. Hirata, M. Aoyagi, Y. Takada, and H. Tohyama

Blood Transfusion Service, Saitama Medical Center, Saitama Medical School, 1981 Tsujido, Kamoda, Kawagoe, Saitama 350, Japan

Abstract

The rates of human leukocyte antigen (HLA) alloimmunization and refractoriness to platelet transfusion in 35 patients who received multiple filtered and/or nonfiltered red cell and platelet products were investigated. Group I ($n = 13$) received at least 1 unit of red cell products without filtration and six (46.1%) developed anti-HLA antibodies, five of which were transient antibodies with narrow specificities. Only one patient developed the persistent anti-HLA antibody with broad specificity, resulting in refractoriness to random donor platelet transfusion. Group II ($n = 10$) received only filtered red cell products associated with filtered or nonfiltered platelet products and two (20%) developed transient but broad anti-HLA antibodies. Group III ($n = 12$) received only filtered red cell and platelet products and three (25%) developed antibodies, all of which were transient. No patients in Groups II and III were refractory to random donor platelet transfusion. The use of leukocyte-depleting filters for red cell products appeared to reduce the rates of alloimmunization and refractoriness to platelet transfusion in multitransfused patients.

Introduction

In Japan, blood component transfusion started in the mid 1970s and has been widely accepted as the blood supply system by which blood could be utilized effectively, although it has serious disadvantages in transfusion-associated infections; three blood components — red cells, platelets, and plasma — from infectious whole blood will possibly infect patients. More recently, the contamination of one blood component, leukocytes, in another blood component has become a problem issue; cellular blood components, concentrated red cells (CRC) and platelet concentrates (PC), contained as many leukocytes as elicit to undesired transfusion reactions. At present, several side-effects associated with the administration of contaminated leukocytes are known. (1) febrile reaction, (ii) the production of alloantibodies, generally inducing febrile reactions and/or refractoriness to platelet transfusion; (iii) transmission of some types of viruses; (iv) graft-versus-host disease; and (v) immunosuppression or immuno-modulation of the recipients.

To avoid these side-effects, red cell and platelet products were depleted of leukocytes by removal of buffy coat or differential centrifugation. Such efforts, however, showed only approximately 1 log reduction of leukocytes in blood products. More recently, leukocyte-depleting filters, which are reported to be potent to 2 or 3 log reduction of leukocytes, have been developed and have been available commercially in Japan for the last 2 years [1–3].

In this chapter, the present status of transfusion practice using leukocyte-depleted blood products in Japan, particularly focused on HLA alloimmunization, is described.

Materials and methods

Patients

The first group of patients comprised 150 patients who underwent gynecologic or orthopedic surgery and received transfusions of standard nonfiltered blood products perioperatively (single transfusion group). Out of 150 patients (40 males and 110 females), 10 patients, all females, already had anti-HLA antibodies preoperatively and the remaining 140 patients were analyzed further.

The second group comprised 35 patients, mostly with hematologic diseases, who received multiple blood and component transfusions (multiple transfusion group). These patients were divided into three groups depending on the nature of the blood products transfused: Group I ($n = 13$) received at least 1 unit of red cell products without filtration; Group II ($n = 10$) received only filtered red cell products but might have received nonfiltered platelet products; and Group III ($n = 12$) received only filtered red cell and platelet products. The number, sex, age, and diagnosis of the patients, and the number of units of blood products transfused in each group are presented in Table 17.1.

Anti-HLA antibodies

The sera of single transfusion group were tested for anti-HLA activity to 12 different panel lymphocytes by a two-stage complement-dependent cytotoxicity test before and 2 and 6 months after operation. The sera from the multiple transfusion group were collected before and monthly until 6 months after operation and were tested for anti-HLA activity as described above.

Blood and components filtration

Whole blood, CRCs, and PCs were filtered according to the manufacturer's instruction at the blood transfusion laboratory immediately before transfusion. Red blood cells

Table 17.1 Background details of the multitransfused patients

	Group I	Group II	Group III
Number of patients	13	10	12
Age	48.3 (5–75)	44.9 (14–67)	57.7 (7–85)
Sex (M : F)	7 : 6	5 : 5	4 : 8
Diagnosis			
Leukemia	9	8	7
Aplastic anemia	1	0	3
Other	3	2	2
Observation time (months)	4.7 (2–6)	4.5 (2–6)	4.0 (1–6)
Units of transfusion			
CRC filter (–)	5.0 (1–12)	0	0
CRC filter (+)	17.6 (3–54)	25.1 (4–66)	23.6 (4–61)
PC filter (–)	160.8 (0–538)	181.9 (20–418)	0
PC filter (+)	150 (0–706)	47.3 (0–374)	280.6 (0–973)

CRC, concentrated red cell; PC, platelet concentrate.

(RBC), white blood cells (WBC), and platelets were counted by the Coulter counter before and after filtration. As the counting limit of WBCs is 100/µl, the residual WBC number after filtration was counted by the manual chamber method using a hemocytometer; 1 volume of the sample was lysed by 4 volumes of the hemolyzing buffer and the number of nucleated cells in the two chambers was counted. One cell in the two chambers corresponded to 2.77 cell/µl.

Results

Residual white blood cells in concentrated red cells and platelet concentrate

The efficiency of leukocyte removal in blood products was tested for five filters: three for the red cells and two for the platelet products. The results are summarized in Table 17.2. A mean of the WBC counts in 2 units of CRCs (400 ml) supplied by the regional Red Cross blood center was 2.2×10^9 (a range of $1.1–4.0 \times 10^9$). After filtration by Sepacell R-500N, the numbers of residual WBCs in 17 (80.9%) of 21 blood samples were reduced to less than 1×10^6, and in only four (19.1%) to more than 1×10^6, yet with a mean of 1.1×10^6. The results of two other filters, Nipro-CF-YR-1 and Pall RC-100D, were similar to that of Sepacell R-500N.

The residual WBCs in 20 units of PC (400 ml) after filtration were also tested. A mean number of WBCs in 20 units of prefiltration PCs was 3.0×10^8 (a range of $1.8–5.6 \times 10^8$). After filtration by Pall PL-100H, the residual WBC number in 46 (64.7%) out of 71 PCs reduced to less than 1×10^6; in 21 (29.5%) to more than 1×10^6, with a mean of 1.6×10^6; and in only four (5.6%) to more than 1×10^7, with a mean of 5.2×10^7.

Table 17.2 Residual white blood cells (WBCs) in 2 units of concentrated red cells (CRCs) and 20 units of platelet concentrates (PCs) before and after filtration

Filter	Before filtration (n)	After filtration (n)
Sepacell R-500N	2.1×10^{9}* (21) ($1.3–3.5 \times 10^{9}$)	1.1×10^{6} (4) $< 1 \times 10^{6}$ (17)
Nipro CF-YR-1	2.4×10^{9}* (15) ($1.5–4.0 \times 10^{9}$)	1.4×10^{6} (3) $< 1 \times 10^{6}$ (12)
Pall RC-100D	2.2×10^{9}* (11) ($1.1–3.0 \times 10^{9}$)	1.3×10^{6} (4) $< 1 \times 10^{6}$ (7)
Pall PL-100H	3.0×10^{8}† (11) ($1.8–5.6 \times 10^{8}$)	5.2×10^{7} (4) 1.6×10^{6} (21) $< 1 \times 10^{6}$ (46)
Sepacell PL-10N	3.5×10^{8}† (5) ($1.7–5.3 \times 10^{8}$)	2.0×10^{7} (1) 2.2×10^{6} (3) $< 1 \times 10^{6}$ (3)

* Mean of WBCs in 2 units of CRCs (400 ml).
† Mean of WBCs in 20 units of PCs (400 ml).

The efficiencies of leukocyte depletion by filters were more than 3 log reduction for 2 units of CRCs, with the residual WBCs of less than 1×10^{6}, and more than 2 log reduction for 20 units of PCs, with the residual WBCs of less than 1×10^{6} in 95% of filtrations.

Antihuman leukocyte antigen antibody in the single transfusion group

One hundred and forty patients received an average of 7 units of whole blood or CRCs. Anti-HLA antibodies at 2 months postoperation were detected in one (2.5%) of 39 males and 16 (16.1%) of 99 females, respectively. The difference was statistically significant ($P < 0.05$). At 6 months postoperation, the antibodies were detected in none of 25 males and six (7.8%) of 76 females (Table 17.3). The overall analysis indicated that 15 (14.5%) out of 103 developed anti-HLA antibodies transiently; the antibodies were either positive at 2 months or at 6 months postoperation. Only eight (7.7%) patients, all females, developed persistent anti-HLA antibodies throughout the observation time.

Table 17.3 Human leukocyte antigen alloimmunization in the single transfusion group

Patients	2 months postoperation	6 months postoperation
Male	1/39 (2.5%)	0/25 (0%)
Female	16/99 (16.1%)	6/76 (7.8%)

Antihuman leukocyte antigen antibody in the multiple transfusion group

The patients in Group I received an average of 5 (range 1–12) units of nonfiltered CRCs in the early transfusion period and 17.6 (3–54) units of filtered CRCs. Six out of 13 patients developed anti-HLA antibodies against more than 10% of the panel lymphocytes, five of which were transient (not more than 2 months) antibodies with narrow specificities (positive against less than 50% of the panel lymphocytes). The remaining one developed the persistent anti-HLA antibody with broad specificities resulting in refractoriness to random donor platelet transfusion (Fig. 17.1). Two of 10 patients in Group II developed transient but broad anti-HLA antibodies against more than 50% of the panel cells. Three of 12 patients in Group III developed antibodies, all of which were transient. Most of the patients who developed transient antibodies showed temporary lower platelet increments during a short, antibody-positive period, but they were not low enough to be called refractoriness; they either continued to show good platelet increments or responded to platelet transfusion after the antibody disappeared. The only patient in Group I who developed the persistent anti-HLA antibody was refractory to platelet transfusion. The frequencies of developing antibodies and refractoriness to platelet transfusion between the three groups were not statistically significant (Table 17.4).

Summary

It is well known that repeated transfusions of red cell products alone, or associated with PCs, lead to alloimmunization, notably production of anti-HLA antibodies in a mean of 43% (31–50%) [4–7]. The presence of anti-HLA antibodies in patients usually results in refractoriness to random donor platelet transfusion. Management of such patients is difficult and expensive, requiring single donor HLA-compatible platelet products. Experimental and clinical transfusion practices have indicated that leukocytes in blood products were responsible for stimulating HLAs to the patients. Efforts to prevent alloimmunization have thus been directed at reducing the number of leukocytes in blood products, either by centrifugation or by filtration. In fact, reduction of residual leukocytes in blood products by filtration reduced the rate of alloimmunization to 16% (12–21%) in multitransfused patients. The results were diverse but consistent in the reduction in rate of alloimmunization, although the number of residual leukocytes in blood products used in each experiment varied considerably from 5×10^6 to 6×10^7. Thus, the reduction of leukocytes in red cell products at the level of 2 log (99%) leads to a significant reduction in the rate of alloimmunization.

In our study, we used filtered red cell products which contained an average of less than 1×10^6 leukocytes. The rate of alloimmunization in Group I was 46.1% (6/13), which was comparable to the rate of hitherto reported results, while those in Group II and Group III were 20% (2/10) and 25% (3/12), respectively; both groups received

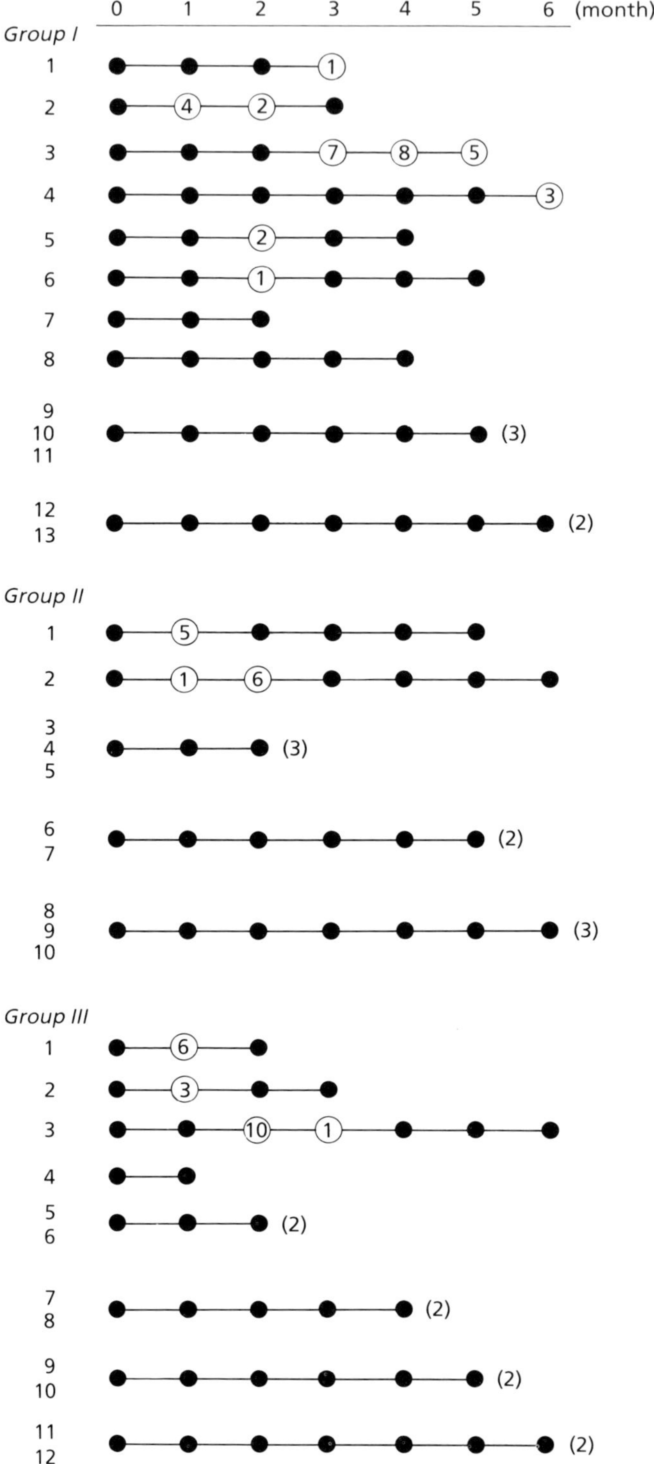

Table 17.4 Human leukocyte antigen alloimmunization in multitransfused patients

Group	No. positive/ no. of patients (%)
Group I	6/13 (46.1%)
Group II	2/10 (20.0%)
Group III	3/12 (25.0%)

only filtered red cell products. Although the number of cases is small, our data support the previous results that the use of leukocyte-depleted red cell products by filtration reduced the rate of alloimmunization in multitransfused patients. More strikingly, only one patient in Group I became refractory to platelet transfusion, and none of Group II and III who received filtered red cell products did so, indicating that leukocyte-depleted red cell products should be used in patients who are to receive multiple blood products, especially platelet products. Practically, the patients would tolerate well random donor platelet products and may be rather easily managed by the filtration technique.

The efficacy of the filters depleting leukocytes in platelet products was not proven in this study, since the rates of HLA alloimmunization and refractoriness to platelet transfusion were not statistically different between Group II and Group III; the former received nonfiltered platelet concentrates and the latter filtered platelets. Thus, the efficacy of the platelet filters in preventing alloimmunization needs to be established by further experiments.

References

1 Sirchia G, Rebulla P, Parravicini A, Carnelli V, Gianotti GA, Bertolini F. Leukocyte depletion of red cell units at the bedside by transfusion through a new filter. *Transfusion* 1987;27:402–405.

2 Kickler TS, Bell W, Ness PM, Drew H, Pall D. Depletion of white cells from platelet concentrates with a new adsorption filter. *Transfusion* 1989;29:411–414.

3 Sirchia G, Wenz B, Rebulla P, Parravicini A, Carnelli V, Bertolini F. Removal of white cells from red cells by transfusion through a new filter. *Transfusion* 1990;30:30–33.

4 Murphy MF, Metcalfe P, Thomas H *et al.* Use of leukocyte-poor blood components and HLA-matched-platelet donors to prevent HLA alloimmunization. *Br J Haematol* 1986;62:529–534.

5 Andreu G, Dewailly J, Leberre C *et al.* Prevention of HLA immunization with leukocyte-poor packed red cells and platelet concentrates obtained by filtration. *Blood* 1988;72:964–969.

6 Sniecinski I, O'Donnell MR, Nowicki B, Hill LR. Prevention of refractoriness and HLA-alloimmunization using filtered blood products. *Blood* 1988;71:1402–1407.

Fig. 17.1 Antihuman leukocyte antigen (HLA) antibody status in multitransfused patients. Closed circles indicate negative anti-HLA antibodies. Open circles indicate positive antibodies. The number in the open circle indicates the number of positives against 10 panel lymphocytes.

7 Brand A, Class FHJ, Voogt PJ, Wasser MNJM, Eernisse JG. Alloimmunization after leukocyte-depleted multiple random donor platelet transfusions. *Vox Sang* 1988;54:160–166.

Discussion

SHIMIZU: Were all the 35 patients who showed the antibody production after repeated transfusions female?

MAEDA: No.

JUJI: (Tokyo University): In your presentation, you said that two patients developed antibodies in spite of the use of filters. Were they female?

MAEDA: Yes, but one of them has no history of pregnancy.

JUJI: There may be such cases, but I suppose small quantities may be enough to sensitize recipients having a history of pregnancy. Therefore, it is better to consider this point, isn't it?

MAEDA: Generally, the antibody becomes positive after a certain period, perhaps 1 month after the transfusion. We learned that it was positive when we tested, not when blood transfusion was performed. Therefore, we noticed the increase in CPI without knowing when it occurred. I think the use of filters will reduce the occurrence of refractoriness.

JUJI: Dr Handa has observed the disappearance of antibody after successive platelet transfusions and this was also our experience. That is to say, there were some cases in which the antibody titers fell and could not be detected during the repeated transfusions of standard, unfiltered blood components.

SHIMIZU: Does this mean that there are not only cases where antibodies disappear with filtered blood but also where they disappear with unfiltered blood?

MAEDA: In the case of the study on platelet filtration, a transient production of antibody was observed, meaning that platelet transfusion itself may act by unknown mechanism, in addition to the possibility that it affects lymphocyte and the immunosystem.

KIYOKAWA (Fukuoka Red Cross Blood Center): We could not find any differences in the incidence of production of anti-HLA antibodies, but the antibody titers were significantly low when we transfused the buffy coat-free RBC components on the order of 1×10^8 prepared by the centrifugation method.

MAEDA: We did not measure the antibody titers, but they seemed to be low because the antibodies temporarily disappeared.

SHIMIZU: Does the high antibody titer suggest that it is the secondary response?

KIYOKAWA: Without filtration or removal of buffy coat, transfusion may induce antibody production. My question is whether there is a difference in titer between your case and the patients receiving blood products having 1×10^8 of leukocytes.

MAEDA: I suppose that the antibody titers were not so high because they disappeared transiently. They disappeared after about 1 month, and I suggest the possibility that the antibody decreased due to the disappearance of immunostimuli, or that it may induce a suppresser of antibody production.

HANDA: When we do a follow-up survey of the production of anti-HLA alloantibodies in acute leukemia patients in a short period, we should carefully observe the reduction of the antibody titer because, generally, transfusion of blood components such as platelet products is repeated only while there exists bone marrow suppression by chemotherapy, that is to say, while remission-induction therapy is being performed. Thus, if we succeed in the therapy, there will not be allosensitization for a while after that.

MAEDA: In this study, there is no case. If the patients receive such a second treatment, it will be possible to follow them up.

18 · Prevention of immunologic and infectious complications of transfusion by leukocyte depletion

I. Sniecinski

Department of Transfusion Medicine, City of Hope National Medical Center, 1500 East Duarte Road, Duarte, California 91010-0269, USA

Abstract

The decade of the 1980s has focused on the development of new approaches for the treatment of hematologic and oncologic diseases. Bone marrow transplantation has become the therapy of choice for treatment of leukemias and aplastic anemia. Significant growth of solid organ transplantation created a need for more intensive and specialized transfusion therapy.

Convincing evidence exists that blood transfusions are associated with deleterious effects caused by the residual leukocytes in blood components. These include alloimmunization to histocompatibility antigens, transmission of viruses, graft-versus-host disease, and increased susceptibility to cancer recurrence and postoperative infection. There is growing evidence that leukocyte depletion of blood components would prevent or ameliorate some of these harmful effects. The results of small-scale clinical trials showed marked reduction in alloimmunization and refractoriness to platelet transfusion. Moreover, preliminary observations suggest that the routine provision of leukocyte-depleted blood components for patients with hematologic malignancies is cost-effective.

Several studies have shown that the transfusion-transmitted cytomegalovirus (CMV) infection can be prevented by leukocyte depletion. CMV-seronegative recipients of CMV-seronegative bone marrow, kidney, heart, or liver transplants clearly benefit from the preferential use of CMV-negative blood support. The large demand for CMV-seronegative blood components in transplant patients places considerable stress on the community blood centers to maintain adequate inventories of these components and determine priorities for the distribution of a limited resource. Thus, management of transplant patients with leukocyte-depleted blood components may provide a practical alternative. The magnitude of leukocyte depletion with the newer filters may be sufficient to eliminate the risk of transmission of CMV and other viruses.

At present, it is debatable whether only selected or all patients who require transfusions should receive leukocyte-depleted products. In the future, however, if the results of the small-scale studies are confirmed by the ongoing multicenter trials, transfusion of every patient with leukocyte-depleted blood components should be considered to avoid the risk of viral transmission and alloimmunization.

Introduction

During the 1980s, rapid advances were made in the treatment of hematologic and oncologic malignancies. More potent chemotherapeutic regimens and broader indications for bone marrow transplantation were introduced. Development of unrelated marrow donor registries in many countries and international collaboration between these organizations has established the unrelated donor marrow transplantation. Similarly, there has been a significant expansion of the solid organ transplantation programs.

These advances and the promise of further scientific developments in the next decade created the challenges for transfusion medicine. During the 1990s, one can expect two dominating trends in transfusion practice: (i) improved safety of transfusion therapy, and (ii) increased utilization of specialized blood components. Consequently, research efforts will be focused on the development of technologies for the preparation of purer blood products.

Transfusion of cellular blood components is associated with the potential of immunologic and infectious complications. Among the immunologic problems, human leukocyte antigen (HLA) alloimmunization represents a major risk to patients requiring numerous blood transfusions during the course of their therapy. Patients with HLA antibodies become refractory to platelets and susceptible to repeated nonhemolytic transfusion reactions which limit the benefits of platelet transfusion therapy.

Among the infectious complications related to intensive transfusion support of patients with hematologic and oncologic malignancies treated with bone marrow transplantation, CMV infection is a devastating one. The significance of transfused leukocytes as vectors of CMV or stimulators of reactivation of the endogenous CMV in the recipient has been appreciated recently.

Several clinical trials have demonstrated the effectiveness of leukocyte-poor blood components in reducing the incidence of these immunologic and infectious complications (Tables 18.1 and 18.2). The current research effort is focused on the premise that routine practice of transfusing leukocyte-depleted blood components could

Table 18.1 Transfusion of filtered blood components: comparison of efficacy and rates of alloimmunization

Authors	Mean residual leukocytes in:		Incidence of alloimmunization:	
	Platelets	Red cells	Controls	Study
Andreu *et al.* (1988) [1]	$0.5{-}1.5 \times 10^8$	6×10^7	11/35 (31%)	4/34 (12%)
van Marwijk Kooy *et al.* (1991) [2]	$< 5 \times 10^6$	$< 5 \times 10^6$	11/26 (42%)	2/27 (7%)
Myllylä *et al.* (1986) [3]	1×10^5	1×10^5	1/18 (6%)	0/21 (0%)
Saarinen *et al.* (1990) [4]	4×10^4	1×10^5	12/17 (71%)	0/18 (0%)
Sniecinski *et al.* (1988) [5]	6×10^6	5×10^7	10/20 (50%)	3/30 (15%)

Table 18.2 Leukocyte-poor trials to prevent cytomegalovirus (CMV) infection

Authors	No. of patients	Diagnosis	CMV seroconversion: no. and (%)	
			Control	Leukocyte-poor
Gilbert *et al.* (1989) [6]	72	Newborns	9/42 (21%)	0/30 (0%)
Murphy *et al.* (1988) [7]	20	Hematologic malignancy	2/9 (22%)	0/11 (0%)
De Graan-Hentzen *et al.* (1989) [8]	145	Hematologic disease/ cardiac surgery	10/86 (12%)	0/59 (0%)
Bowden *et al.* (1989) [9]	65	Allo- and auto-BMT	7/30 (23%)	0/35 (0%)
Verdonck *et al.* (1987) [10]	29	BMT		0/29 (0%)
DeWitte *et al.* (1990) [11]	28	Hematologic malignancy		0/28 (0%)

BMT, bone marrow transplantation.

eliminate the multiple risks associated with leukocytes. The practical problems of this approach are: (i) the limits of leukocyte depletion that are required for reducing the alloimmune response and viral transmission; (ii) the consistency of various methods to achieve the desirable level of leukocyte depletion; and (iii) the cost-effectiveness of providing leukocyte-depleted blood products for all transfusions.

In the present study, we have evaluated the performance characteristics of various filters designed for leukocyte depletion of packed red blood cells, pooled random donor, and plateletpheresis concentrates. In addition, we examined the cost of transfusion therapy with leukocyte-depleted blood components as it relates to prevention of HLA alloimmunization and morbidity caused by recurrent febrile transfusion reactions. Finally, we compared the cost of CMV-seronegative blood transfusion support with the cost of transfusion therapy with leukocyte-depleted blood.

Methods

Packed red blood cells and random donor platelet concentrates were prepared from whole blood donations using the standard technology. Plateletpheresis concentrates were prepared using the Fenwal CS-3000 (Fenwal, Deerfield, IL, USA), Cobe Spectra (Cobe, Denver, CO, USA), Haemonetics V-50 (Haemonetics, Braintree, MA, USA), and Fresenius AS-104 (Fresenius, Germany) cell separators. The following filters were used for leukocyte depletion of red cell concentrates: Imugard-500 (Terumo, Japan), RC-100, RC-50, and BPF-4 (Pall, Glen Cove, NY, USA), Cutter Leukotrap II (Cutter, West Haven, CT, USA), and Sepacell R-500 (Asahi, Japan). One filter was used for filtration of single red cell concentrate.

Plateletpheresis products were leukocyte-depleted using the PL-50 filter. Random donor platelet concentrates were leukocyte-depleted using the following filters: Imugard 500 (Terumo, Japan), PL-50 (Pall, Glen Cove, NY, USA), and PL-10A

(Terumo, Japan). One filter was used to process a pool of six random donor platelet concentrates or one plateletphercsis concentrate. The effectiveness of leukocyte removal by filtration was determined using the counting technique which allowed detection of a low number of leukocytes in the red cell and platelet concentrates. We used two manual counting chambers; the Hausser chamber with the detection limit of 3.1 white blood cells (WBC)/μl and the Nageotte chamber with a detection limit of 0.2 WBCs/μl. Manual counts were validated by flow cytometric counting with the detection ability of 0.05 WBCs/μl. The flow cytometry method was a modification of that of Bodensteiner [12] and it was based on reducing the platelet to leukocyte ratio with the lysing agent and staining the remaining WBC nuclei with a lytic stain reagent composed of RNase, sodium citrate, P-40, and thiazide orange. Fluorescein beads were added to the final mixture to calculate the volume analyzed.

The cost of transfusion therapy with leukocyte-depleted blood components was studied in a group of patients with acute leukemia. Patients were randomized to receive standard cellular blood products (standard group) or filtered blood products (filtered group). The evaluable patients were monitored for alloimmunization and refractoriness. All febrile reactions occurring during or immediately following platelet transfusions were assessed and documented. A febrile reaction was defined as an elevation of body temperature of $>1\,^{\circ}\mathrm{C}$ and/or chills without an identifiable medical cause. Hemolysis was excluded by the recipient's posttransfusion direct antiglobulin test and bacterial contamination was excluded by Gram stain as well as culture of the residual component.

In another group of patients, we enumerated the number of febrile transfusion reactions in response to either red cell or platelet transfusions during a 3-year period. After individual patients developed two febrile transfusion reactions, they were considered to be at high risk for subsequent reactions and thereafter received only leukocyte-poor blood products. Transfusion reaction rates were calculated for red cell, random platelet pool, and plateletpheresis concentrates according to the standard formula.

In addition, in a group of bone marrow transplant patients, we compared the cost of leukocyte-depleted hemotherapy versus provision of CMV-seronegative blood products.

Results

The results of WBC removal by various types of filters from the red cell concentrates and random platelet pools are shown in Tables 18.3 and 18.4. Results are expressed as the log of WBC removal and the mean of residual WBC counts in the filtered concentrates. Red cell filters demonstrated an efficiency of WBC removal from 1.9 to 3.4 logs. The numbers of residual leukocytes in the filtered red cell concentrate varied from 4.0×10^7 when the Imugard G-500 filter was used to 6.4×10^5 when red cells were processed with a Pall BPF-4 filter.

Table 18.3 Levels of leukocyte depletion from red blood cell concentrates

Log	Filter	Per unit
1.9	Imugard-500 (Terumo)	5.0×10^7
2.3	Imugard E (Terumo)	1.7×10^7
2.5	Cutter Leukotrap II	1.35×10^7
2.9	RC-50 (Pall)	3.0×10^6
3.0	RC-100 (Pall)	2.0×10^6
3.1	Sepacell R-500 (Asahi)	1.5×10^6
3.4	BPF-4 (Pall)	6.4×10^5

Table 18.4 Levels of leukocyte-depletion from platelet products

Log	Filter	Per pool of 6 units
1.9	Imugard-500 (Terumo)	6.0×10^8
2.2	PL-50 (Pall)	9.7×10^5
2.5	PL-100 (Pall)	7.5×10^5
2.9	PL-10A (Sepacell)	6.0×10^5

Similarly, the efficiency of WBC removal by platelet filters varied between 1.9 and 2.9 logs and the residual number of leukocytes in the filtered pool of six platelet concentrates varied between 6.0×10^5 for PL-10A filter and 6×10^8 for the Imugard filter. The leukocyte content in plateletpheresis products before and after filtration using the PL-50 filter is shown in Table 18.5. As can be seen in this table, there were differences between the various cell separators relative to the number of WBCs contaminating the platelet concentrates they produced. These differences were maintained after preparation of leukocyte-depleted plateletpheresis products by filtration.

Table 18.5 Levels of leukocyte-depletion from plateletpheresis products

Cell separator	Prefiltration leukocytes	Postfiltration leukocytes	Log
Fenwal CS-3000	2.2×10^8	3.3×10^6	1.9
Fenwal CS-300 Plus TNX-6			
ID Offset 6	5.5×10^6	5.0×10^4	2.2
ID Offset 10	1.1×10^7	1.0×10^5	2.0
Haemonetics V-50	1.9×10^8	1.9×10^6	2.0
Cobe Spectra	2.4×10^7	3.4×10^5	1.8
Fresenius AS-104	1.4×10^7	2.0×10^5	1.9

Filtration was performed with the PL-50.

Table 18.6 Cost-effectiveness of platelet filtration

	Standard group	Filtered group
Number of patients	20	20
Study period (months)	22	22
Number of platelet transfusions/patient per month	9.14	5.75
Cost of platelet support/patient per month	$2468*	$1553*
Cost of platelet support/patient per month, including cost of filtration	$2468	$1639–1898†

* Calculated using $45/platelet unit and $270/platelet transfusion (pool of 6 units).
† Calculated using a range of $15–60/filtration procedure.

Table 18.6 shows the cost differential of platelet transfusion therapy in a group of acute leukemia patients randomized to receive either filtered or standard blood components. Twenty patients in each group were studied for 22 months. The difference is shown in the number of platelet transfusions per patient, which is lower for the filtered group.

When we derived the cost of platelet support per patient per month, there was a substantial difference between the filtered and control group. That difference was maintained even when the cost of the filter was added. The cost differential was magnified when we computed the cost associated with the refractory state. The additional cost of providing single donor HLA-matched platelets per month was $4400 for a refractory patient in a standard group, as compared to $3200 for a refractory patient in a control group. Table 18.7 shows the cost associated with the number of transfusion episodes complicated by the febrile transfusion reaction. There was an appreciable difference between the study and filtered group. Table 18.8 demonstrates the incidence of febrile transfusion episodes over a 3-year period. Again, there was a significant difference in the transfusion reaction rates between recipients of filtered and nonfiltered red cell and platelet concentrates.

Table 18.9 compares the cost related to provision of CMV-seronegative blood components with the cost of provision of filtered blood components for patients undergoing bone marrow transplantation. Filtered blood components from donors of

Table 18.7 Cost of morbidity related to recurrent febrile transfusion reactions due to alloimmunization

	Standard group	Filtered group
Number of transfusion episodes/patient per month accompanied by febrile reaction	5.5	0.8
Cost of morbidity related to transfusion episodes with reaction/patient per month	$1650–5500	$240–800

Calculated using $300–1000 per transfusion reaction.

Table 18.8 Febrile nonhemolytic transfusion reactions from January 1988 to December 1990

	Pools of platelet concentrates		Plateletpheresis concentrates		Red cell concentrates	
	Unfiltered	Filtered	Unfiltered	Filtered	Unfiltered	Filtered
Transfusions	2141	8036	847	9500	10 907	10 563
Reactions	88	30	3	8	45	10
Reaction rate/ transfusion (%)	4.1	0.4	0.4	0.08	0.4	0.09

Table 18.9 Comparison of costs related to prevention of transmission cytomegalovirus (CMV)

	CMV-seronegative	Filtered
Cost of red blood cell support	$17.30 \times 16 = $277	$36 \times 7 = $252
Cost of platelet support	$17.30 \times 27 = $467	$36 \times 12 = $432
	$570 \times 12 = $6840	$45 \times 72 = $3240
Total cost	$7584	$3924

(based on assumption that 56% of donors are seropositive)

Average number of red blood cell transfusions/BMT patient = 7

Average number of platelet transfusions/BMT patient = 12 SD or 72 RD

Cost of RD plateletpheresis concentrate = $45.00
Cost of SD plateletpheresis concentrate = $570.00
Cost of CMV test = $17.30

BMT, bone marrow transplantation; RD, random donor; SD, single donor.

unknown CMV status appear to provide a less costly alternative as compared with CMV-seronegative blood support because it allows the use of platelet concentrates prepared from random blood donations.

Summary

Procedures for preparation of blood components have improved considerably during the last decade. Removal of WBCs from red cell and platelet concentrates has been more widely used in order to prevent or delay nonhemolytic transfusion reactions and HLA immunization in polytransfused patients. Reports have been published on the use of leukocyte-poor blood components to reduce CMV infection. At present, filtration appears to be the best method available for leukocyte-depletion. Recently, third-generation filters have become available that are highly effective in the removal of leukocytes from blood components and are easy to handle. These filters are capable of decreasing the number of leukocytes by 3–4 logs and produce blood components delivering fewer than 10^6 WBC per transfusion. The limits of leukocyte depletion that are required to prevent the occurrence of alloimmunization and the spread of

Table 18.10 Guidelines for the use of filtered blood components

---

- To prevent febrile transfusion reactions in patients with recurrent reactions
- To prevent or delay the onset of alloimmunization in multitransfused patients
- To prevent refractoriness to platelet transfusions in patients requiring long-term platelet transfusion support
- To prevent transfusion-transmitted cytomegalovirus infection in immunocompromised patients

---

transfusion-transmitted CMV infection are unknown. Several small-scale studies reported that the incidence of alloimmunization can be significantly lowered with transfusions of blood containing more than 10^6 residual white cells [1,5]. Also, the transmission of CMV infection was reported to be prevented in patients receiving leukocyte-depleted blood products containing more than 10^6 leukocytes. However, it would be prudent to infuse less than 1×10^6 leukocytes during each transfusion in order to avoid primary HLA alloimmunization and viral transmission. In our study, using more sensitive methods for the enumeration of leukocytes in filtered red cell and platelet concentrates, we demonstrated that such a level of leukocyte depletion could be achieved. Therefore, we are recommending the use of filtered blood components for all patients requiring long-term transfusion therapy (Table 18.10). Opponents of this policy have frequently used economic arguments to support their view. However, our cost and benefit analyses demonstrated that filtration of blood components was indeed cost-effective for prevention of HLA alloimmunization and platelet refractoriness and morbidity caused by recurrent transfusion reactions. In addition, preparation of blood components by filtration was found to be cost-effective in relation to prevention of CMV transmission.

With the expectation that the rapid growth of bone marrow and solid organ transplantation will continue throughout the 1990s, it is likely that there will be an increased need for specialized blood components. Important areas of research on the preparation of blood components will include improved methods for leukocyte-reduction and bacterial and viral inactivation. The new technologies for leukocyte removal hold the promise of a more practical and less expensive approach that could be implemented for all patients requiring blood transfusions.

References

1 Andreu G, Dewailly J, Leberre C *et al.* Prevention of HLA immunization with leukocyte-poor packed red cells and platelet concentrates obtained by filtration. *Blood* 1988;72:964–969.

2 van Marwijk Kooy M, van Prooijen HC, Moes M, Bosma-Stants I, Akkerman J-WN. Use of leukocyte-depleted platelet concentrates for the prevention of refractoriness and primary HLA alloimmunization: a prospective, randomized trial. *Blood* 1991;77:201–205.

3 Myllylä G, Ruutu T, Oksanen V, Rasi V, Kekomäki R. Preparation and properties of leukocyte-free platelet concentrates. 19th Cong Int Soc Blood Transfusion, Sydney, Australia, 1986.

4 Saarinen UM, Kekomäki R, Siimes Ma, Myllylä G. Effective prophylaxis against platelet refractoriness in multitransfused patients by use of leukocyte-free blood components. *Blood* 1990;75:512–517.

5 Sniecinski I, O'Donnell MR, Nowicki B, Hill LR. Prevention of refractoriness and HLA-alloimmunization using filtered blood products. *Blood* 1988;71:1402–1407.

6 Gilbert GI, Hayes K, Hudson IL, James I. Prevention of transfusion-acquired cytomegalovirus infection in infants by blood filtration to remove leukocytes. Neonatal Cytomegalovirus Infection Study Group. *Lancet* 1989;1:1228–1231.

7 Murphy MF, Grint PCA, Hardiman AE, Lister TA, Waters AH. Use of leukocyte-poor blood components to prevent primary cytomegalovirus (CMV) infection in patients with acute leukemia. *Br J Haematol* 1988;70:253–4.

8 DeGraan-Hentzen YC, Gratama JW, Mudde GC *et al.* Prevention of primary cytomegalovirus infection in patients with hematologic malignancies by intensive white cell depletion of blood products. *Transfusion* 1989;29:757–760.

9 Bowden RA, Sayers MH, Cays M, Slichter SJ. The role of blood product filtration in the prevention of transfusion associated cytomegalovirus (CMV) infection after marrow transplant. Transfusion 1989;29(suppl):57S.

10 Verdonck LF, DeGraan-Hentzen YC, Dekker AW, Mudde GC, De Gast GC. Cytomegalovirus seronegative platelets and leukocyte-poor red blood cells from random donors can prevent primary cytomegalovirus infection after bone marrow transplantation. *Bone Marrow Transplant* 1987;2:73–78.

11 DeWitte T, Schattenberg A, van Dijk BA, Galama J, Olthuis H, van der Meer JWW, Kunst VAJM. Prevention of primary cytomegalovirus infection after allogeneic bone marrow transplantation by using leukocyte-poor random blood products from cytomegalovirus-unscreened blood-bank donors. *Transplantation* 1990;50:964–968.

12 Bodensteiner DC. A flow cytometric technique to accurately measure post-filtration white blood cell counts. *Transfusion* 1989;29:651–653.

Discussion

WHYTE: Thank you for that lovely detailed work, particularly on the costing. The costings are done from the laboratory perspective. As I read it, your costs for the filters do not include overheads in the hospitals where the costs for the platelets, for example, include labor time and costs in the blood center. Can you tell me what the relative effect is because, for example in France, where it is all done centrally, that cost would need to be built in and therefore the cost of filtering would be higher than you have quoted.

SNIECINSKI: That is true. At our institution, all the filtration is performed in the transfusion laboratory that issues blood components for transfusion; none of the filtration is performed at the bedside. And it is true that in the cost of the filtration I have not included the labor and overheads, as you mentioned. It wouldn't be a very marked additional cost because, first of all, filtration with the new filters does not take an appreciable time. Second, it does not require highly trained individuals, for example, it does not require medical technologists. You could train other individuals whose labor is not as expensive. But this is a very good point, I can't argue with it.

MERYMAN: To your list of infectious agents that may be dealt with by filtration, I think we may be able to add *Yersinia*, which is a new problem being taking very seriously in the States. Claus Högman from Sweden has recently obtained data showing that artificially contaminated units which are then filtered do not grow *Yersinia* with subsequent storage, which implies that this may be an effective way of avoiding the problem.

SNIECINSKI: Yes, exactly.

SHIBATA (Toranomon Hospital): By your guidelines for red cell concentrates, half the patients use unfiltered and half use filtered blood. Do you use filtered blood for patients who show febrile reactions?

SNIECINSKI: You wonder why almost all the platelet transfusions are filtered and only half of the red blood cell transfusions have been filtered. This is the number of filtered blood components used at the institution, not only for hematology and oncology patients but also for surgical patients. The red cell transfusions that were not filtered were predominantly used by patients undergoing elective surgical procedures. As platelet transfusions are used by hematology–oncology patients, it is a uniform policy that all hematology patients receive filtered blood components. The difference between the percentage of filtered blood components in the two groups is the result of providing those components for patients other than those in hematology.

WOODFIELD: Could you tell me why you are not doing the filtration at the bedside? We have found that the clinical staff, if supervised and trained, can do it just as effectively as in the laboratory and it's more convenient.

SNIECINSKI: I think it has been a choice of our institution basically for the reason of quality control of the filtration and it's just an individual preference. It just works better at our institution by doing filtration in the laboratory rather than at the bedside. But there is no question you can train the nursing staff and you can organize the quality control with bedside filtration. And the cost of labor that we were just discussing a few minutes ago would be decreased because it would just be for replacing the standard filter that is part of the transfusion process.

STIENSTRA: Shouldn't the responsibility for the blood products that you deliver to the clinicians be in the blood bank so that you deliver blood products, the contents of which you know and thus do not give further responsibility to the clinicians?

WOODFIELD: I think clinicians are often very competent and as long as we are sure that the filter is satisfactory and it's quality-controlled to a certain degree, and that we can do random sampling, I see no reason not to use the filters at the bedside. It is not logical to think that we can do filtration better than the trained clinical staff, and we can certainly do quality control from time to time.

STIENSTRA: It's not the skill; I'm thinking only about the effect of quality control, responsibility for which should theoretically be in the blood bank. I would also like to make another point on that. My feeling is that it's better to filter red blood cells when they are rather young. Young blood cells are more easily filtered than older blood cells, in which I found more stiffness in the outer membrane so that there is more debris, more fragments, after filtering older red blood cell units.

19·Role of leukocyte depletion from platelet concentrates in reducing HLA alloimmunization and platelet refractoriness in polytransfused patients: a prospective multicenter randomized study in Japan

M. Handa *et al.**

Abstract

A prospective multicenter randomized trial was conducted in order to evaluate the efficacy of leukocyte-depleted platelet concentrates prepared with a newly developed second-generation polyester filter in preventing human leukocyte antigen (HLA) alloimmunization in patients receiving multiple transfusions. Patients with hematologic cancers requiring multiple platelet transfusions were randomly assigned to either of two study groups: one group received standard platelet concentrates (control group) and the other received leukocyte-depleted platelet concentrates (filtered group). All the patients received leukocyte-depleted red blood cell products. Of 96 randomized patients, 53 were evaluable; 21 in the control and 32 in the filtered group. The groups were comparable with regard to age, sex ratio, diagnosis, previous exposure to alloimmunogens through transfusion or pregnancy, actual transfusion regimens, and follow-up time. There were significant differences with regard to the HLA alloimmunization rate (8/21 = 38% in the control versus 2/32 = 6% in the filtered group; $P < 0.01$) and in the manifestation of refractoriness to platelet transfusions from

* M. Handa, Blood Center and Department of Internal Medicine, Keio University; Y. Ikeda, Blood Center and Department of Internal Medicine, Keio University; Y. Kurata, Department of Blood Transfusion, Osaka University; K. Tsubaki and A. Horiuchi, Departments of Blood Transfusion and Internal Medicine, Kinki University; K. Furihata, Department of Blood Transfusion, Shinshu University; Y. Kimura and K. Toyama, Department of Internal Medicine, Tokyo Medical College; S. Takamoto, Department of Blood Transfusion, Tokyo Metropolitan Kogagome Hospital; I. Tsukimoto, Department of Blood Transfusion, Toho University; T. Asai, Department of Blood Transfusion, Chiba University; M. Baba, Department of Blood Transfusion, Nihon University; H. Niikura and H. Terada, Department of Internal Medicine, Showa University; K. Ninomiya, Tokyo Metropolitan Fuchu Medical Center for the Severely Handicapped; S. Sekiguchi, Hokkaido Red Cross Blood Center; S. Sasagawa and M. Miyamoto, Central Blood Center of Japan Red Cross; M. Masuda, H. Mizoguchi, M. Takanashi, and M. Shimizu, Departments of Internal Medicine and Blood Transfusion, Tokyo Women's Medical College; and The Leukocyte-depleted Blood Transfusion Therapy Study Group.

random donors (6/21 = 29% in the control versus 1/32 = 3% in the filtered group; $P < 0.05$). These results indicated that leukocyte depletion from platelet concentrates was of great importance in the prevention of HLA alloimmunization and refractoriness to platelet transfusions from random donors.

Introduction

HLA alloimmunization due to contaminated leukocytes in blood products, frequently occurring in polytransfused patients, can be very troublesome, rendering patients refractory to platelet transfusions from random donors [1]. As compared to conventional centrifugation for the removal of contaminated leukocytes, recent studies have clearly indicated that the use of filters to prepare leukocyte-depleted blood products appears to be a simple and effective method of reducing the frequency of HLA alloimmunization in patients with multiple transfusions [2,3]. Since the filters utilized in these studies were developed essentially for whole blood products, and not for platelet concentrates, when they were applied to leukocyte depletion from platelet products, some drawbacks emerged, i.e. extra efforts had to be made to improve platelet recovery by priming and rinsing the filters or by adding platelet antagonists to the platelet products before filtration [4]. Very recently, second-generation filters composed of nonwoven polyester fabric have been developed for platelet products; these filters, which can be used without the above precautions, allow desirable platelet recovery and at least 2 log reduction of the number of contaminated leukocytes [5–8]. However, to date their effectiveness in the clinical setting has remained unproven. Here we describe a summary of the results of a prospective multiinstitutional randomized trial [9], performed from October 1989 through September 1990, in Japan, to evaluate the efficacy of leukocyte-depleted platelet products prepared with a polyester filter, Sepacell-PL, in the prevention of HLA alloimmunization in patients receiving multiple platelet transfusions.

Methods

Patients

Newly admitted patients with hematologic malignancies, who were expected to require frequent platelet transfusions during the clinical course of first-remission induction therapy, were eligible for this study. Ten university hospitals and one city hospital located near Tokyo and Osaka participated in this study. The diagnosis of patients included acute nonlymphocytic leukemia, acute lymphoblastic leukemia, acute phase of chronic myelogenous leukemia, acute transformation of myelodysplastic syndrome, and malignant lymphoma. There were no age restrictions. Patients were not eligible for the study if they had a history of frequent or recent blood transfusions (more than 4 units of either red blood cells or platelet products; or transfusions received within 3 months before entry). At entry, patients who met the inclusion criteria were selected by the attending physician at each institution and were subsequently randomized into the two study groups; i.e. they either received standard platelet concentrates (control group) or they received leukocyte-depleted platelet concentrates prepared by filtration with a polyester filter (filtered group). Written informed consent was obtained from all patients. Randomization was done by an envelope method using random lists for the four strata. Patients were excluded if they had anti-HLA or antiplatelet antibodies in sera collected at entry; if they received an insufficient number of platelet transfusions (less than 3 episodes); if they had a short follow-up time due to early death (death less than 2 weeks after commencement of the study); or if a violation of randomization or the transfusion protocol was revealed.

Transfusion protocol

Patients assigned to the control group received standard platelet products, including platelet concentrates from random or single donors, supplied from a regional blood center of the Japan Red Cross. In some cases, platelet concentrates collected from single donor apheresis at each institution were used. Patients in the filtered group received leukocyte-depleted platelet products prepared by filtration of standard platelet products with a polyester filter, Sepacell-PL. All the patients in both groups received leukocyte-depleted red blood cell products either supplied from a regional blood center of the Japan Red Cross or prepared at each institution by filtration of standard red blood cell products with a polyester filter, Sepacell-R. There were no restrictions on the use of fresh frozen plasma. Granulocyte transfusions were not allowed in either group.

Preparation of blood products

Platelet concentrates from random donors were prepared and stored by a regional blood center of the Japan Red Cross. One unit of platelet concentrate was derived from 200 ml of whole blood collected with citrate phosphate dextrose by routine blood donation. Whole blood was subjected to centrifugation at 550 g for 5 min and the resultant platelet-rich plasma was then centrifuged at 650 g for 15 min. After platelet-poor plasma was separated, 20 ml of platelet concentrates was stored for 24 h at room temperature, with gentle agitation. Platelet concentrates from a single donor were also prepared by the Red Cross, or at each institution using blood cell processors. The leukocyte-depleted platelet concentrates were prepared by filtering the standard platelet concentrates with a polyester filter, Sepacell-PL. The filtration procedure was carried out according to the manufacturer's instructions. In brief, the platelet concentrates, stored for up to 72 h, were directly applied to the filter, which had been prerinsed with 30 ml of saline, and were allowed to flow through by gravity. Residual

Table 19.1 Quality of platelet concentrates from random donors before and after filtration with Scpacell-PL (mean ± s.d.)

	Platelet concentrates per 10 units $(n = 105)$	
	Prefiltration	Postfiltration
Volume (ml)	221 ± 24	202 ± 35
Platelet count ($\times 10^{11}$)	2.70 ± 0.04	2.52 ± 0.04 (94.6 ± 3.7% recovery)
Leukocyte count ($\times 10^{6}$)	150 ± 100	4.20 ± 6.70 (95.8 ± 3.7% elimination)

platelets in the filter were recovered by rinsing with 30 ml of saline. Prerinsing of these filters can be omitted and thus filtration could be performed at the bedside. To evaluate the quality of the leukocyte-depleted platelet concentrates, each institution determined the numbers of leukocytes and platelets in the product before and after filtration, using an automated cell counter. Table 19.1 shows the quality of the leukocyte-depleted platelet concentrates derived from random donors. The efficacy of the filter for platelet concentrates from single donors was shown in the rates of contaminated leukocyte removal and platelet recovery, which were 83.9 ± 9% and 89.0 ± 10.7% (mean ± s.d., $n = 8$), respectively. The leukocyte-depleted red blood cell concentrates were prepared and stored by the Red Cross, using standard procedures consisting of conventional centrifugation and subsequent filtration with leukocyte-depletion filters. The product derived from 200 ml of whole blood (1 unit) contained an average of 2.5×10^{6} leukocytes.

Evaluation of alloimmunization and refractoriness to platelet transfusion

Serum for the determination of anti-HLA antibody and antiplatelet antibody was obtained at entry and at 2-week intervals after the first platelet transfusion. The sera were usually followed up for 12 weeks but sera obtained after this time from some patients were also included for evaluation. Anti-HLA antibody was assayed by a modified leukocyte cytotoxic test method using antihuman globulin (AHG-LCT) with a panel of 10 lymphocytes. A mixed passive hemagglutination test (MPHA) was used for the detection of antiplatelet antibody. Anti-HLA antibody was considered positive when the serum reacted with 20% of the paneled cells. For confirmation, positive serum was tested again on another occasion. To determine the clinical effectiveness of platelet transfusions, the percentage of expected platelet recovery 12–18 h after every transfusion was calculated based on the following formula:

$$\% \text{ Recovery} = \frac{\text{blood volume} \times \text{platelet count increase} \times 100}{\text{number of platelets transfused} \times 0.67}$$

Patients were considered refractory to random donor platelets when the value of a 12–18-h posttransfusion platelet recovery, without any clinical factors, such as active bleeding, disseminated intravascular coagulopathy, high fever, or splenomegaly, that affect platelet recovery being present was below 20% on two successive transfusions.

Statistical analysis

Groups were compared by Student's t-test for continuous variables and chi-square test for categoric variables. All tests of significance were two-tailed. To analyze differences in the rates of HLA alloimmunization, Kaplan-Meier survival curves were constructed for the two study groups and these were compared by Wilcox on statistical analysis.

Results

Patients

Between October 1989 and December 1990, 96 patients with hematologic cancers participated in this study (Table 19.2). Of the 96 patients, 48 were randomly assigned to the control group, and 48 to the filtered group. A total of 53 patients, 21 in the control group and 32 in the filtered group, were considered evaluable. The clinical characteristics of all patients entered are summarized in Table 19.2. There were no significant differences between the two groups with respect to age, sex, diagnosis, or history of prior sensitization to alloimmunogens by either transfusion and/or pregnancy. As shown in Table 19.3, the actual transfusion regimens and the follow-up time for antibody detection were also well balanced between the two groups, although in the filtered group all the values were greater than in the control group. One unit was defined as the amount of platelet products derived from 200 ml of donated blood.

Efficacy of filtered platelet concentrates in preventing HLA alloimmunization and refractoriness to platelet transfusion from random donors

The overall incidence of HLA alloimmunization was compared in the two study groups, as shown in Table 19.4. There was a significant difference between patients in the control and filtered groups in the risk of being alloimmunized to HLA antigens (8/21 = 38% versus 2/32 = 6%; $P < 0.01$). Of 21 patients in the control group, five had persistent antibodies, as compared with one of 33 in the filtered group, this difference

Table 19.2 Patients profile 1

	Control	Filtered	
Number of patients entered	48	48	
Number of patients evaluable	21	32	
< 15 yr	20	29	
≥ 15 yr	1	3	NS
Mean age (range)	41 (8–66)	40 (2–74)	
< 15 yr	43 (16–66)	45 (18–74)	
≥ 15 yr	8 (8)	6 (2–15)	
Sex ratio (M/F)	7 : 14	12 : 20	NS
Diagnosis			
Acute nonlymphocytic leukemia	11	20	NS
Acute lymphoblastic leukemia	5	8	
Chronic myelogenous leukemia	4	1	
Lymphoma	2	3	
Number of patients			NS
with prior sensitization			
Transfusion	2	6	
Pregnancy	3	6	
Transfusion + pregnancy	0	1	

NS, not significant.

Table 19.3 Patient profile: transfusion regimen and follow-up time: mean (range)

	Control	Filtered
Platelet concentrate		
Days with transfusion	8 (1–17)	14 (3–52)
Duration of transfusion episodes (days)	52 (11–120)	63 (5–150)
Number of transfusion (units)	109 (12–280)	177 (21–660)
Red blood cell product		
Number of transfusion (units)	19 (0–158)	21 (0–124)
Follow-up time for antibody detection (days)	69 (15–132)	100 (21–231)

was also significant (5/21 = 24% vs. 1/32 = 3%, $P < 0.05$). The incidence of refractoriness to platelet transfusions was significantly lower in patients in the filtered group than in those in the control group (1/32 = 3% vs. 6/21 = 27%, $P < 0.05$). All the patients had anti-HLA antibodies, and one patient in the control group who was temporarily positive for antibody was in the refractory state during the time the

Table 19.4 Overall incidence of alloimmunization

	Control	Filtered	
Number of patients			
with human leukocyte antigen antibodies	8/21 (38%)	2/32 (6%)	$P < 0.01$
Number of patients refractory			
to platelet transfusion	6/21 (29%)	1/32 (3%)	$P < 0.05$
Preexposure to alloantigen	2/8	0/2	NS
Transfusion	1	0	
Pregnancy	1	0	
Transfusion and pregnancy	0	0	
Number of days			
to alloimmunization: mean (range)	47 (1–132)	42 (21–62)	NS
Number of platelet transfusions			
before antibody detection: mean (range)			
Episodes	9 (1–17)	11 (8–13)	NS
Units	142 (20–280)	182 (104–260)	NS
Number of red blood cell transfusions			
before antibody detection: mean (range)			
Units	29 (0–158)	10 (10–10)	NS

antibody was present. Antiplatelet antibody was detected in only one patient in the filtered group, who was negative for anti-HLA antibodies and did not become refractory to platelet transfusions. On the basis of the Kaplan-Meier product-limit estimates of the probability of becoming alloimmunized, the rates of occurrence of alloimmunization as a function of time were analyzed and compared for the two groups (Fig. 19.1). Within 6 weeks, 10 of 11 patients (91%) were immunized; only one patient in the control group became immunized later, 145 days after the first transfusion. There was a significant difference between the two groups regarding the rate of alloimmunization 48 days after the initial transfusion ($P < 0.01$).

Summary

The results of this clinical trial showed, firstly, that the use of platelet products depleted of contaminated leukocytes was very effective in preventing the development of HLA alloimmunization in patients receiving multiple platelet transfusions, and, secondly that the use of a second-generation polyester filter in the preparation of leukocyte-depleted platelet concentrates was simple and effective, yielding high-quality products. In the past 10 years, a number of clinical studies have been conducted to determine the clinical efficacy of leukocyte depletion from blood products in the prevention of alloimmunization [2,3,10–13]. Comparisons of patients

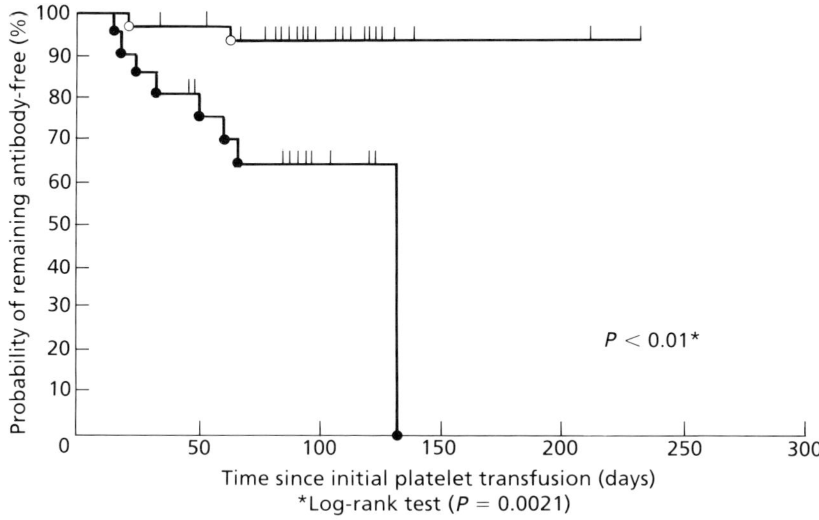

Fig. 19.1 Kaplan-Meier product-limit estimate of the probability of patients receiving multiple platelet transfusions remaining antihuman leukocyte antigen antibody-free. ● control; ○ filtered.

receiving standard red blood cells and platelet concentrates and patients receiving leukocyte-depleted red blood cells and platelet concentrates were made between two study groups with regard to the rate of alloimmunization and the incidence of refractoriness to platelet transfusion from random donors. All the studies, except one [10], concluded that leukocyte-depleted blood products were significantly useful. However, the nature of the transfusion protocols in these studies precluded the clarification of the individual role of leukocyte depletion from red blood cells and platelet concentrates in the prevention of alloimmunization. During the preparation of data from the present study, van Marwijik Kooy *et al.* published their report indicating that leukocyte depletion from platelet concentrates was necessary to reduce the rate of alloimmunization in patients receiving frequent platelet transfusions [4]. Table 19.5 is a summary of the results of prospective randomized studies so far reported, including ours, which utilized filtration methods to prepare leukocyte-depleted blood products [2–4,9]. It should be noted that all four studies yielded a similar incidence of HLA alloimmunization in both control (31.4–50%) and filtered (6–11.7%) groups, although Sniecinski *et al.* [2] and Andreu *et al.* [3] evaluated the effects of leukocyte depletion from both red blood cells and platelet concentrates while van Marwijik Kooy *et al.* and ourselves compared the effects of leukocyte depletion from platelet concentrates only. Early in our trial, seven patients in the control group were excluded because standard red blood cells had been transfused owing to a misunderstanding of the study protocol. Of these seven, three (43%) developed anti-HLA antibodies, indicating that leukocytes contaminated in the platelet concentrates have an important role in raising alloimmunization in polytransfused patients.

Table 19.5 Prospective randomized studies showing efficacy of leukocyte-depleted blood products prepared using filtration methods

| | Blood products | | | | Human leukocyte antigen immunization rate | | |
| | Platelets | | Red blood cells | | | | |
Study	Control	Filtered	Control	Filtered	Control		Filtered
Sniecinski et al. (1988) [2]	Standard	Imugard IG-500	Standard	Imugard IG-500	10/20 (50%)	versus	3/20 (6%)
						$P < 0.01$	
Andreu et al. (1988) [3]	Standard	Imugard IG-500	Standard	Imugard IG-500	11/35 (31.4%)	versus	4/34 (11.7%)
						$P < 0.05$	
van Marwijik Kooy et al. (1991) [4]	Standard	Cell select	Cell select	Cell select	11/26 (42%)	versus	2/27 (7%)
						$P < 0.04$	
Present study	Standard	Sepacell-PL	Filtered*		8/21 (38%)	versus	2/32 (6%)
						$P < 0.01$	

*Leukocyte-depleted products supplied by Japan Red Cross or prepared by filtration with Sepacell-R at each institution.

Our study was the first clinical trial to use a special filter for platelet concentrates [9]. As compared with the Imugard IG-500 [2,3] and Cellselect filters [4], which were essentially designed for whole blood products, this second-generation filter, Sepacell-PL, needed less than 100 ml of saline for priming and yielded a better leukocyte depletion rate and platelet recovery [5]. In addition, this filter can be used at the bedside without being rinsed before and after filtration. Thus, second-generation platelet filters would appear to be the first choice for the leukocyte depletion of platelet products in clinics [13].

References

1 Murphy MF. Platelet transfusion, the problem of refractoriness. *Blood Rev* 1990;4:16–24.

2 Sniecinski I, O'Donnel MR, Nowicki B, Hill LR. Prevention of refractoriness and HLA-alloimmunization using filtered blood products. *Blood* 1988;71:1402–1407.

3 Andreu G, Dewailly J, Leberre C et al. Prevention of HLA immunization with leukocyte-poor packed red cells and platelet concentrates obtained by filtration. *Blood* 1988;72:964–969.

4 van Marwijik Kooy M, van Prooijin HC, Moes M, Bosma-Stants I, Akkerman JWN. Use of leukocyte-depleted platelet concentrates for the prevention of refractoriness and primary HLA alloimmunization: a prospective, randomized trial. *Blood* 1991;77:201–205.

5 Miyamoto M, Sasakawa S, Ishikawa Y, Ogawa A, Nishimura T, Kuroda T. Leukocyte-poor platelet concentrates at the bedside by filtration through Sepacell-PL. *Vox Sang* 1989;57:164–167.

6 Bock M, Heim MU, Weindler *et al.* White cell depletion of single-donor platelet preparations by a new adsorption filter. *Transfusion* 1991;31:333–334.

7 Kickler TS, Bell W, Ness PM, Drew H, Pall D. Depletion of white cells from platelet concentrates with a new adsorption filter. *Transfusion* 1989;29:411–414.

8 Patel S. Preparation of leukocyte-poor platelet concentrates. *Transfusion* 1989;29:562–563.

9 Handa M. The Leukocyte-depleted Blood Transfusion Therapy Study Group. Efficacy of leukocyte-depleted platelet products prepared with a second generation polyester filter in preventing HLA-alloimmunization in patients receiving multiple platelet transfusions: a prospective multi-center randomized study. (In preparation.)

10 Schiffer CA, Dutcher JP, Aisner J, Hogge D, Wiernik PH, Reilly JP. A randomized trial of leukocyte-depleted platelet transfusion to modify alloimmunization in patients with leukemia. *Blood* 1983;62:815–820.

11 Saarinen UM, Kekomaki R, Siimes MA, Myllylä G. Effective prophylaxis against platelet refractoriness in multitransfused patients by use of leukocyte-free blood components. *Blood* 1990;75:512–517.

12 Oksanen K, Kekomaki R, Ruutu T, Koskimies S, Myllylä G. Prevention of alloimmunization in patients with acute leukemia by use of white cell-reduced blood components — a randomized trial. *Transfusion* 1991;31:588–594.

13 Sekiguchi S, Takahashi TA. Leukocyte-depleted blood products and their clinical usefulness. In: Brozović B, ed. *The Role of Leukocyte Depletion in Blood Transfusion Practice*. Proceedings of the International Workshop. London: Blackwell Scientific Publications. 1989:26–36.

Discussion

OHTO (Fukushima Medical School): Your data show that almost 10% of patients developed antibodies. Can the incidence of production of alloantibodies be reduced to zero if we decrease the residual leukocytes to as close to zero as possible?

HANDA: I doubt if we can prevent the production of alloantibodies completely by decreasing the absolute number of residual leukocytes in platelets. It is reported from foreign laboratories that the incidence of platelet refractoriness could be decreased to zero by reduction of the residual leukocytes to the 10^4 level.

OHTO: Even if leukocytes are thoroughly removed HLA antigens are still expressed on the platelets. Don't they cause allosensitization?

HANDA: This is one of the basic problems. It is known that immunologic function does not work in the absence of Class II antigen. Although I have no data, I think platelets themselves are not immunogenic.

IKEDA: It is reported from examination of rats in the 1980s that allosensitization against HLA Class I antigens does not occur only by platelet transfusion. I suppose it is reasonable to think that HLA sensitization does not occur without Class II mediated response.

OHTO: With autologous transfusion, a man who has no history of allogenic transfusions developed anti-HLA antibody. I think that the fibrinogen used in the operation must have been the immunogen and that it was not the passive immunization by the γ-globulin products. Then I suppose some people may develop alloantibodies without intact cells.

IKEDA: There may be such cases. Other than the experiment with rats that I mentioned, we have also performed a rat experiment. We transfused lymphocytes that had lost their viability by freezing and thawing into another rat, but we could not observe any antibodies. The production of anti-HLA antibodies may not occur without intact cells. Of course, there is some possibility that HLA sensitization may exist as a result of repeated sensitization to dead cells or other factors.

OHTO: There is a case in which an Rh(–) donor had anti-Rh(+) antibody as a natural antibody. This phenomenon can be explained by the grandmother theory. The same mechanism possibly exists in the reaction between HLA antigen and anti-HLA antibody.

YOKOYAMA (Kyoto Red Cross Blood Center): It is desirable for blood centers that plateletpheresis products with high unit numbers and filtration are used for platelet concentrate transfusion. Actually, the demand for HLA-matched platelets is decreasing in the Kyoto Blood Center.

SEKIGUCHI: Whether blood centers should provide leukocyte-depleted blood products is an important question. As for red blood cell products, I think there is no difficulty. We can perform 1 log reduction of white cells by removing buffy coat and we can decrease this to 10^6 when we use filters. But with regard to platelets, I wonder if we can issue the leukocyte-depleted platelet concentrates practically in routine work. We filter 20 units of platelet products with only one filter at the bedside now. Is it economic to use one filter to each platelet component prepared from a 200 ml blood collection? I think we can produce leukocyte-depleted platelets if we filter at least 5 units with one filter. Therefore, as Dr Yokoyama stated, I think, as a practical policy, we should usually issue a high number of units of platelet products and when a request for the leukocyte-depleted products comes we can filtrate and deliver them.

MERYMAN: I think it's extraordinary that all of the studies that you summarized there and your study and our study, all done on different patients and with different ways of leukocyte depletion, all end up with the same answer — somewhere between 40 and 50% in controls and somewhere around 7% in the depleted. That says to me that probably the leukocyte depletion that is necessary for red cells is equally effective for platelets and the residual alloimmunization is coming from somewhere else.

HANDA: Exactly, I agree with you. Actually the studies are very heterogeneous all over the world but the outcome is very similar.

20·Leukocyte depletion of blood and blood components: current problems and solutions

B. Brozović

North London Blood Transfusion Centre, Colindale Avenue, London NW9 5BG, UK

Abstract

We now know how the allogeneic "passenger" leukocytes, present in the transfused blood, may cause immunization in the recipient against human leukocyte antigens (HLAs), immunosuppression, graft-versus-host disease (GvHD), and may serve as a vehicle for transmission of resident viruses. However, laboratory issues, such as evaluation of methods used for counting low concentrations of leukocytes as well as the cause of filtration "failures" (where the expected leukocyte depletion following filtration has not been achieved), have yet to be solved. In addition, clinical outcome measures for patients receiving leukocyte-depleted blood and blood products still await to be defined. Without the definitions it is not possible to formulate clear policies on the selection of patients likely to benefit from receiving leukocyte-depleted blood.

These issues are illustrated and discussed in this chapter. Firstly, it is concluded that the filtration provides the means for reducing the number of leukocytes in blood and platelet concentrates below the level required for HLA immunization of almost all the recipients. Secondly, the mechanism of leukocyte retention by the filter most likely involves expression of leukocyte cell adhesion molecules (CAMs) and their function. Finally, an agreement on measures of the clinical outcome in patients receiving leukocyte-depleted blood and blood products will allow comparisons between studies and enable evaluating strategies for prevention of HLA immunization.

Introduction

Since the 1950s, when it was recognized that the allogeneic "passenger" leukocytes present in transfused blood can sensitize the recipient and subsequently cause a nonhemolytic febrile transfusion reaction (NHFTR), we have learned that leukocytes in the blood and cellular blood components can also cause platelet refractoriness [1], immunosuppresion [2,3], GvHD [4,5], and may serve as a vehicle for transmission of viruses which reside in them [6,7] (Table 20.1). However, it must be borne in mind that only some recipients will suffer from one of the adverse consequences. Although we have no means of predicting who will be affected, we know that the factors which will determine the type and severity of the reaction are, on the one hand, the absolute

Table 20.1 Adverse consequences which may occur following the transfusion of allogeneic leukocytes

---

Alloimmunization
Nonhemolytic febrile transfusion reaction in patients receiving red cell transfusions
Platelet refractoriness in patients receiving platelet concentrates
Rejection of transplanted tissues or solid organs

Immunosuppression
Diminished prospects of cure in patients with malignancy
Increased susceptibility to infection

Graft-versus-host disease
In immunocompromised patients
In immunocompetent patients

Transmission of viruses (resident in the leukocytes)
Cytomegalovirus
Epstein–Barr virus
Human immunodeficiency virus types 1 and 2*
Human T-cell leukemia virus (HTLV) types I and II
Human herpes virus 6
JC virus
BK virus?

---

* Transmitted by blood and all noncellular blood components.

number of leukocytes transfused, and on the other hand, the inherited characteristics of the recipient (for example, enhanced immune responsiveness of individuals who possess HLA DRw2) and his or her acquired properties (for example, immunosuppression due to cytotoxic treatment or sensitization by pregnancy).

In spite of the immense improvement in understanding of the action of allogeneic leukocytes on the recipient made in recent years, several laboratory and clinical problems still remain to be solved.

In the laboratory two issues of particular importance are still awaiting solutions. First, methods used for the determination of low leukocyte counts should be properly evaluated, compared, and standardized. Second, accurate methods for leukocyte counting will provide the means to establish the size, if not the cause, of the filtration "failures" where the expected leukocyte depletion following filtration has not been achieved. Evidence available so far suggests that it is unlikely to be due to a defect in the manufacturing process of the filter, and that a search for the cause of the failure should be directed toward the individual variability of leukocyte surface adhesion proteins.

On the wards, the first of the issues is the definition of clinical outcome measures for measuring the patient's response to filtered (or leukocyte-depleted by other means) red cells and platelet concentrates; for example, will the presence of HLA antibodies, their titer, or their clinical manifestation define their significance? Once the clinical outcome measures are agreed upon it will become possible to define the criteria for the selection of patients most likely to benefit from receiving leukocyte-depleted blood and platelet concentrates.

Laboratory issues

Counting leukocytes in red cell preparations is more difficult than in platelet concentrates: the red cells have to be hemolyzed before the count is carried out, which may introduce error and decrease in accuracy (specificity). Furthermore, at the same concentration of leukocytes, the smaller volume of platelet concentrates increases the precision (sensitivity) of counting by one order of magnitude ($\log_{10}$). That has been found in all methods described for counting leukocytes in low concentrations: automated hematology cell counters, manual counting in standard or large-volume chambers, flow cytometry, cytospin technique and the polymerase chain reaction (PCR). It is also illustrated in Figure 20.1 and reviewed elsewhere [1,8]. In addition, the accuracy of the leukocyte count may be affected by the age of the sample, presence of leukocyte fragments, denuded leukocyte nuclei, and the presence of intact red cells and reticulocytes. The sensitivity of manual counting, flowcytometry and cytospin techniques can be enhanced by 1 or 2 $\log_{10}$ by staining nuclei with

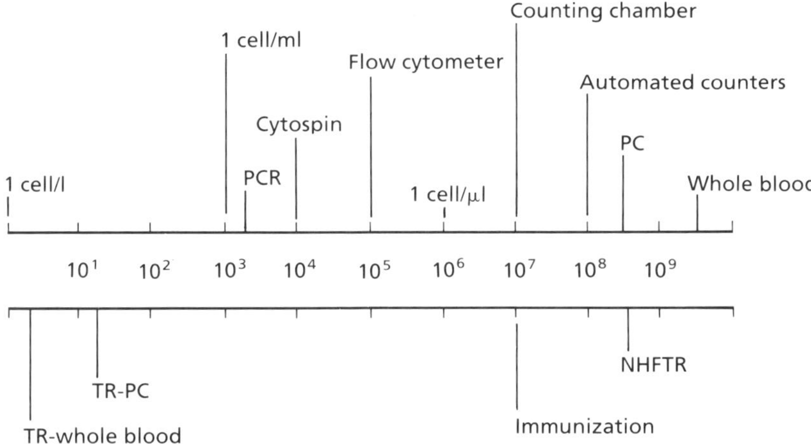

Fig. 20.1 Methods available for counting low concentrations of leukocytes and absolute numbers of leukocytes required for some clinical manifestations. The upper scale represents the concentration of leukocytes. The sensitivity of the available methods may be increased by 1 or 2 $\log_{10}$ by enhancement of the sensitivity of each method (for details, see text). The lower scale represents the minimum absolute number of leukocytes required for some clinical manifestations. NHFTR, nonhemolytic febrile transfusion reaction; PC, platelet concentrate; PCR, polymerase chain reaction; TR-PC, transmission of viruses by leukocytes in a unit of platelet concentrate; TR-whole blood, transmission of viruses by leukocytes in a unit of whole blood.

propidium iodide or by immunofluorescent labeling of leukocyte membrane antigens [9–11]. Although the differential count of leukocytes remaining after filtration has been described, the immunogenic potential of different leukocytes is not known [12–14]. It can be seen from Figure 20.1 that we are able to prevent by filtration NHFTR and HLA immunization in almost all patients receiving multiple transfusions of blood and platelet concentrates [15–17] but we are far from being able to prevent by filtration GvHD for which, at least in theory, engraftment of one live lymphocyte would be sufficient, or to prevent transmission of a disease caused by one leukocyte carrying the viral genome. Fortunately, not all live lymphocytes would be able to engraft, and only a few leukocytes may carry the viral genome (in the case of cytomegalovirus probably about 1 in 10 000 lymphocytes carries the virus).

Filter "failures," where the expected reduction of leukocytes following filtration was not achieved in all the filtered units of blood or platelet concentrates, have been seen in almost every study on filtration. Although double filtration has been suggested as a remedy for the filter failure by Friedman *et al.* [13], who also studied in detail the residual leukocytes, little is known of its cause. However, the following case and the review of previously published observations from the author's laboratory may provide a clue to that phenomenon.

> A unit of AB Rh-positive blood, donated by a 23-year-old woman on March 17, 1986, was filtered with a Sepacell R-500 filter 3 days later and sent to the hospital requesting filtered blood. A sample of filtered blood was retained and the leukocyte concentration subsequently determined was 7.0×10^9/l. At the receiving hospital the decision was made to filter the blood again, using an Imugard IG-500 filter. Following the second filtration the residual leukocyte count was 2.7×10^9/l. We recalled the donor who presented herself a week after donation in perfect health, without a history of disease in the recent past and with normal hematologic parameters including the leukocyte count of 5.1×10^9/l and a normal differential count. At that time we were unable to provide even a hypothetic explanation for this observation.

In 1989 the failure of filtration of blood donated by donors who possess hemoglobin-S trait (HbAS) has been reported by Mijović and Kruse [18]. They found that the average number of white cells in the product filtered with the Sepacell R-500 filter was 0.6×10^9 — 30 times higher than the value obtained with donations with adult hemoglobin (HbAA). A review of the original data revealed that out of 31 units of HbAS blood, seven blocked the filter, 17 had more than 0.2×10^9 leukocytes, and only seven had less than 0.2×10^9 leukocytes after filtration (Figs. 20.2 and 20.3). That is a remarkable observation since filters from that batch performed as expected when used for the filtration of blood with HbAA.

It seems to me most unlikely that the manufacturing process could be responsible for the filtration failure. In my view there is sufficient indirect evidence to indicate that

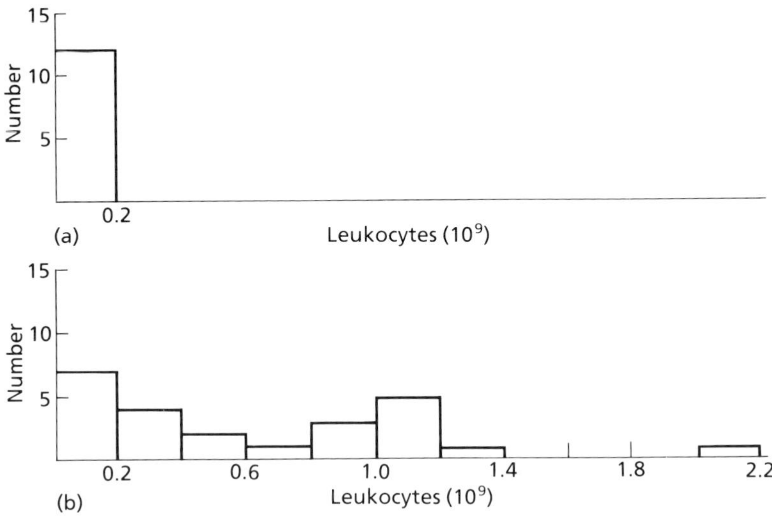

Fig. 20.2 Leukocyte depletion using the Sepacell R-500 filter in units of blood given by donors with (a) HbAA (n = 12) or (b) HbAS (n = 24).

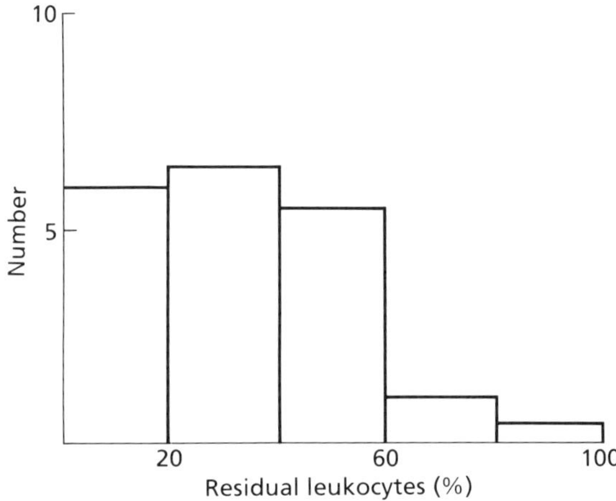

Fig. 20.3 Leukocyte depletion using the Sepacell R-500 filter in units of blood given by donors with HbAS.

the interaction between the leukocyte adhesion molecules and the chemically modified surface of the filter fibers will determine the overall capacity of the filter to retain leukocytes as well as proportions of different residual leukocyte (lymphocyte) subsets. The individual variability and/or loss of CAMs may be responsible for the loss of "stickiness" seen in some leukocytes. The natural model illustrating the role of CAMs, listed in Table 20.2 and reviewed elsewhere [19,20], is the syndrome of congenital

Table 20.2 Cell adhesion molecules (CAMs) (after Albelda and Buck [19] and Springer [20])

Integrins — heterodimeric molecules, including LFA-1
CAMs of the immunoglobulin superfamily
Cadherins — Ca^{2+}-dependent homophilic molecules
Lec-CAMs — lectin-like domains on blood cells and endothelial cells
Homing receptors on lymphocytes

leukocyte adhesion deficiency (LAD) caused by homozygous inheritance of mutation in the β_2 subunit of integrin lymphocyte function-related antigen (LFA-1), presenting clinically with recurring infections, often fatal in childhood, and with abnormal leukocytes which fail to adhere to the endothelium.

The above observations will have a major impact, first, on the evaluation of strategies for the prevention of HLA sensitization of recipients of multiple transfusions of blood and platelet concentrates, and second, on the research and development of the next generation of leukocyte-depleting filters, and finally, on the understanding of the role of LAMs in individuals with HbS.

Clinical issues

In my view the two clinical issues which deserve consideration are, firstly, the diversity of definitions used to describe the clinical outcome of multiple transfusions of allogeneic leukocytes, and secondly, the need for cost–benefit analysis in addition to cost–efficiency analysis before formulating clinical protocols for the use of filtered blood and platelet concentrates.

For example, the diversity of definitions used to describe immunization to HLA antigens is illustrated in Table 20.3. Using only two sets of criteria — the presence of the HLA antibodies and platelet refractoriness — Brand *et al.* [15] were able to describe several categories of immunized patients. It would be difficult to set the target and

Table 20.3 Presence of human leukocyte antigen (HLA) antibodies and platelet refractoriness as measures of clinical outcome in 335 patients receiving platelet concentrates (modified from Brand *et al.* [15])

Number (%) of patients	HLA antibodies*	Platelet refractoriness
266 (79)	Absent	No
18 (5)	Transient	No
20 (6)	Weak (25%)	No
31 (10)	Strong (86%)	Yes

*By lymphocytotoxicity test (% of the panel reactive).

Table 20.4 Chance of developing platelet refractoriness in 209 patients receiving platelet concentrates (after Brand *et al.* [15])

	Human leukocyte antigen phenotype	
Previous pregnancy	DRw2-positive	DRw2-negative
Yes	80% (12/15)	36% (14/39)
No	28% (13/46)	13.7% (15/109)
All	41% (25/61)	19% (29/148)

compare the achievement of the protocols for the prevention of immunization established in different departments without generally accepted agreement on definitions for immunization.

Administration of filtered blood and platelet concentrates will prevent immunization to HLAs in most of the patients receiving multiple transfusions [1,15,16,21]. That policy is expensive and would confine benefit to only a small number of patients (Table 20.3). However, by selecting those patients most likely to become immunized for transfusion with filtered blood and platelet concentrates one would maximize the benefit at a modest cost. That approach to the selection of patients has now become possible following the study by Brand *et al.* [15]. These researchers have found in a group of 209 patients receiving multiple platelet transfusions that the HLA DRw2 phenotype (inherited factor) and previous pregnancy (acquired factor) each doubled the likelihood of platelet refractoriness (Table 20.4). It certainly is true to say that the cost–benefit analysis could and should be carried out for all adverse consequences caused by transfusion of allogeneic leukocytes (listed in Table 20.1).

Conclusions

It is well established that filtration can reduce the number of leukocytes present in blood and platelet concentrates below the level required for HLA immunization of patients receiving multiple transfusions of blood and platelet concentrates.

The mechanism of leukocyte retention by the filter is not yet fully understood. Further studies to improve available methods for counting low concentrations of leukocyte on the one hand, and to unravel the cause of filtration failures on the other hand, are required.

An agreement on measure of the clinical outcome in patients receiving multiple transfusions of red cells and platelet concentrates will allow comparisons between studies performed at different centers. Measures of the clinical outcome should also be used for evaluating strategies in the prevention of HLA immunization. The financial burden of preventing HLA immunization by filtration (or by any other means) should be assessed using a cost–benefit analysis.

References

1 Meryman HT. Transfusion-induced alloimmunization and immunosuppression and the effects of leukocyte depletion. *Transfus Med Rev* 1989;3:180–193.

2 Brunson ME, Alexander JW. Mechanisms of transfusion-induced immunosuppression. *Transfusion* 1990;30:651–658.

3 Alexander JW. Transfusion-induced immunomodulation and infection. *Transfusion* 1991;31:195–196.

4 Voglesang GB. Transfusion-associated graft-versus-host disease in nonimmunocompromised hosts. *Transfusion* 1990;30:101–103.

5 Otsuka S, Kunieda K, Kitamura F *et al.* The critical role of blood from HLA-homozygous donors in fatal transfusion associated graft-versus-host disease in immunocompetent patients. *Transfusion* 1991;31:260–264.

6 Gilbert GL, Hayes K, Hudson IL, James J. Prevention of transfusion-acquired cytomegalovirus infection in infants by blood filtration to remove leukocytes. *Lancet* 1989;i:1228–1231.

7 Okochi K, Sato H. Transmission of adult T-cell leukemia virus (HTLV-1) through blood transfusion and its prevention. *AIDS Res* 1986;3:3157–3161.

8 Friedman LI, Sadoff III BJ, Stromberg RR. White cell counting in red cells and platelet: how few can we count? *Transfusion* 1990;30:387–389.

9 Sadoff BJ, Dooley DC, Kapoor V, Law P, Friedman LI, Stromberg RR. Methods for measuring a 6 $\log_{10}$ white cell depletion in red cells. *Transfusion* 1991;31:150–155.

10 Dzik WH. White cell-reduced blood components: should we go with the flow? *Transfusion* 1991;31:789–791.

11 Dumont LJ. Sampling errors and the precision associated with counting very low numbers of white cells in blood components. *Transfusion* 1991;31:428–432.

12 Vakkila J, Myllylä G. Amount and type of leukocytes in 'leukocyte-free' red cell and platelet concentrates. *Vox Sang* 1987;53:76–82.

13 Friedman J, Blanchette V, Hornstein A *et al.* White cell depletion of red cells and pooled random-donor platelet concentrates by filtration and residual lymphocyte subset analysis. *Transfusion* 1991;31:433–440.

14 Wenz B, Burns ER. Phenotypic characterization of white cells in white cell-reduced red cell concentrate using flow cytometry. *Transfusion* 1991;31:829–834.

15 Brand A, Claas FHJ, Gratama JW, Eernisse JG. Leukocyte-depleted blood components prevent primary HLA immunization in the majority of patients receiving multiple blood transfusions. In: Brozović B, ed. *The Role of Leukocyte Depletion in Blood Transfusion Practice.* Oxford: Blackwell Scientific Publications, 1989:4–7.

16 Sirchia G, Rebulla P, Parravicini A, Carnelli V, Bertolini F. Prevention of non-haemolytic transfusion reactions by a simple, effective and economical procedure. In: Brozović B, ed. *The Role of Leukocyte Depletion in Blood Transfusion Practice.* Oxford: Blackwell Scientific Publications, 1989:8–17.

17 Masse M, Andreu G, Angue M *et al.* A multicentre study on the efficiency of white cell reduction by filtration of red cells. *Transfusion* 1991;31:792–797.

18 Mijović V, Kruse A. Filtration of blood from donors with HbS: an unexpected problem. In: Brozović B, ed. *The Role of Leukocyte Depletion in Blood Transfusion Practice.* Oxford: Blackwell Scientific Publications, 1989:48–50.

19 Albelda SM, Buck CA. Integrins and other cell adhesion molecules. *FASEB J* 1990;4:2868–2880.

20 Springer TA. Adhesion receptors of the immune system. *Nature* 1990;364:425–434.

21 Oksanen K, Kekomaki ER, Ruutu T, Koskimies S, Myllylä G. Prevention of alloimmunisation in patients with acute leukemia by use of white cell-reduced blood components — a randomized trial. *Transfusion* 1991;31:588–594.

Discussion

MERYMAN: In the situation where the HbAS blood passed the leukocytes through, one possibility you did not mention was that perhaps the red cells are adhering to the filter and permitting the white cells to pass through as well as reducing the flow rate. Did you look at any filters after this?

BROZOVIĆ: Yes, that was the first thing we did. We found two things. The first one is that the recovery of red cells is not impaired, so we have the same recovery in HbAA as in HbAS blood. When we started to trace sickle cells in the system we could not demonstrate their presence in the filters. So I don't think that we can blame the presence of sickle cells for the leukocytes which are coming through. However, I must say that the times which were required for the cells to come through were quite high. The time required for the unit to be filtered was proportional to the age of the unit stored at 4°C. We looked at different age groups for about 14 days and found that with 14-day-old cells, for hemoglobin AS, you really need a good number of minutes to get the units through.

IKEDA: Did you have any chance to test lymphocyte filtration failure for mixed lymphocyte culture or some other immunologic parameters?

BROZOVIĆ: No, we haven't tested it. I can't comment.

IKEDA: You mentioned the possibility that those leukocytes or lymphocytes have some failure of the adhesion molecules.

BROZOVIĆ: That is a possibility.

SNIECINSKI: Coming from an institution that cares mainly for patients with hematologic and oncologic malignancies, and those undergoing bone marrow transplantation, I clearly see the need for the uniform provision of leukocyte-depleted blood products for those patients, and I think my standpoint may be different from that of other investigators in regard to the incidence of clinical refractoriness in patients who are not receiving such blood products. This incidence has been much higher in our studies compared to the studies of others. I deal on a daily basis with such refractory patients so I'm appreciative of the tremendous effort being made to provide adequate platelet transfusion therapy to them. I see very clear indications for decreasing the load of the leukocytes, even at increased cost, if we consider all the factors that are related to the provision of those components. So, when you state that perhaps only a small percentage of patients really do require leukocyte-depleted transfusions, I have a hard time agreeing with that.

BROZOVIĆ: I totally accept your comment. The problem, of course, lies in the cost, and if you have comparatively small costs or a small difference in cost. And it's frightfully expensive to provide HLA-matched platelets. In that case you can consider filtration. On the other hand, if your costs are differently structured, then you might find that it is very difficult to please the administrators, to get them to release more money for a procedure which might not be so obviously justified. So I think that what we have to look at is the cost–benefit analysis, and say yes, we do accept that it is going to cost more or that it is better, providing that we get clear benefits which are acceptable to the administrators, or should I say managers.

MERYMAN: You mentioned the possible use of ultraviolet (UV) irradiation as an alternative to filtration and I would like to observe that UV-B irradiation is one very effective way to inhibit the presentation of the accessory signal from the APC, which probably explains why UV-B is known to have an immunosuppressive effect. We have to be very careful about UV-B as a treatment for blood cells, since we may be preventing one problem and creating another.

BROZOVIĆ: Thank you. That's a perfect comment.

Concluding remarks

B. Brozović

I feel privileged to be given the task by Dr Sadayoshi Sekiguchi, the cochairman, of providing the concluding remarks for this symposium on leukocyte depletion and its clinical consequences.

The clinicians and researchers speaking at the symposium have shown, firstly, how complex has become the field on leukocyte depletion — nowadays it spans the range from the production of filters to the study of diverse pathologic consequences caused by administration of allogeneic leukocytes to patients requiring multiple transfusions of red cells and/or platelet concentrates. Secondly, the presenters revealed novel ways of using existing methods for counting low concentrations of leukocytes on the one hand, and interpreting the information provided by clinical studies on the other hand. Their presentations have opened up new routes for research and development in the future. Finally, it has become clear from the discussions which followed the presentations that all the participants of the symposium, whether they are working in the USA, Europe, or Japan, share the same interests and often use similar approaches to solve the current problems.

Dr R. Richter has presented an overview on the clinical importance of leukocyte depletion of red cells and platelet concentrates for patients awaiting organ transplantation. Mr M. Masse, Dr S. Stienstra, and Dr T.A. Takahashi presented different ways of using a combination of human resources and sophisticated technology for counting low concentrations of leukocytes with equal success.

Mr H. Cullis has described the design and performance of the new CS-3000 blood cell separator (Baxter Healthcare) used for the collection of platelets, with its TNX-6 separation chamber. I have provided a hypothetical explanation for the "filter failure" observed in many studies on filtration, and have addressed the question of a cost–benefit analysis for protocols on the usage of leukocyte-depleted blood products in the clinical setting.

Dr H. Meryman has presented an elegant study on the mechanism of immunization against human leukocyte antigens by allogeneic leukocytes and Dr I. Sniecinski has presented her experience in using filtered blood and platelet concentrates in her hospital. She has also provided a most illuminating analysis of cost for such a program for leukocyte-depletion of blood and platelet concentrates. Dr I. Handa has remined us all, in his presentation on the efficacy of leukocyte-depleted platelet concentrates in the prevention of alloimmunization in patients receiving multiple platelet transfusions, how successful are multicenter studies on a large number of patients at providing clear conclusions.

Finally, Dr G. Whyte presented an informative study on the beneficial effect of leukocyte removal on high molecular weight multimers of von Willebrand factor which remain in the blood stored at 4°C.

CONTENTS

LIST OF TABLES

LIST OF FIGURES

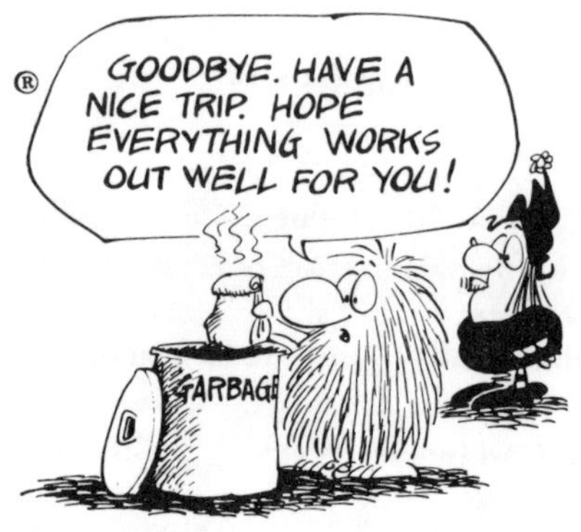

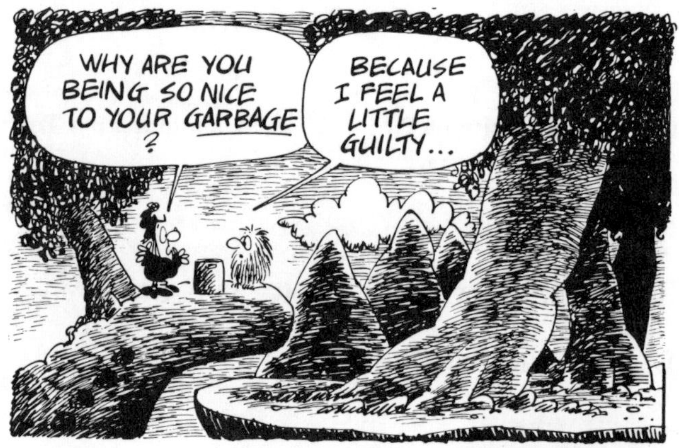

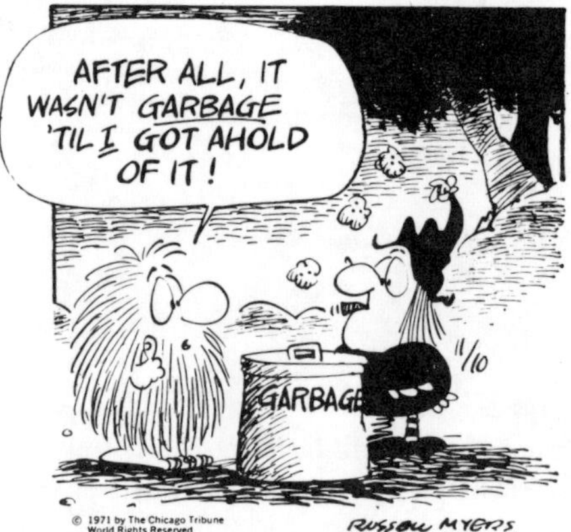

Reprinted through the courtesy of the Chicago Tribune-New York News Syndicate, Inc.

Chapter I

INTRODUCTION

Important changes in the organization of refuse collection may be in the offing in various places around the country. Many cities are in difficulty, some in periodic crisis, over the problem of removing accumulated refuse from residential dwellings and commercial and industrial establishments. Costs spiral, sanitary conditions of neighborhoods deteriorate, allegations are made that services are distributed unfairly, interruptions in service occur. At the same time, the demand for refuse collection service increases, partly because of a growing population, partly because increasing affluence leads to greater volumes of discarded material, and partly because concerns about the natural environment (e.g., air pollution) have transferred the demand for other waste removal options (such as incineration) to demand for collection and, ultimately, sanitary landfill disposal.

While cities ponder their collection problems, the private solid waste collection industry has come of age. The day of the lowly "garbageman" who drove an old truck and earned a marginal living picking up trash and salvaging what he could is rapidly disappearing. Garbage is becoming big business. Although one-truck or two-truck firms are still important, firms are growing larger, by merger and internal growth, and are modernizing their operations.[1] Many firms have expanded vertically into equipment manufacture, operation of disposal sites, and so on. Some firms have expanded operations into several separated geographic locations, while others have "gone public" in ownership.

This youthful and vigorous industry is seeking public recognition and protection. Its spokesman feel that the industry can contribute significantly to solving the problems of urban solid waste management. While this may be so, the proposed changes in the economic organization of local solid waste collection favored by some in private industry will have to be scrutinized carefully from the point of view of the public interest. In some places private industry is seeking to replace public collection. In other places, the industry wants to eliminate competition and have prices and service standards

1

controlled through a public utility type of arrangement. While such proposals may offer short-run benefits, it is perhaps more important to consider the longer run implications. This requires a basic understanding of the operating incentives that cause performance to improve or deteriorate over time. This paper therefore focuses on the <u>dynamic</u> behavior of alternative modes of organization. Thus, for example, although we will be concerned with cost per se, we will be more interested in what happens to costs over time.

In the United States at the present time, cities have chosen to organize garbage collection in a variety of ways. We begin our analysis by reviewing the choices that American cities have made and the relationship between these choices and the cities' economic and demographic characteristics. We then investigate how the supply of refuse collection should be organized economically from the standpoints of efficiency and stability. Finally, we discuss how demand should be organized; this involves the issues of financing and public decision making and criteria of general resource allocation and equity in providing the service. As we discuss these matters we develop a series of conclusions which broadly define the nature of a desirable organizational arrangement for refuse collection.

Unfortunately, the success of a waste removal program depends not only on a well-designed collection system but also on social and economic conditions, which vary from place to place. Refuse accumulation, for example, is often a symptom of more fundamental social problems -- as when a high incidence of crime in a neighborhood discourages the practice of proper sanitation methods (e.g., storage cans may be stolen, or they may be located in dangerous places). Tax laws and other economic factors may result in low levels of dwelling maintenance and underinvestment in storage or other waste treatment facilities. Lack of community pride or cohesion may weaken social restraints against unsanitary refuse accumulation or dumping in public areas such as streets or alleys. For these and other reasons, we cannot expect a given type of organizational arrangement to work equally well in all places. Individual cities have their own peculiarities and their own degrees of common economic and social problems. The motivations and attitudes of citizens, workers, and public officials vary from place to place by virtue of culture and tradition. Clearly, though, the organizational arrangements make an important difference, as they determine incentives to which residents, managers, laborers, and other important parties must respond. If the incentives associated with a given mode of organization encourage high productivity and fair treatment, and discourage wasteful practices, then we can expect improvement in performance, social conditions notwithstanding.

Chapter II

HOW REFUSE COLLECTION IS CURRENTLY ORGANIZED

In the array of public services, refuse collection displays perhaps the greatest variety of organizational practices. Here we will describe the principal types of organization and, using available survey data, see what kinds of cities tend to use these different arrangements.

In some places, refuse collection is entirely private and is still unfettered by public regulation or franchise restrictions. In cities in Oregon, such as Eugene, or in unincorporated areas of Los Angeles County, for example, collectors are required only to obtain a license to operate. No limits are set on the number of licenses issued, nor are prices or service specifications publicly controlled. Such free competition is more common for commercial and industrial waste collection than for collection in residential areas. In some cities, such as Los Angeles and Washington, D.C., commercial collection is freely competitive while residential collection is not.

In other places, collection is performed privately, but the number of collection firms is artificially (and usually severely) restricted by a regulatory agency. Within the restricted entry framework, firms may be nominally free to compete directly for accounts. The form of the regulatory body differs from place to place. In Colorado it is a public utility commission, in New York City (commercial collection) it is a bureau within the city's Department of Consumer Affairs, and in Portland, Oregon, it is nominally the city government but in reality the Teamsters local to which all collection firm owners and workers belong. The regulatory practices also vary. Colorado plans to administer prices for collection, although it currently does not. New York City establishes maximum prices. Portland collectors determine their own price schedule, subject to city approval.

Frequently, franchises to private collectors are granted on an _exclusive_ basis. Under this system, other private firms are barred from operating in an area where an exclusively franchised firm holds a certificate. In such cases, price and service regulation is usually imposed. San Francisco, which has two enfranchised companies that operate in separate areas of the city, is perhaps the best known example, but the practice is not uncommon. Exclusive franchises can be essentially permanent, as in San Francisco, or may be periodically renewable.

In the latter case, the system approaches that of a contractual arrangement between the government and private firms. Seattle, Washington, provides residential collection this way, contracting the northern half of the city to one firm and the southern half to another. Contract specifications are drawn up by the city (e.g., the Seattle Garbage Utility) and are let out to bid on a five-year basis. Revenues are collected by the city and distributed to the contractors according to the population-based formula specified in the contract. Although Seattle levies direct user charges for collection services, this is not always the case under a contract arrangement; the government may pay the contractor directly out of general revenues. In the special garbage disposal districts in unincorporated areas of Los Angeles County, the county finances contract services by additions to the property tax. Contractors in turn are paid according to a formula based on the number of electric light meters in the district (a proxy indicator of refuse collection levels).

An interesting aspect of the Seattle operation is the fact that the agency which administers the contracts (the Seattle Garbage Utility) is an independent, business-type entity, financed and administered separately from other agencies of city government. This is also the case in Tacoma, Washington, where the refuse collection system is one step closer to full public control. The Tacoma utility is also a separate municipal corporation, which performs all residential and commercial collection itself. Private collectors are not permitted to operate within the city limits. The services are supported by user charges, allowing the utility to be financially self-sustaining. Prices are regulated by the Tacoma city council in the manner of a public utility.

Finally, many cities provide refuse collection through local government itself. New York City, Los Angeles, Washington, D.C., and Denver all provide some proportion of residential collection under the auspices of a department of sanitation. Often this service is limited to certain classes of residential structures -- for example, those with fewer than a certain number of dwelling units. Financing is often through general taxes but sometimes through service charges.

While available surveys do not provide much detail on refuse collection organization in individual cities, they do furnish an overall (if simplified) picture of how practices are distributed. The 1968 National Survey of Community Solid Waste Practices[2] canvassed a significant proportion of local communities throughout the country, asking (among other questions) whether the community operated a public collection system, and what proportions of the volume of refuse was picked up by public or by private agencies. These data (which must be viewed with caution because of their poor technical quality) indicate a strong correlation between organizational practice and the size of a community, the region in which it is located, and whether it is urban or rural. In particular, the data indicate that public collection is more intensively used in urban areas and in larger communities in every region but the South, and that there are large regional differences in the use of public and private collection -- the South, Southwest, and Mid-Atlantic regions using public collection most intensively, and the Northeast, North Central, and West using it least.

The American Public Works Association survey of 1964[3] provides further detail. Table 1 shows that the exclusive use of a single arrangement – municipal (public), contract, or private -- declines as cities get larger, while the use of combinations of public and private operations increases.

Table 2 displays some additional characteristics of cities using different practices, for the sub-sample of cities in the 1964 APWA Survey with 1960 populations of 25,000 or more.[4] The results here confirm that the South leads in its preference for municipal (and municipal plus contract) collection and makes little use of private collections. The West shows the strongest preferences for private (and contract) collection and little preference for municipal service. With certain exceptions, the "pure" alternatives (municipal, contract, or private) seem to have more favor with cities that are less dense, less heavily commercial, and more heavily single-family in residential areas. The same biases seem to hold for cities favoring service charges over general tax financing.

Table 3 indicates a fair amount of stability in the distribution of practices over the years. The most outstanding change is a 10 point drop in the use of exclusively municipal collection between 1955 and 1964. On the other hand, Western City magazine,[5] in its surveys of western cities in 1958 and 1964, reports a dramatic increase in the proportion of cities using municipal collection (from 24 to 42 percent), and a significant decline (from 41 to 22 percent) in the proportion using contract services. While admittedly incomplete and outdated, the available data do suggest that urbanization and regional tradition (state law, the relative vigor of the local public and private sectors, and so on) significantly affect the choice of organizational practice for refuse collection. Within the framework of regional convention, cities have apparently tried to cope with solid waste problems brought on by urbanization by relinquishing their reliance on a single method (public, contract, or private) and favoring combinations of practices.

Little material is available on how the different arrangements affect performance. Although beyond the scope of the present paper, a very careful empirical analysis of costs and other variables would be extremely useful. Such a study will not be easy in view of the many service-quality and other factors that affect performance. Hirsch is to be commended for having included an organizational variable in his regression studies,[6] but his analysis was inconclusive, partly because it failed to account for important variations within his broad categories of "private" and "municipal" service.

Perhaps the first step is to understand how the different arrangements actually work, and how their performance tends to evolve over time. That is the focus of this paper.

TABLE 1

Proportion of Cities of Different Sizes
Using Different Collection Arrangements*

APWA Survey of 995 Cities in 1964

Method	Population in 1000's							Total No. of Cities	Proportion of Total
	5-10	10-25	25-50	50-100	100-1000	1000 and more	Not Stated		
Municipal	.47	.48	.46	.35	.37	--	.27	446	.45
Contract	.22	.19	.15	.13	.09	--	.09	175	.18
Private	.20	.12	.10	.12	.04	--	.27	130	.13
Municipal and Private	.06	.13	.14	.23	.44	.80	.27	151	.15
Municipal and Contract	.00	.03	.06	.08	.01	--	.09	33	.03
Municipal, Contract, Private	.01	.01	.03	.01	.01	.20	--	16	.02
Contract and Private	.03	.04	.06	.07	.04	--	--	44	.01
Total No. of Cities	246	359	199	97	78	5	11	995	0

*Proportions may not add up to 1.0 due to rounding errors.

TABLE 2

Cities by Basic Characteristics and Organizational Practices

- 1964 APWA Survey - Cities of Population Over 25,000 -

Characteristics of Cities Where Practice Is Used*	Organizational Arrangements: Municipal Collection	Contract Collection	Private Collection	Municipal & Private	Municipal & Contract	Contract & Private	Municipal, Contract & Private	Financing: Service Charges	General Taxes	General Taxes & Service Charges
Median Population (Thousands)	44.0	43.0	49.0	85.0	51.0	48.0	47.5	45.0	57.5	47.0
Median Family Income (a) (Dollars)	5970	6781	7018	6091	6506	6735	5862	6390	6087	6455
Median Population Density (b) (Population Per Square Mile)	4100	4048	4192	5024	4913	5334	5092	3913	4946	5141
Ratio of Commercial to Residential Establishments (c) (Median Value)	0.0379	0.0339	0.0295	0.0371	0.0398	0.0336	0.040	0.03551	0.03761	0.03561
Proportion of Housing Units That are Single Family (d) (Median Value)	0.774	0.819	0.802	0.714	0.828	0.751	0.691	0.823	0.712	0.790
Region Where Probability of Use is Highest (e)	4	9	9	6	4	8	1	7	1	4
Region Where Probability of Use is Lowest	9	7	1,3,4	4	2,7,8	3,4,7	3,4,6 7,9	1	7	6
Type of Government for which Probability of Use is Highest (f)	3	3	2,3	1	1	2,3	1	3	1	1
Type of Government for which Probability of Use is Lowest	2	2	1	3	3	1	3	1	2	3

*See Notes on Following Page.

NOTES
TO
TABLE 2

(a) 1960 Census.
(b) 1960 Census.
(c) Census, 1960 Housing, 1963 Commercial Establishments.
(d) Census, 1960 Housing, 1963 Commercial Establishments.
(e) Department of Health, Education and Welfare Regions.

REGION	STATES
1	Connecticut, Maine, Massachusetts, New Hampshire, Rhode Island, Vermont
2	Delaware, New Jersey, New York, Pennsyvania
3	Kentucky, Maryland, North Carolina, Virginia, West Virginia, District of Columbia
4	Alabama, Florida, Georgia, Mississippi, South Carolina, Tennessee
5	Illinois, Indiana, Michigan, Ohio, Wisconsin
6	Iowa, Kansas, Minnesota, Missouri, Nebraska, North Dakota, South Dakota
7	Arkansas, Louisiana, New Mexico, Oklahoma, Texas
8	Colorado, Idaho, Montana, Utah, Wyoming
9	Alaska, Arizona, California, Hawaii, Nevada, Oregon, Washington

(f) International City Manager's Association Master File, 1965

Code: 1. Mayor-Council; 2. Council-Manager; and
3. Other: Town Meeting, Commission, etc.

TABLE 3

American Public Works Association Surveys

Type of Collection Agency Used by Cities in 1939, 1955 and 1964.*

Collection Agency	A 1939 Survey		B 1955 Survey		C 1964 Survey	
	Number of Cities	%	Number of Cities	%	Number of Cities	%
Municipal	105	55	494	55	446	45
Contract	34	18	134	15	175	18
Private	20	11	95	11	130	13
Mun. & Private	20	10	51	6	151	15
Mun. & Contract	4	2	72	8	33	3
Mun., Con., Private	–	--	26	3	16	2
Contract & Private	7	4	21	2	44	5
Total	190		893		995	

*Percentage may not add to 100% because of rounding.

Chapter III

THE ECONOMIC FRAMEWORK FOR REFUSE COLLECTION SUPPLY

What kinds of agencies should deliver refuse collection services, and under what economic ground rules should these agencies operate? The alternatives are private, governmental, or nonprofit collection firms operating within competitive or regulatory frameworks of different kinds. The choices hinge primarily on three criteria: efficiency, quality control, and stability. We aim for a system that will deliver services at as low a cost as possible while maintaining quality and presenting an acceptable risk of service discontinuity. These criteria, and their organizational implications, are discussed below. The questions of what the level and quality of services should be, and how these should be determined, are dealt with separately in Chapter Four which focuses on the organization of "demand" for refuse collection.

OPERATIONAL EFFICIENCY

The major portion of solid waste management effort -- about 80 percent of expenditures for solid waste collection and disposal[7] -- is devoted to collection. Especially in our large cities, lagging productivity in collection is an outstanding problem.

The major item of expenditure in the budgets of solid waste collection agencies is labor. In Washington, D.C., for example, labor costs (not including management personnel) amounted to approximately 85 percent of the total cost of collecting trash, garbage, or ashes, or cleaning streets in fiscal year 1969.[8] In Fort Worth, Texas, <u>total</u> labor expenses were 66 percent of the sanitation division budget,[9] while in New York City labor expenses amounted to 78 percent of total refuse collection costs[10] in that year. Although these figures are not perfectly comparable to one another, they do serve to indicate that labor is the major cost component.

This fact has great implications for the future of refuse collection, as labor continues to become more expensive. A University

13

14

of California report for the Public Health Service, for example, warns
of systematic failures in solid waste collection systems unless lower
"labor to output ratios" are achieved.[11] This is evident. In New York
City, the productivity of labor in collection activity from fiscal year
1959 to fiscal year 1969 has shown almost no net change over the
period, while direct expenses of collection increased 13.4 percent <u>per
year</u>.[12] In Fort Worth, productivity increased from 422 tons per man
in fiscal year 1965 to 469.3 in fiscal year 1970, an increase of 11.2
percent. Personnel expenditures per employee, on the other hand,
increased by 33.4 percent in the same period.[13]

There are three conceivable avenues of relief for this lagging
productivity: (1) increase worker motivation and productivity
directly, (2) improve management decisions regarding the use of
equipment, labor and new technology, and (3) adjust external constraints
which limit management's prerogatives or inhibit the exploitation of
potential economies of density and scale in collection. Organizational
arrangements for refuse collection should directly address the third
measure, while providing positive long-run incentives for the first
two. These three factors and their implications for refuse collection
organization are discussed below.

Organizational Implications of Personnel Systems

To improve labor productivity, a personnel management system
should provide: incentives for workers to perform their daily routines
efficiently and conscientiously; opportunities to discipline recalcitrant
worker behavior and to reward outstanding work; and benefits and
working conditions of sufficient quality to attract and maintain a
stable and competent work force. The first two of these objectives
are highly dependent on the ability of management to deploy and
supervise workers. The second objective also depends on the degree of
discretion allowed to management in dealing with personnel. The
third objective depends on the resources available to the collection
agency and the opportunity structure within that agency, as well as on
the motivation, sensitivity, and flexibility of management in dealing
with labor's requirements. These various elements in turn depend on
organizational factors, such as the size of the agency and whether it
is public or private.

To encourage good performance on a day-to-day basis, employees must be rewarded in some immediate way for completing their collection routines quickly and conscientiously. The incentive can (and often does) consist of increased leisure time gained by completing a designated workload (e.g., truckloads, or, preferably, complete servicing of a given route) in less than the nominal workday. In principle, a leisure-time incentive system should allow the gains achieved by increased worker efficiency to be shared by both the workers and the public. The workers should receive benefits in the form of increased leisure, while the public should gain from lower costs per unit of output. This requires proper supervision to ensure that quality is maintained (i.e., that no corners are cut in completing assigned tasks) and periodic reevaluation of workload assignments to keep the actual length of working days at an efficient level. To ensure that workers do not consume all of the gains in the form of increased leisure, a portion of every hour saved by increased worker efficiency must be "taxed" away through workload revisions to provide savings to the public.

Periodic workload reevaluation is also necessary to accommodate changing service demands and crew capabilities along routes. Thus, successful workload assignment requires management's interest in efficiency, both to prevent workers from usurping more than their share of the gains, or from being overloaded to a point where incentives for efficiency dissolve.

Effective supervision of work crews also depends on the size of the organization.[14] A collection agency must be small enough to permit close ties between workers and foremen, and foremen and management. If every foreman has to oversee fifty crews or if the management executive has to keep tabs on a hundred foremen or go through several layers of middle managers to find out what is happening in the field, then the visibility of the crews and the ability to supervise is lost. The importance of supervision as an efficiency factor implies that the size of the collection agency should be limited. This does not necessarily preclude large firms or government bureaus, but if collection is performed by large organizations, route management operations at least should be decentralized. (Functions like billing and accounting on the other hand, are more efficiently performed centrally.)

Any system of personnel management will offer opportunities for abuse by workers. Some benefits, for example, such as sick leave, are especially subject to misuse. Incentive methods exist for minimizing such abuse, but these again require a vigilant management. For example, the "collapsing system" of personnel deployment discourages absenteeism. Under this system, alternative work schedules, corresponding to different levels of absenteeism, are drawn up. On a day when worker attendance is high, the work plan will allow completion of routes early in the day. On low attendance days, fewer crews will have to cover more territory, resulting in a longer day's work. On a normal day, crews would finish in the nominal amount of time. Group pressure is thus created among workers to minimize lost work days. Just as for the leisure time incentive system of daily workload allocation, the collapsing system plan must be carefully administered to avoid workloads that are frequently too light or too heavy.

Abuse by personnel can result from too much occupational security. If it becomes very difficult to discipline an errant worker, or terminate his employment when necessary, then problematic workers can exert a drag on the system. Conversely, if it is difficult to reward outstanding workers, opportunities will be lost for improving operations. Thus, an efficient personnel system must provide reasonable flexibility in hiring and firing, awarding promotions and raises, and taking disciplinary actions. The important organizational consideration here is whether the civil service or private industry model is preferable.[15] The private industry employment model has far greater flexibility than civil service. The latter tends to be rigid and impersonal. Fixed rules govern decisions on pay and promotion. Formal procedures are often required for requests, appeals, or complaints. Many decisions are made by a separate civil service commission, apart from the public collection agency's immediate management staff. The results may work at cross-purposes to the service agency's objectives. Advancement of workers, for example, may be through civil service examinations, putting men with manual work at an unfair disadvantage and failing to reward them for good performance on the job. Furthermore, supervisory positions may be appointed "from out of the ranks" based on cross-departmental civil service rankings. This practice can create dissension among sanitation workers who feel they deserve promotion. In theory, at least, the private model presents none of these difficulties.

The fault of the private system is the greater risks it presents of arbitrary or capricious decision-making, an abuse that can be held in check by labor unions in any case.

The third personnel objective – to attract and maintain a stable and conscientious work force – is a singularly difficult problem since "garbageman" is generally viewed as a low prestige occupation. Several traditional factors are essential to developing "professional pride" among refuse collectors, including respectable salaries, fringe benefits, reasonable working conditions, security, and prospects for advancement. In short, the service should offer the chance of a good career, in contrast to a day-to-day piecework system of employment. While some would argue the folly of establishing a seemingly more expensive career service for sanitationmen (since "anyone can empty a can of garbage"), collection agencies must have the means to attract good workers from the available labor pool. How attractive the job of the sanitation man needs to be made will depend, of course, on general conditions in the labor market as well as on what quality of service is demanded. In any case, there are certain organizational parameters that will affect the collection agency's ability to provide desirable job characteristics.

Perhaps the most important of these is organizational size. Very small agencies will be unable to offer very attractive career benefits because of the costs involved and the limited opportunities for advancement. Very large agencies will of course be able to offer generous benefits and advancement opportunities. Civil service, in particular, may provide fringe benefits and advancement opportunities unparalleled for such an occupation. At some point, however, large size necessarily means depersonalization and contributes to a sense of powerlessness on the part of the worker. A logical outcome of large size is the emergence of unions to represent the workers in their individual dealings with the employers.[16] A middle-sized collection agency seems desirable for providing attractive employment opportunities, especially if effective worker representation is lacking.

Another factor in attracting good workers and promoting efficiency is the workers' stake in the financial success of the collection business. Laborers could conceivably be provided financial interest through profit-sharing, stock ownership, or other such plans. In San Francisco the original partners (or their beneficiaries) who banded together to form the two large companies, Sunset Scavenger and Golden Gate Disposal, each own a share of the business. The current shareholders are collectors as well, route foremen in particular. But the apparent experience under that arrangement is that shareholders as well as hired workers press for increases in <u>wages</u> (through the union), rather than returns from ownership. This may, however, be partly because the regulatory arrangement for collection in San Francisco restricts allowable profits.

Our discussion thus far has dealt with personnel considerations in terms of management's policies toward its employees as individuals. We have found that the size of the organization should be moderate -- small enough to offer proper supervision and avoid excessive depersonalization, but large enough to permit attractive benefits and advancement opportunities. We have also found that a private career service offers more management flexibility than does a civil service structure, implying a disadvantage to collection by a government bureau. Throughout, we have noted how important it is for management to be concerned about worker efficiency.

Management, however, deals with workers not only as individuals but also as a group, through labor unions. The incentives and capability of management to deal effectively with unions, especially in contract negotiations, are particularly crucial to collection efficiency. This has important organization implications, as we shall see below.

Labor Unions and Collection System Organization

Unionization of workers is a factor to be reckoned with in both public and private refuse collection. The Teamsters Union most often represents private agency sanitation workers but also represents some in the public agencies, while the American Federation of State, County, and Municipal Employees has organized a significant portion of public agency work forces.[17]

As we observed earlier, one reason for worker organization is that depersonalization in large collection agencies makes it difficult for workers and management to negotiate their concerns and settle their differences. Unions ease this problem by providing a communications channel and a negotiating representative for labor. Even in the public collection agencies, where civil service traditionally performed these communications and judicial functions, unions are beginning to play a major role.[18]

Clearly another reason workers choose to organize is their belief that unionization will result in higher wages and benefits and better working conditions than they can achieve by negotiating as individuals. The validity of this proposition hinges in part, on the organization of collection as an industry. If refuse collection is provided by a government bureau, an exclusively franchised private collector, a cartelized multi-firm industry, or some other non-competitive arrangement, the employer will have a certain degree of monopsony power in the labor market and workers may be at a competitive disadvantage. Both public and private agencies may tend to exploit this power, consciously or implicitly, but for different financial reasons -- the private firm for profit, and the public agency for pressing claims to the government budget in other areas. Following Galbraith's hypothesis of countervailing power, strong unions will emerge in these circumstances to offset the employer's advantage.[19]

In a competitive collection industry, on the other hand, labor will be offered competitive wages and benefits. The process of unionizing will be more difficult and the rewards less certain in these circumstances. Unless most firms in the industry can be union-ized, worker demands for greater benefits will only jeopardize their employer's competitive position and threaten the security of their jobs.

From the viewpoint of a local collection industry not yet unionized, the organizational implications are clear. Smaller, less impersonal firms in a competitive environment will discourage unionization and its potential effects on increasing the costs of collection. Assuming pervasive unionization of workers, however, management must be willing and able to effectively negotiate with labor unions.

Management's incentive to control costs and produce services as efficiently as possible will lead to aggressive negotiation. But, a second factor is management credibility; management must be convincing when it indicates that no more than a certain level of increase in wages or benefits is possible. Credibility requires that the collection agency's financial picture (balance sheet) be as clear and unambiguous as possible, so that labor and management both understand what is and what is not feasible. A government agency is at a substantial disadvantage in this regard, because of its accounting practices and access to the public purse; to a lesser extent very large private firms may be also.

Even for small or moderate sized firms, however, simply showing a clear balance sheet is not sufficient to prove credibility. On the basis of its cost/revenue picture a firm may argue that if labor demands become too severe it will be driven out of business and labor will have "killed the goose that laid the golden eggs." This is too simple a view, however, in light of the various formal and informal arrangements through which firms in the industry may act in unison to negotiate with labor or determine prices. A firm's ability to survive in the face of increased labor costs depends on its ability to pass the increases along to the consumer. While the overall demand for garbage collection is probably highly inelastic, the demand for the services of a particular firm is clearly much more elastic. The small firm that tries to raise its rates individually will risk financial losses. But if the industry as a whole raises rates, individual firms will not measurably suffer. Hence, if the industry acts collectively, labor will not be swayed by a "golden goose" argument.

The foregoing suggests that credibility in negotiations is possible only with a competitive collection industry. One may object that with a union monopoly of the labor supply, individual firms in a competitive industry (unless they are very small and can operate without hired help) are at a distinct disadvantage unless they too act collectively in negotiating labor contracts. Yet as Wellington and Winter ably point out, it is the very noncompetitiveness of provision that permits a union to exploit the inelasticity of total demand for a public service:

> ... the inelasticity of demand for governmental services
> does not necessarily mean excessive wages for governmental
> employees, any more than the inelasticity of demand for

some agricultural products means excessive income for
farmers. It is the lack of competition - monopoly -
that permits producers to take advantage of an inelastic
demand schedule.[20]

On a related point, it is interesting to note that a single union may
not dominate a local collection industry, even if all workers are
organized. In particular, different unions may represent workers in the
public and private sectors. This suggests an additional possibility for
controlling labor demands. If agencies in different sectors compete
with one another, in both input (labor) and product markets, then
agencies in the sector with the lower labor costs will be at a competitive advantage. Pressure will then fall on the union for that sector
to trim its demands for fear of losing jobs for its membership. In
fact, the very existence of another sector, even if it does not compete
for the same business, is threatening to a union whose members
belong only to one sector. The aggressive opposition that public
employee labor unions exhibit toward the option of "contracting
out" is a demonstration of this.[21] The concept of inter-sectoral
competition is further developed later where we deal with public nonprofit agencies.

Finally, if the collection agency has an efficiency-motivated
management and a fairly unambiguous cost/revenue picture and is
competitive, its success in negotiations will still depend on its
vulnerability to economic and political pressure from unions.
Perhaps only very small firms can sustain the economic burden of
a strike. In a one-truck or two-truck firm the owner-laborers can
work overtime, and with the possible assistance of a friend or
relative can manage to operate without hired help. Bigger firms or
agencies would be immobilized. If a strike reaches such proportions
as to substantially immobilize total refuse collection in a city,
political pressure enters the picture and gives unions additional
leverage for bargaining, especially against a public collection agency.[22]
Public officials know they will be blamed for service interruptions
and so may be more malleable in negotiations. This, plus the direct
political muscle of a union that represents a large number of voters
and has a significant political lobby, gives unions extra leverage
against a public agency.

If collection is private the union may still use political leverage if collection is concentrated in the hands of a few firms, or if firms in the industry act in unison in labor negotiations – through a trade association, for example. Under these conditions, the threat or execution of a strike may bring union-inspired governmental pressure to bear on the few identifiable management figures whose firms are assumed to serve in the public trust. Nevertheless, political pressure is not easily applied to private executives whose jobs are not dependent upon election.

In summary, collection agency effectiveness in labor negotiations requires financial credibility and minimum vulnerability to economic and political pressure. These requirements are best met by moderately sized nongovernmental agencies in a competitive environment. In our ensuing analysis of management incentives, we discuss the various economic environments for collection. The questions of agency size and competition will again be especially significant.

Management Motivation

Management decisions have by far the most crucial bearing on the efficiency of a collection operation. We have already observed the importance of management vigilance in maintaining good supervision, adjusting workload schedules, developing enlightened personnel policies, and negotiating with labor unions. In addition, management must make decisions about new technology and equipment and other matters. If these decisions are to be made in the interest of efficiency, management must have a constant concern with minimizing the costs of a given quality of services. This motivation stems largely from the economic nature of the collection agency and from the ground rules under which it operates.

The types of agencies we will consider are the private firm, the government bureau, and the public nonprofit corporation. These agencies may conceivably operate in a variety of economic environments – particularly the private firm, which we shall discuss first. We shall indicate the incentives and behavioral tendencies that characterize the different organizational arrangements, rather than present a perfectly representative picture of present performance in U.S. cities.

<u>*Economic Organization of Private Collection.*</u>

Beginning with open competition we will consider arrangements which progressively display more and more governmental involvement.

<u>Open Competition</u>. Where refuse collection is left essentially to the forces of the marketplace, anyone can enter the field, providing he meets the necessary health and safety standards required to obtain a license. In this situation, firms solicit individual residential and commercial accounts, and prices and service levels are determined by the impersonal forces of supply and demand. Management is motivated to produce the services desired by customers at minimum cost, for this permits increased profit margins per unit of output (tons collected) or increased <u>total</u> profits by allowing a firm to lower prices and increase its market share. As a result, firms tend to operate efficiently and to lower prices to the point where profit levels no longer attract new firms to the industry.

An exception to this behavior might occur if a very large firm were to engage in price discrimination. For example, a firm operating in two locations could lower its prices below cost in the location where it faced the strongest competition and raise its prices in the other location in an attempt to drive its competitors out of the first area and create a local monopoly there. It can then charge monopoly prices and also have a less pressing incentive to minimize costs. However, this is unlikely to succeed in refuse collection because one-truck or two-truck firms can operate with great economy and can enter or leave the industry with relative ease. If the very small firm cannot face up to discriminatory pricing by a larger one (and there is reason to believe it can), it or others like it can re-enter quickly once monopoly prices are imposed. Of course, the ease of entry (and exit) depends on the stringency of public standards imposed on collection equipment, and on the market for used garbage trucks. High equipment standards entail more expensive and more specialized trucks and containers. The result is higher entry costs because of greater initial investment and higher exit costs due to capital losses in selling used equipment in a restricted market. However, assuming fairly lenient equipment standards and a local collection industry large enough to support an active market in used equipment, smaller firms will be an integral part of an openly competitive situation.

Open competition is a hazardous environment. Firms in the industry feel constantly insecure about their customers, not only because of present competition but also because of potential competition due to the ease of new entry. One thing that existing competitors agree on is their distaste for additional competition, and this may induce existing firms to work together for tough restrictions on entry. In the past, cruder techniques have been used to "discourage" new competitors, but the control of entry now is normally accomplished under local or state governmental auspices through issuance of "franchises." (Licenses are granted to anyone meeting minimum standards of qualification; franchises are issued in very limited numbers regardless of the number of qualified applicants.) Thus, competitors may organize, usually through a trade association, to lobby for governmental restrictions which make it very difficult for new firms to enter.[23]

Competition Under Restricted Entry. There are, conceivably, four different ways that new entry can be achieved. The most common of these is to buy out an existing firm. (Under restricted entry, the sale price of a firm might be anywhere from 10 to 25 times its monthly revenue, whereas without entry control, the value would be much less, perhaps only 5 or 6 times the monthly revenue.) But this is not really new entry, for the number of franchised firms does not increase. (The total number will actually decrease if one franchised firm buys another.)

A second method of entry is to convince the controlling governmental agency that the new entry is required for "public necessity and convenience." The would-be entrant must demonstrate that the particular locale for which the franchise application is made currently receives inadequate service. He may also have to prove that the currently franchised firms either can't or won't provide better service. The entrant's attempt to prove "public necessity and convenience" may take place at a public or an administrative hearing where he will normally be opposed by the industry. The public rarely gets involved, and few new franchises are granted.

A variation of this procedure, perhaps slightly less biased against the new applicant, requires the new firm to sign up enough customers to prove consumer desire for a change of collector or to prove its financial viability.

On the basis of the customer affidavits or petitions, a hearing may be held and a new franchise awarded. In practice, this is a very difficult and expensive procedure for the would-be entrant. Customers may be reluctant to sign for fear of reprisal from their current suppliers, franchised collectors will try to discredit the customer petitions, and the controlling agency, accustomed to working with industry representatives, may not be very sympathetic to a new applicant.

Finally, new entry may be accomplished by having the government periodically put up the existing franchises for rebidding. We will set this case aside for the moment, since the behavior of firms may be substantially different if franchises are not "permanent."

Assume, therefore, that entry is severely restricted and that new entry is only possible by purchasing an existing business or by persevering through the rigors of proving "need and necessity." In such a situation existing competitors will feel quite secure from the incursions of new entries, and they will find it more practical and more attractive to cooperate with each other in certain respects. It becomes possible to obtain tacit agreement on prices and market areas, free from the fear that new competitors will attempt to undercut them. It also becomes attractive for firms to trade customer accounts thus consolidating their individual operations spatially and making it cheaper for all to operate. In essence, except in competition for new accounts, the nominally competitive industry begins to act, under restricted entry, like a cartel. Management is no longer faced with the same cost-reducing imperatives since a basic source of competition has been eliminated. The cartelization process has its limits, however, for if fixed-price levels get too far out of line, incentives for breaking the tacit agreements will increase.

Furthermore, over the long run what is left of the competitive structure under restricted entry may tend to dissolve through mergers. Firms in contiguous georgraphic areas will tend to combine, and eventually only a few large firms will be left. This is what appears to be happening in Portland, Oregon, for example, which is losing five firms a year to agglomeration. Such a result seems almost inevitable, if sometimes slow in evolving, unless arbitrary restrictions are imposed on firm size and on spatial distribution of accounts.

In summary, restrictions of entry in a nominally competitive collection industry will ease management incentives for efficiency by providing opportunities for tacit interfirm cooperation. However, as we point out later, efficiency may actually increase in the <u>short run</u> because of the spatial sorting out of routes that takes place, despite the dulling of incentives. In the long run, the industry may be reduced to a few monopolistic firms through the merger process, and managements incentives to minimize costs may deteriorate accordingly.

<u>Rate and Service Regulation.</u> In a cartelized industry or where, by evolution or design, private firms have obtained exclusive or semi- exclusive franchises for collection in local areas, some form of public price control is usually imposed for the avowed purpose of avoiding monopoly exploitation. This control normally entails prescribed service standards and a requirement to serve all customers within the area of franchise. Hence, equilibrium problems (e.g., shortages) are not at issue since firms cannot restrict output or arbitrarily raise prices, as an unregulated monopolist can. Price and service regulation is administered through a utility commission, an administrative bureau, or a local legislature.

In an exclusive franchise situation (or where there are only a few large franchised firms) rates will be established by the regulatory body, with increases normally considered upon application by the collection firm itself. Rate-making is based on an analysis of the firm's costs. As a rule, rates are set to allow the firm a "fair" rate of profit. For example, a cost-to-revenue "operating ratio" of 95 percent may be set, allowing a 5 percent profit margin. The stated rationale for this procedure is to ensure a profit level that is equitable both to the ownership of the firm and to the public and is sufficient to induce a satisfactory level of investment in the collection industry. However, even assuming that profit levels are set to satisfy these concerns, this "cost-plus" rationale defeats another important function of profit – to provide incentives for efficiency.[24]

A straight cost-plus policy clearly fails to provide a firm with productivity incentives, since an increase in cost will result in increased absolute levels of profit. Conversely, cost reductions will reduce profit levels. There are some compensating factors, however, one of which is the "regulatory lag" resulting from the slow and discontinuous nature of the rate-making process. If the regulated firm experiences a cost increase, it may be months before a rate increase is actually granted. In the interim, the firm must "tighten its belt" until a revenue increase can relieve the financial pressure. Conversely, if the firm develops a technical innovation that increases its productivity and lowers its costs, it may keep the increased profits until the regulatory body gets around to revising the rate structure. Hence regulatory lag provides an incentive for management efficiency. Another compensating factor is that under cost-plus regulation, a loss of patronage will mean a loss in profit. While demand for refuse collection may be inelastic, alternatives to garbage collection _do_ exist -- including on-site incineration, use of garbage disposals, or illicit collection by unauthorized parties. As collection becomes more expensive relative to these alternatives, some corresponding decline in its usage will result, providing incentives for efficiency even within the cost-plus framework of monopoly regulation.

Despite compensating factors, the cost-plus mode of price setting on balance does not seem to encourage management efficiency. While this may be an inevitable part of regulating monopoly franchises, there is reason to believe that positive efficiency incentives can be built into the rate setting process.[25] In principle, this would entail correlating a firm's rate of profit to its efficiency. At present, rate-making bodies make sporadic and unpredictable attempts at this when they feel that costs are getting too high or that certain cost items are inappropriate. In such cases a firm might be penalized on an _ad hoc_ basis by a cut in the profit rate, or in the base to which the profit rate is applied. But there are no examples of regulation that incorporate a uniform policy of incentive rate-making. Such a policy would penalize inefficiency by dropping allowed profit rates to levels that would lower the market value of the firm and would reward efficiency by raising profit levels to increase the firm's value. Such a system requires an ability to measure the costs attributable to management and to establish a credible norm from which deviations can be rewarded or penalized. This requirement could conceivably be met through the use of statistical techniques (e.g., regression analysis) to compare the performance of different regulated firms in the industry and to isolate differences attributable to factors under management control.[26] The difficulties in setting up a workable method are not to be minimized. In addition to the technical problems, commissions or legislatures usually lack the analytical capability to undertake the task. Yet the comments of

Professor Trebing in 1963 still apply:

> Given the potential gains, there seems to be little excuse for delay on the part of the commissions in sponsoring concerted research in the area of incentive regulation. Possibly the best organization to initiate such an effort might be the National Association for Railroad and Utilities Commissioners. Certainly in an age characterized by massive research programs on the part of governmental and private agencies as well as non-profit foundations, it does not seem inappropriate that the NARUC should assume such a responsibility.[27]

This would seem particularly relevant in view of NARUC's current interest in exploring the possibility of bringing solid waste management under the utility umbrella.[28]

The problems of regulating a multi-firm collection industry under restricted entry differ somewhat from those associated with regulating in a monopoly setting. For one thing, it is simpler to set rates directly for a few firms then for a large number of firms. In the latter case, the regulatory agency must try to identify the characteristics of a "typical" firm and gauge the rates accordingly. Any set of uniform rates is bound to be more favorable to some firms than others. Those with inherently low costs will benefit, and those with unusually high costs will suffer. To avoid "unnecessary hardships" to firms, rate-making bodies may specify a maximum rate structure, which sets upper limits on what firms may charge, but such a policy ignores the chance to build efficiency incentives into the rate structure through interfirm comparisons. In particular, one can conceive of setting rates according to the costs of the most efficient firms. This would "simulate" competition and cause inefficient firms to improve or fall by the wayside. Of course, there would be technical difficulties in developing such a system, since rates would have to be normalized for interfirm cost differences not attributable to management. Again, a sophisticated statistical regulation method would need to be developed. The alternative practice of setting uniform maximum rates, based on a conservative evaluation of the costs of a typical firm, provides little in the way of efficiency incentives to management.

This is not to say, however, that efficiency incentives will be absent under such a system. In fact the stipulated maximum rate will tend to

remain above the prevailing rate charged by firms because of the
vestiges of competitive behavior that remain in a cartelized industry.[29]
Specifically, since firms will be tempted to break the cartel agreement if
the prevailing price becomes excessive (because the opportunities for a
quick profit at the expense of competitors will become more and more
irresistable as the price gets higher and higher) the stable cartel price
quite conceivably may be below the maximum regulated rate.
Secondly, the cartel price may be kept in check by customers' options
to do their own solid waste management because at some point this
becomes worthwile, especially for large commercial establishments.
Finally, cartel agreements may not encompass new customer accounts.
If a lucrative new business or residential structure is built, the competition for its refuse collection account may be intense. The bargained
rates in such cases may exert a downward influence on the prevailing
set of established rates.

In summary, management efficiency incentives do exist within
a cartelized multi-firm (restricted entry) collection industry under
regulation, but these incentives are related to the vestiges of competition that remain, rather than the regulatory mechanism itself.

Regulation of refuse collection may be administered by a bureau
in the executive branch of local government, by an independent
commission of appointed or elected members, or by a local legislature
(or one of its committees). Whatever its nature, the regulatory
agency should be expert in the economic analysis required to set
rates and service standards for industry efficiency, and should be
motivated by its accountability to the general public rather than to
the industry alone. On the first count, all three types of agencies,
given sufficient resources, could afford the expertise required for
intelligent economic decision making. Only with a commission or
a bureau, however, is there a reasonable chance that the decision
makers themselves will have professional competence. Unfortunately,
as a matter of history, this competence has been slanted heavily
toward law and accounting rather than toward economics. Regulatory commissions especially tend to operate like courts rather
than administrative or policymaking bodies. As a result they make
decisions on a case by case basis, relying on precedent rather than

well conceived general policy and using legal rather than economic analysis.[30] This process of making economic decisions on a judicial basis has fundamental implications for efficiency. Decisions will be influenced by the relative exhuberance with which adversaries on an issue pursue their respective cases. And as Roger Noll observes:

> Most regulatory issues are of deep interest to regulated industries, with a very substantial amount of income for these industries riding on the decisions. The stake of the general public may in the aggregate be even higher, but it is diffused among a large number of unorganized individuals. Issues of regulation are likely to be extremely important to the welfare of the individuals in a regulated industry; however, to society at large any given regulatory issue is likely to be far down the list of concerns. The motivation of a single firm to fight an unfavorable regulatory decision is very high, while a regulatory decision unfavorable to the general public is unlikely to generate enough interest to cause a general public issue to be raised.[31]

The preference for amicable rather than efficient solutions puts regulatory decision making at a distinct disadvantage relative to competitive supply, since the latter, operating through impersonal market forces, reverses these priorities.

On the matter of accountability, the independent commission form of regulation falls notoriously short. Commissioners are normally appointed by an elected official, such as a governor. Election of commissioners lessens the likelihood of professional competence. On the other hand, appointed commissioners are substantially independent and isolated from the pressures of public opinion. Their only accountability is to the legislature, usually at the state level. They are not, however, so independent of the collection industry. First, the industry lobby is usually an effective influence on the legislature, which in turn can exert pressure on the commission for favorable decisions in particular cases. The medium of deliberation for a commission is the public hearing, and whereas the consuming public is rarely organized to present a coherent viewpoint, quite the opposite is true for the collection industry. Even when the industry consists of many firms, these firms often represent themselves in a unified manner through their trade associations. Aside from hearings, representatives of the industry are in touch with the commissioners on a day-to-day basis. A relationship is established between industry and the commission to facilitate the work of both. Yet in the process, without any improper behavior having occurred, the industry and the commission accommodate each other to the exclusion of the consuming public. As a result, management may become fairly relaxed about efficiency considerations.

Some of the problems with commission regulation of refuse collection might be solved by moving responsibility from the state to the local level, where public opinion can vie on more nearly equal terms with industry lobbies. There is little reason, however, to proliferate local commissions when regulation can be performed as well through the executive branch of local government. While subject to some of the same criticisms as independent commissions, executive bureaus would seem at least as liable to act in the public interest. A bureau is accountable, through the executive, to the local voting public. The voters more strongly influence an administration that must be re-elected than they do an independent commission despite the fact that the commission is accountable to the legislature. And, aside from outright corruption or dishonesty, which can manifest itself under any form of regulation, a bureau seems less subject than a commission to being dominated by the industry or harassed by industry-oriented legislators.

Theoretically, therefore, the administrative bureau has the best potential for properly balancing professional expertise and accountability to the general public. Admittedly this is an imperfect solution, for local government agencies are not generally renowned for either their outstanding competence or their integrity. However, the problem of finding a satisfactory regulatory agency indicates the precariousness of the regulatory process itself, even aside from the technical problems that would face the most competent and honest of regulatory authorities.

Collection by Contract. So far in our discussion of the various competitive and noncompetitive arrangements possible under private collection, we have assumed that collection firms provide services over an indefinite time period, subject to market forces or the good graces of governmental agencies, or both. We have concluded that unless entry is unrestricted, competition will become ineffective in providing incentives for efficiency, and that this situation is unlikely to improve under regulatory supervision. One additional option for having collection performed privately under restricted entry is to limit the time period for enfranchisement and to make the acquisition of franchises competitive. Under such an arrangement, franchises would be put up for bid periodically, with service specifications and contractor requirements drawn up in advance by the local government. Bids would be made in terms of the fee for basic service (e.g., once per week, front of house pickup) with payments made for incremental services above the basic level according to a formula specified in the contract. Since price and service specifications would be set by contract, franchises would be exclusive (no competitive function could be served by having franchise areas overlap).

As with some of the other systems we have discussed, collection by contract is a delicate arrangement, but it is also one that seems ultimately more perfectible. A contracting system involves the following stages: design of contract specifications by the public agency; bidding by the competing contractors; selection of the successful bidder; monitoring compliance with contract terms; adjustment of contract terms to accommodate unforeseen circumstances during the life of the contract. In the design stage, perhaps the trickiest problem related to efficiency is compiling specifications that are sufficiently general to attract a reasonable number of bidders but restrictive enough to discourage bidding by incompetent or disreputable collection firms. Once it has drawn up specifications, the public agency is obliged to choose the lowest qualified bidder. If it does otherwise, it may become involved in long and costly legal proceedings. Specifications design is crucial, therefore, because low bid or not, an inept or disreputable contractor may become very expensive as a result of administrative effort required to maintain compliance with contract stipulations, and also of damages caused by unsatisfactory performance. There is a high premium on weeding out the losers at the start.

One common practice for minimizing the risk of bad contractors is to require "performance bonds." Such a bond makes the financing institution responsible, up to the amount of the bond, for carrying out collection in the event that the bonded contractor fails to abide by the terms of the contract. While the execution of a performance bond (in the event of a contractor problem) can be a cumbersome matter, the bond is a valuable device, since financial institutions will presumably be unwilling to underwrite irresponsible firms.

In the bidding process itself, competing firms will attempt to slightly undercut the lowest bid competitor. An "optimal" bid is one that would win the contract yet maximize revenues within that constraint. The process can be viewed as a game, with all the temptations of industrial espionage and the prospect of collusion among bidders if opportunities arise (such as multiple contract offerings) for competitors to "fix" the bids and "split the take." Such distortions are minimized by increasing the number of bidders, for illicit activities become much more difficult to execute in a multi-firm situation. The desirability of having many bidders raises some interesting organization-related questions, such as: (a) Into how many geographic subareas should a given jurisdiction be divided for purposes of contracting? (b) Should contracts be let on all areas simultaneously or should they be staggered over time? (c) How many subareas should a given contractor be allowed to service at any one time? (d) How long a period should elapse between successive bidding opportunities?

The more contract areas there are, the greater the number of individual contractors the jurisdiction will support, hence the greater number of contractors will be available for bidding. If, however, all subarea contracts go out for bid at the same time, the competition will be diffuse and the opportunities for collusive dealing will be enhanced. Hence a staggering of the bidding process seems desirable. Some restriction should be placed on the number of subarea contracts allowed to a single contractor, for the holding of simultaneous contracts by one firm reduces the number of contractors and potential bidders a jurisdiction will support. Also, holding simultaneous contracts reduces the competitive edge in the bidding process because fewer bidders are enfranchised. Thus, to maintain the competitive edge more outside bidders would have to be sought. Unfortunately, such outside firms are typically at a disadvantage because they lack familiarity with the local territory.

On the other hand, too severe restriction on the number of contracts allowed per firm may decrease the aggressiveness of presently enfranchised firms. Finally, to preserve competitive bidding, the period between bidding opportunities should be kept relatively short so that unsuccessful bidders will not lose interest in bidding again. Loss of interest can be avoided, without making the life of an individual contract too short, if the bidding on different contract areas is staggered over time.

Once the successful bidder is awarded a contract, the problems of monitoring and compliance come to the fore. Three considerations are important at this stage: (a) possible laxity on the part of the successful bidder over the life of the contract; (b) problems of contractor compliance because of unwitting or intentional underbidding; and (c) problems of contractor compliance caused by circumstances unforeseen at the beginning of the contract period.

Awarding a contract is akin to granting an exclusive franchise, if only for a limited time. As such, the job of the public agency monitoring the contract is similar to that of a regulatory agency, except that policy decisions on price and service are already specified in the contract. It remains for the monitoring agency to enforce the terms. The tools of enforcement consist of the government's ability to withhold payments or to put a lien on payments if the firms do their own billing, and ultimately to void the contract if the firm's performance becomes intolerable. While these are drastic steps, these prerogatives put government in a position of strength to effect compliance.

The length of the contract may also determine whether the contractor becomes lax in performing his tasks. If the contract period is too long, it may give the contractor too great a feeling of security and may seriously weaken the competitive pressure which a shorter enfranchisement is supposed to provide. On the other hand, a very short contract period would diminish the attractiveness of the franchise and so decrease the number of bidders. A period of five to seven years seems appropriate since it would permit the contractor to write off his equipment over a reasonable period of time without excessive cost to the public.

Despite the safeguards of carefully drawn contract specifications and the requiring of performance bonds, contracts may sometimes be underbid. This is especially likely if the contractor believes that he can renegotiate parts of the contract after he has "bought in" and has operated under the original terms for a while. Thus, although underbidding may be a matter of mistaken calculations, it can also happen by design.

On the other hand, unforeseen circumstances can occur which threaten the viability of the contract and legitimately require adjustment (e.g., inflation or drastic changes in local demand for collection). All the better if these contingencies can be anticipated and if adjustment mechanisms, such as a cost-of-living clause, can be built into the contract. But since this is not always possible, a dilemma arises. Disallowing interim adjustments may cause serious contractor problems and threaten disruptions of service; but allowing adjustments too easily will undermine incentives for accurate bidding and efficient operation over the contract period. Any automatic adjustment based directly on cost overruns or increases in the prices of factors of production -- such as a fixed formula for sharing cost increases between the government and the contractor – will merely be reflected in the contractor's bidding and his bargaining for labor and equipment. This would seemingly make cost over-runs inevitable. In addition, with such adjustment procedures, the government would have to maintain an elaborate surveillance system to monitor contractor costs. This would bring the contracting arrangement closer in design to traditional regulation, an alternative which we have discovered is not terribly attractive. An effective compromise would be to make midterm contract adjustments possible but very difficult to obtain. For example, legislation could be required before adjustment of contract terms were permitted. If adjustment is difficult enough, contractors will be motivated toward efficiency, for any savings achieved or losses incurred will accrue directly to themselves, as they do in the case of a uniform regulatory lag.

In summary, a workable contract system for refuse collection would entail a carefully constructed set of contract specifications to attract a sufficient number of competent bidders; a performance bond requirement on collection firms; division of the governmental jurisdiction into a number of contract areas, each large enough to economically support a single collector; a maximum on the number of contracts allowed to a single firm at any given time; letting of contracts for subareas on a staggered basis over time; five to seven year life to each contract; a governmental capability to monitor contract compliance; and a very stringent procedure for permitting midterm adjustments of contracts.

Existing contract systems do not always measure up to these requirements. But contracting seems to be the one system for fully private collection which can maintain the proper efficiency incentives and avoid the diseconomies of open competition (which we discuss later).

Collection by a Government Bureau.

Private collection, as we have observed, may take place in a variety of economic environments. Collection by a government bureau, such as a department of sanitation, is more restricted. The bureau, as an administrative agency of local government, is accountable through the executive, to the local legislature. It normally operates as a monopoly supplier to whatever class of accounts it services (such as residential), although there are minor exceptions to this rule.[32]

There are several important problems with government bureau collection. Many of the difficulties stem from the bureau's inherent non-market orientation. Anthony Downs describes the situation this way:

> Unlike most other large organizations, bureaus are economically one-faced rather than two-faced. They face input markets where they buy the scarce resources they need to produce their outputs. But they face no economic markets on the output side. Therefore, they have no direct way of evaluating their outputs in relation to the costs of the inputs used to make them. This inability is of profound importance to all aspects of bureaucratic behavior . . . . Thus, there is no direct relationship between the services a bureau provides and the income it receives for providing them. Instead, it receives an allocation of resources from the central budgeting agency of a large institution of which it is a part . . . . If the bureau is part of a government, that government collects taxes from citizens who may benefit, not benefit, or be adversely affected by the bureau's activities. There is no mechanism for matching the taxes paid by each citizen with the utility he receives from government activity, whether we consider total or marginal taxes and utility.
>
> For all practical purposes, there is a complete separation of each bureau's income from its expenditures. As a result, the bureau's ability to obtain income in a market cannot serve as an objective

guide to the desirability of extending, maintaining or contracting the level of expenditures it undertakes. Nor can it aid the bureau in determining how to use the resources it controls, or in appraising the performance of individual bureaucrats. In short, the major yardsticks for decision-making used by private non-bureaucratic firms are completely unavailable to men who run bureaus.[33]

In short, bureaus have no yardstick and no profit objective by which to measure and motivate performance. Even if they did, bureaus are limited in their discretion to adjust revenues and expenditures to carry out rational economic decisions. They cannot use surplus revenues to invest in service improvements, for budget surpluses must be turned back to the treasury. Deficits are prohibited, so that potential red ink results in deteriorated services.

In addition, under bureau provision refuse collection is subject to a number of political distortions. This service has low priority on government agendas compared to police, education, fire protection, and so on. This "last in line for the tax dollar" status hampers current operations and may also preclude timely capital investments to improve productivity in future years.

The bureau's inherent shortcomings are aggravated by its monopoly position, which eliminates immediate threats to job security and agency survival. Although the legislature may threaten to cut the budget or to replace the bureau with another type of collection agency, these actions require mounting severe political pressures. Furthermore, the legislature is not apt to be effective in detecting or correcting inefficiency. As we have previously noted, legislatures are traditionally short on technical expertise and lack the time to explore technical matters in depth. Thus, except for checking by the executive budget agency, the bureau is effectively insulated from external pressure to improve productivity.

But suppose the bureau were deprived of its monopoly and were made to compete with private firms? This would stimulate the bureau's will to survive and would thus help to solve its motivation problem. Either revenues or service patronage could serve as indicators of performance. However, it is difficult to establish a regime under which a government bureau would compete fairly and efficiently with private firms. A key difficulty is to ensure that the bureau's decisions on output (and pricing and bidding, if these are involved) are based on accurate estimates of costs. It is not a simple matter for a bureau to identify the true costs of its output. Part of the cost of general governmental administration must be allocated to refuse collection. In addition, expenditures attributable to refuse collection are often intertwined with those of other departments or functions and must be separated from the other departmental budgets -- and vice versa. Even a well-designed "program budget" may fail to resolve the problem of cost separation satisfactorily.

Second, the issue of separation between revenues and expenditures remains. As long as the bureau operates on a fixed budget allocated by the legislature, its incentives to set prices or distribute outputs on rational economic grounds, will be weak. One answer to this problem is to finance the bureau out of its own revenues, an option which moves the bureau in the direction of an independent self-financing enterprise. (If collection is subsidized by government, the subsidies would of course have to be administered by an agency separate from the collection bureau.) Even with this arrangement, as long as the bureau remains a subordinate part of the local government administration, it will still be subject to political intrusions. There will be pressure to divert sanitation revenues to other priorities. Industry will press local politicians to moderate the bureau's aggressiveness in competition, and citizens may urge the government to undercut its private competitors by drawing on public resources.

These problems limit the attractiveness of collection by a government bureau in a competitive environment, although this prospect does seem more desirable than government monopoly. But the problems involved in governmental competition are reduced if the bureau is established as an independent public non profit corporation separate from the formal government structure.

Collection by a Public Nonprofit Corporation.

In the present context the public nonprofit corporation is an independent agency chartered by general local government to provide refuse collection services within the government's jurisdiction. The corporation's financial accounts are kept completely separate from those of the general government, and the corporation is required to pay the full costs of all inputs it utilizes. Revenues come from service charges or <u>explicit</u> subsidies (per unit of service rendered) from general government. The corporation operates on a business basis, with revenues required to match expenditures, except for borrowing. The corporation is managed by a salaried professional staff accountable to a board of directors appointed by public officials.

Like a private firm or a government bureau, such a corporation can also operate on a monopoly basis, whether under legislative commission or bureaucratic regulation. In this mode it would be stronger than a bureau because of its apolitical nature and greater market orientation. It would be less dynamic than a private monopoly because of its lack of a profit motive and its inherent immobility. In particular, the public nonprofit corporation is not able to grow by seeking new business outside its own political jurisdiction or in other fields of commerce.

Unlike the government bureau, however, the public nonprofit corporation could be made to compete satisfactorily with private firms, since it does not face the cost identification and revenue/expenditure separation problems or the political pressures that distort competition by a government bureau.

As with other organizational forms, the public nonprofit corporation is likely to perform best under competition, either directly for individual accounts or for contracts. The corporation's will to survive or to grow would motivate its performance in such an environment. But what purpose would such competition serve? Envision a situation of "intersectoral" competition in which a public nonprofit corporation competes with a few private firms within its jurisdiction. As a creature of the local government, the nonprofit corporation would provide a standard for measuring the performance of the private firms. As a provider of services, on the other hand, it would itself be disciplined by the market. Advantages from intersectoral competition in the labor market would, as we mentioned earlier, accrue if unions for the public (nonprofit) and private employees were distinct. In any case, intersectoral competition would exhibit the advantages of competition in general, relative to labor negotiations and management efficiency. Moreover, intersectoral competition, even with restricted entry of private firms, would be less likely than purely private competition to deteriorate into noncompetitive forms over the long run, since there would be a <u>sectoral barrier</u> to interfirm cooperation. Thus, an attractive prospect emerges: vigorous competition made viable over the long run, even under conditions of limited entry.

So far, we have concluded that motivation for efficient refuse collection is best supported by competition. We have noted that private competition, unless entry restrictions are lenient, tends to deteriorate into noncompetitive forms over the long run. However, a carefully designed system of competitive contracting or a system of competition between private and public nonprofit firms would provide alternatives for viable competition over the long run, when entry is severely limited. How far competition should be limited by restricted entry and when collection should be performed under exclusive contracts are issues that turn principally on the cost structure for collection in different localities.

The Basic Cost Structure of Collection

In refuse collection, some economies are gained by increasing the density of refuse pickups. In addition, certain economies and diseconomies of scale are associated with the size of collection firms. These and other factors set important bounds on the extent to which competition can be effective.

<u>Economies of Collection Density.</u>

The cost of collecting a ton of refuse has two basic components — labor costs and truck operating cost.[34] Each of these is inversely related to the density of pickups (i.e., the number of collection route miles needed to collect a ton of refuse). There are four types of paid labor time: pickup time — the time which collectors and drivers actually spend traveling the collection route and loading refuse into the truck; haul time — the time spent taking the full truck to the disposal point and returning empty to the collection route or garage; off-route time — the paid labor time spent off the job; and site time — the time spent unloading at the disposal point. Only the first of these components, pickup time, is affected by density of refuse along the collection routes. Hence, in characterizing labor cost per ton in the following formula, the other components are not depicted explicitly.

Labor Cost/ton = effective wage rate [(pickup time + effective haul time) per ton],

or

$$C_L = W[P(d) + H], \text{ where } d = \text{density in tons per collection route mile.}$$

Off-route time is subsumed in the effective wage rate W, which gives wages per productive working hour. Hence W is inflated to account for vacation, sick leave, retirement, as well as meal and slack times during a working day. W also includes a factor for overhead and supervision. Effective haul time H includes site time.

A graph approximating the relationship $P(d)$ between the pickup time and the density of pickups is given in Figure 1, developed in an empirical study of thirteen California cities by the University of California in 1951.[35] (The figures and numerical values used here are only for illustration and apply in concept but not in magnitude to all collection situations.) The graph may be converted to a man-minutes per ton versus tons per mile basis by multiplying the abscissa by average tons per service and the ordinate by average man-minutes per ton. The graph illustrates that density is inversely related to labor cost per ton, with the rate of labor cost savings declining rapidly at moderate densities.

Truck cost per ton has three components -- depreciation, interest, and operation (including maintenance and repair) -- each of which is also inversely related to collection density. For example, depreciation cost per ton is,

$$C_D = \frac{\text{Initial Cost per truck}}{\text{Miles/Truck-life}} \ (\text{Miles/Ton}),$$

$$= \frac{I}{M} \left(\frac{1}{d} + h \right),$$

where I is initial cost per truck, M is miles per truck life, d is tons

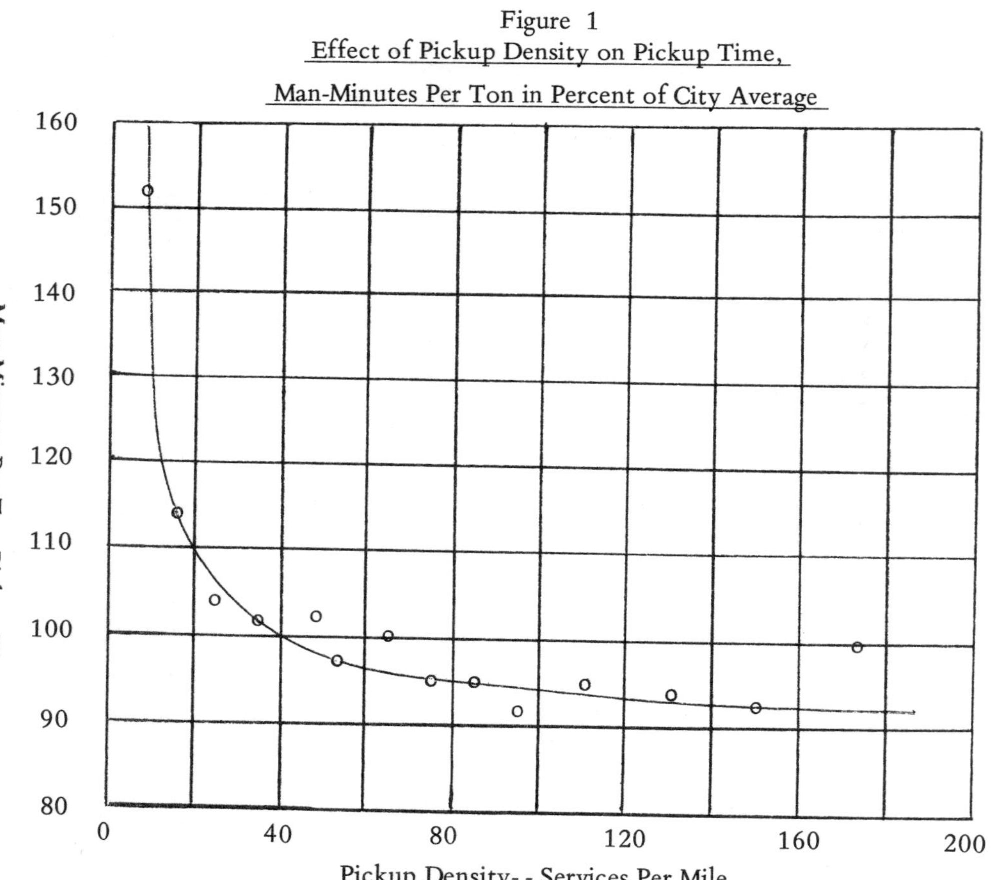

Figure 1
Effect of Pickup Density on Pickup Time,
Man-Minutes Per Ton in Percent of City Average
Man-Minutes Per Ton Pickup Time
Percent of City Average
160
150
140
130
120
110
100
90
80
0
40
80
120
160
200
Pickup Density- - Services Per Mile

per collection route mile, and h is haul miles per ton.

Similarly, we may obtain the interest cost per ton,

$$C_{INT} = \frac{I}{m} \left(1 + \frac{m}{M}\right) \frac{i}{2} \left(\frac{1}{d} + h\right) ,$$

where m is the number of miles per truck per year and i is the interest rate.[36] Finally, the operation cost per ton is:

$$C_O = c_m \left(\frac{1}{d} + h\right) ,$$

where c_m is the operating cost per mile (including fuel, maintenance, repairs, etc.).

Adding C_D, C_{INT}, and C_O, the truck operating cost per ton may be expressed as:

$$C_T = \left\{ c_m + I \left[\frac{1}{M} + \frac{i}{2m} \left(1 + \frac{m}{M}\right)\right] \right\} \left\{\frac{1}{d} + h\right\} ,$$

showing clearly the inverse relationship to density d. Thus, total cost per ton $C = C_L + C_T$ is also inversely related to d.

As an illustration, consider the following "typical" values for the parameters in the formulas:

Parameter Value	Based On
Average tons per service = .04	3 lbs. per person per day; 4 persons per service; 1 service per week
Average man-minutes per ton pickup time = 60	3 tons per hour; 3 men per truck
H, effective haul time, man-minutes per ton = 22.5	5 ton truckloads; 80% load factor or 4 tons/haul; roundtrip haul time 30 minutes; 3 men per truck

Parameter Value	Based On

W, effective wage rate
  = \$ 7.15/man-hour
  = 11.9¢/man-minute
	\$4 per hour basic wage; 25% for vacation, sick leave, and retirement; additional 25% for overhead and supervision; 1 hour out of 8 for non-productive time per working day.

I, initial cost per truck = \$20,000 i, interest rate = 6% M, miles per truck life = 100,000 m, miles per truck per year = 20,000	Equivalent to 5 year/100,000 mile truck life
c_m, operation cost per mile = \$.50	Equivalent to \$3 per hour, assuming 300 days/yr.; 7 hours per day; 10 miles per day.
h, haul miles per ton = .74	4 tons per trip; 2.8 miles per (round) trip.

[Note: No claim is made for the generality of the particular values used here. The example is solely for illustration. Guidelines for some parameters are given by Dair.][37]

Using these values, Figure 2 illustrates the labor, truck, and total cost per ton as a funtion of density d. It is evident that once moderate collection densities are reached (approximately 1.6 tons per collection route mile for this example) the rate at which additional economies of density are achieved diminishes rapidly.

One additional note is in order at this point. We have simplified the density discussion by ignoring the independent effect on cost per ton of the parameter "tons per service." As individual accounts become larger and larger the number of stops and the amount of labor time required to load a ton of refuse decreases even if the overall density in tons per mile remains constant. The effect of this is to lower the total cost curve of Figure 2, leaving its shape substantially

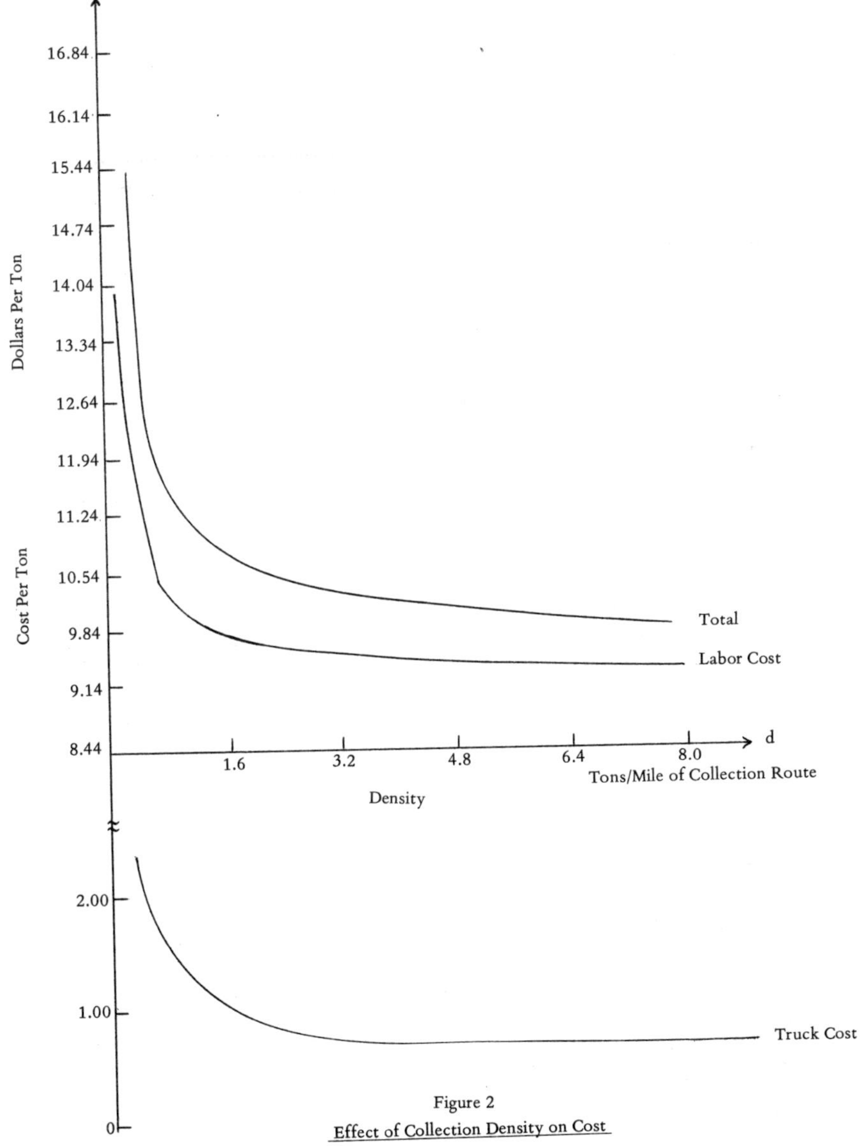

Figure 2

Effect of Collection Density on Cost

unaffected (i.e. at a given density of accounts, costs decrease as account size increases). Thus, the average tons per pickup may be viewed as a parameter affecting the height of the cost per ton versus density curve. Raising the value of tons per service lowers the curve, while increasing tons per service raises it. At some critical value of tons per service, it becomes economical to introduce a new technology – such as containerized pickup – to replace conventional loading and to lower costs even more.[38] Thus, curves in the upper range of the tons per service parameter will represent containerized pickup, while curves in the lower range will represent conventional collection methods. Services in commercial areas will be represented by points on the higher density end of curves in the upper tons per service range, while light residential services will be represented by points on the lower density end of curves in the lower tons per service range.

Economies of Scale.

Given the density of refuse along collection routes (and the size of individual accounts), the cost per ton may also be affected by the total tonnage collected by a single collection agency. Larger volumes of collected refuse require firms with more trucks and more employees. The question, therefore, is what sized firms are most efficient.

Clear empirical evidence on this question is not available.[39] What we need is a comparative cost analysis of different sized firms which isolates the effect of scale from the contributions of other independent factors that influence cost, such as density of accounts, size of individual accounts, hauling distances to disposal points, and quality of services offered. One may speculate that something is revealed about efficient size by the existing distribution of firm sizes. By this standard, small firms dominate. According to the 1971 survey,[40] 57 percent of private collection firms have three trucks or less while only 16 percent have ten trucks or more. But at the same time, firms with three trucks or less collect only 11 percent of the tonnage while those with ten or more trucks collect 68 percent, with firms in the 10 to 50 truck range accounting for 51 percent of collected tonnage. In addition, as we noted earlier, the average number of packer and nonpacker trucks per firm has increased from 3.15 in 1965 to 4.88 in 1971. These data suggest some economies of scale, but if firms are increasing in size under noncompetitive conditions, that growth reveals little about efficiency.

A priori reasoning suggests that both very small (one to three trucks) and fairly large firms (ten or more trucks) are relatively efficient. Middle-sized firms are too small to take advantage of expensive new equipment, management techniques, and so on, and too large to significantly reduce overhead as owners of small firms do by contributing their own labor. But in a very large firm, diseconomies of scale set in because of problems of supervision and control. Under these assumptions, the short-run average cost curves of firms constrained to different sizes, and the long-run average cost curve which reflects removal of that constraint, would look like those of Figure 3.[41]

Organizational Implications.

Economies of density indicate that the tons collected per route mile should be maintained above a certain minimum level. For a given collection agency, the density of collection is determined by two factors — the total tonnage of refuse generated along a collection route, and the share of the total which the given agency picks up. Thus, if several collection agencies are competing directly in a given area where their accounts are not spatially segregated, it may be efficient to limit their number to keep the density of accounts for each firm from becoming unreasonably diluted. In high-density areas, or in areas with a substantial number of high-volume commercial accounts, several overlapping competitors can be supported without much sacrifice in economy. Hence, a system of limited direct competition between private and nonprofit firms seems desirable for this case, since, as we have seen earlier, it provides greater incentives for efficiency than do other collection arrangements, without much loss from route overlap. In low-density residential areas such direct competition will not be efficient. Here, contract competition between private and nonprofit agencies or between private agencies alone, seems preferable. Such an arrangement is not affected by density economies, because contracts are awarded on a spatially exclusive basis.

Given a system of limited direct competition, or competition for spatially exclusive contracts, how large a geographic area should franchised collectors be allowed to service? Scale economies are important here. Franchise areas ought to be large enough to allow

Figure 3
Short-Run (SRAC) and Long-Run (LRAC) Average Cost Curves

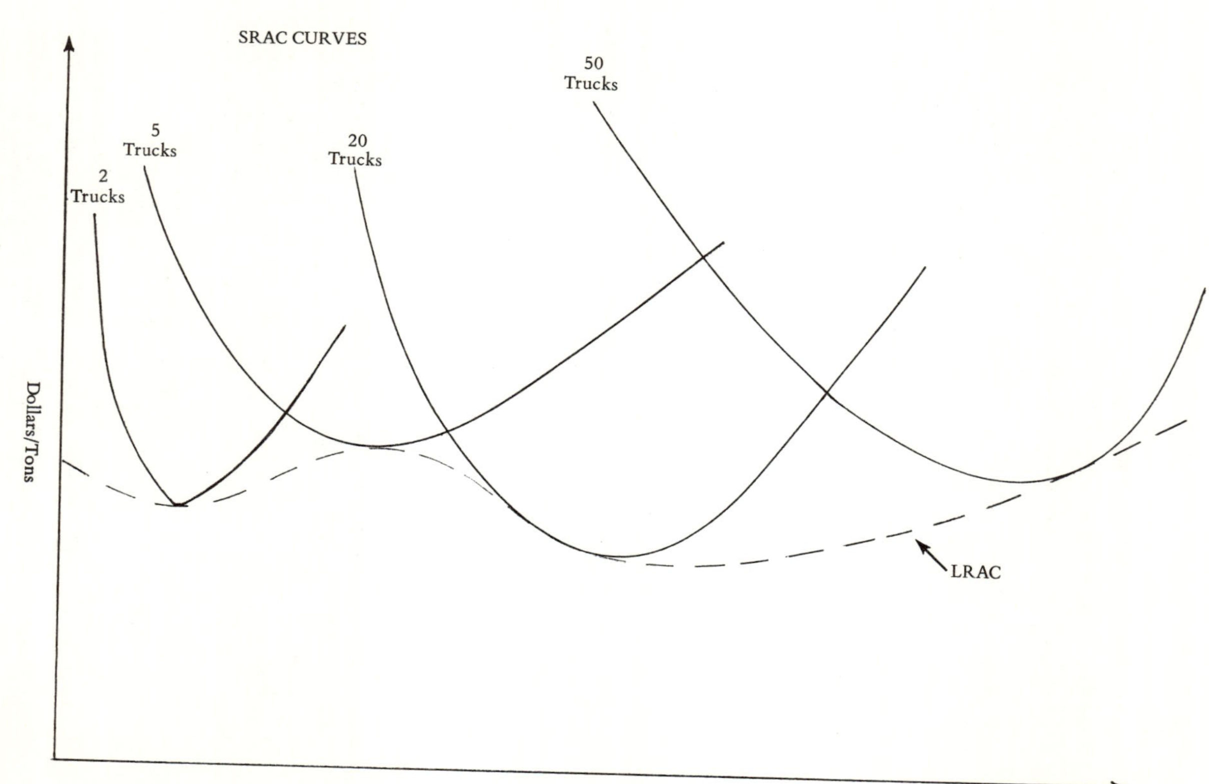

relatively large firms with ten or more trucks to operate economically, but small enough to avoid diseconomies of very large scale. For example, suppose we want franchise areas to be large enough to support a ten-truck firm but not large enough to support a 40-truck firm. Using figures from our example, if the collection density is 3.2 tons per mile and we assume that a truck hauls eight tons per day (two trips per day, four tons per trip) six days per week, with service once per week, then a 10-truck firm can serve an area with $8 \times 10 \times 6/3.2 = 125$ miles of collection route; a 40-truck firm under the same conditions will serve 500 miles of route. If we assume five blocks per mile in a square grid pattern then the lower limit would be about 10 square miles and the upper limit 50 square miles.

The minimum desirable size of the franchise areas will differ, of course, between direct competition and contract competition. Under direct competition, franchise areas must be larger, since the volume of collection per firm is diluted by that competition. Using our example, if density is 3.2 tons per mile, a ten-truck firm, under contract, would require ten square miles. If that firm shares the business within its franchise area on an equal basis with another firm, however, the effective collection density will fall to 1.6, still dense enough to achieve density economies (for our illustration) but requiring twenty square miles to occupy ten trucks.

The rationale for delineating franchise areas will also differ between systems of contract versus direct competition. Under a contract arrangement, a system of compact nonoverlapping areas should be set up. Under direct competition franchise areas must be allowed to overlap or coincide with each other as long as the distribution of competitors permits density economies to be achieved in any given neighborhood.

QUALITY CONTROL

To maintain collection efficiency also means maintaining the quality of collection. That is, lowering the costs of services, cannot be said to improve efficiency unless the quality of those services is preserved. The option to switch collection firms is probably the most effective quality control from the consumer's point of view. However, arrangements that do not involve direct competition for accounts do not permit consumers to express their dissatisfaction with service quality by switching patronage from one supplier to another. And, we have recognized that for reasons of efficiency, direct competition is not always desirable. In addition, it is not at all clear that consumer choice is very effective in controlling those aspects of quality which affect a community or neighborhood as a whole. (This issue is addressed in Chapter IV.) If I am satisfied with my collector I will most likely keep him, whether or not my neighbors approve.

Thus, additional mechanisms, namely complaints and inspections, are important in controlling the quality of refuse collection, particularly where consumer choice is absent. Fortunately, the complaint mechanism will be strongest where individual choice is missing -- first, because users have no other options and therefore concentrate their energies on complaining and, second, because it is easier to identify the offender and make him accountable if there is only one collector rather than a number of competitors.[42]

Inspection and follow-up of complaints are the responsibility of a public agency charged with maintenance of health, safety, and protection of the consumer. These functions fit best into a bureau setting in the executive branch of local government. Under a contract system, preference for the bureau setting becomes even more clear; a bureau, having designed the contract specifications and become expert in its nuances, would logically be charged with monitoring contract compliance.

STABILITY

As with police, fire protection, and other essential services, it is crucial that refuse collection be as free as possible from interruptions. Extended service discontinuity may risk public health and safety. The four major sources of instability in refuse collection — labor disputes, contract compliance problems, belligerent competition between collection agencies, and disputes between collectors and customers — are each sensitive to organizational arrangements.

Work Stoppages

In New York City in February, 1968, Memphis in March and April of 1968, and Washington, D.C., in February, 1970, there were union work stoppages by municipal sanitationmen. In these and other cases, refuse accumulation became a major problem.[43]

In our earlier discussion of management effectiveness in labor negotiations, we concluded that collection agencies should be non-governmental and competitive in the labor and product (output) markets. These characteristics are necessary to provide management with motivation, credibility, and minimum vulnerability, especially to political pressure, in labor negotiations. While there is some danger that a management which is strongly efficiency motivated will also be more vociferous in resisting union demands – thus aggravating labor tensions and increasing the probability of a strike – these virtues would, on balance, seem to work toward minimizing the number and seriousness of work stoppages. Competitive arrangements would reduce a union's ability to organize workers initially, to coordinate a strike of all suppliers and bring services to a complete standstill, and to apply leverage during a strike by pressuring public officials.

In line with these observations, direct competition between moderately-sized private and nonprofit firms would be appropriate, as long as the nonprofit corporation was truly independent of government. A system of contract competition, with stringent procedures for midterm contract revision to maintain financial credibility and with multiple contract offerings to preclude dominance of the labor market by any one collection agency, also seems acceptable. However, the political leverage that a union has, in threatening to strike a firm which has an exclusive contract for collection in a particular area, could be troublesome. This difficulty might be eliminated by arranging to have the timing of labor and contract negotiations and contract lifetimes coincide. A firm's bid would thus be made on the basis of more certain estimates of labor costs.

52

In our earlier discussion of contract systems we concluded that
to maintain efficiency incentives, the procedures for permitting midterm
modifications of contracts should be quite stringent. The other side of
this coin is that the more difficult it is to achieve midterm adjustments
the greater risk there is of precipitating a crisis in which a contractor
might abdicate his responsibilities. In the earlier discussion we noted
certain safeguards against this, particularly the requiring of performance
bonds.

Performance bonds help to maintain stability in several ways:
(1) unreliable collection firms have difficulty obtaining bonds if the
guarantee level is set too high; (2) abdication of contract responsibilities
will damage a firm's ability to obtain future performance bonds or
contract jobs; and (3) the terms of the bonding agreement make it
worthwhile for the company issuing the bond to reinstate collection
service with a minimum of delay, once a bond is "exercised."

The first two points decrease the likelihood that a bond will ever
have to be exercised. The third insures that, in such an event, the damage
will be minimized. If a bonding company is liable for collections up to
some $\underline{x}$ hundred thousand dollars, and if in the interim, when it is responsible for collection, after the contractor abdicates but before a new
contract is consummated, the company is penalized a certain amount for
each missed day of collection and, on the other hand, is allowed to
collect the revenue for days that it does provide services, then there will
be a strong financial incentive for the bonding company to have services
quickly resumed. The company may arrange this in any way it likes --
by subcontracting with another collector, or by taking over the original
collection company under a previous agreement between that contractor
and itself. Midterm contract terminations are events to be avoided if
possible. A performance bond arrangement works toward this objective
and at the same time minimizes the hardships if a contract abdication
does occur.

Unstable Competition

Where there is competition with free entry – and to a lesser extent where there are many small firms and restricted entry – there is danger of bitter competition for customers, which could deteriorate into vendettas where the weapons are not only prices. In the harsh environment of free entry, there are few structural inhibitions against aggressive behavior, and this presents opportunities for strongarm tactics and gangster influence. In a restricted entry cartel, the inhibitions are much stronger. On the other hand, the stakes are higher because the routes acquire a higher capitalized value. Hence, one firm might raid another's customers by offering unrealistically low rates and then sell the account for a capital gain once it has been acquired.

The likelihood of price instability or service disruption from these problems is minimized where collection is under contract, for under this system no direct competition for accounts takes place. Under a directly competitive system between private and nonprofit agencies, the accountability of the nonprofit organization to a publicly appointed board would act as a moderating factor. In both cases, the relatively large size of competitors, compared to a free entry or a multi-firm restricted entry situation, would give these firms high visibility. Hence, tighter public supervision could be exercised to prevent belligerent activity.

Customer-Collector Friction

Disputes between customers and collectors, a fourth potential source of instability, usually involve payments for services. The source of disagreement may be the customer's alleged irresponsibility in paying bills, or the collector's inaccuracy in estimating charges. While failure to pay bills may occur for all types of accounts, problems in estimating charges are more often confined to commercial accounts, whose demands are more variable so that proper billing is more dependent on accurate record keeping and accounting. Disputes over payment can deteriorate into situations where collection is terminated and refuse is allowed to accumulate.

Failure to pay bills will not be a problem, of course, if services are tax-financed, but the overall advantages of service charges are not outweighed by this consideration. The simplest means of avoiding service discontinuity in the event of nonpayment is to have government adjudicate the dispute, take over payments in the interim, and later collect the appropriate charges from the liable party through the tax mechanism. Several cities currently employ this kind of arrangement for waste collection, water, and other utilities.

Disputes over collection volume estimates are slightly more troublesome. Without a choice of collectors, or very intensive governmental oversight, the commercial user will be at the mercy of the collector in estimating the quantity of refuse collected. Fortunately, in commercial areas the density of accounts will be great enough to economically support direct competition. The equalization of bargaining power between customer and collector that this allows will discourage dishonesty and minimize disputes. Still, a government inspection authority, capable of auditing collection volumes, is desirable.

Another type of supplier-consumer conflict may arise on accounts which collection firms find unprofitable and thus may prefer not to service. For example, a resident in a remote location may be denied service at _any_ reasonable price because of the high marginal cost that any collector would face in providing that service. This problem is most apt to arise in low density areas where direct competition would be uneconomical. In such areas, collection should be provided under a contract system that would allow the maximum possible density of accounts per firm. Hence, enfranchisement terms could include a requirement for servicing all customers within the franchise area.

In high density areas, where direct competition is sensible, there is still a possibility of service denial by firms that lack other accounts in the location of the customer applicant. But if the area is indeed high in density then one or more firms will be capable of serving the given account without much sacrifice. Indeed, if an even distribution of accounts among firms is maintained over space, then several firms will be in a position to provide the service. These firms could be required to accept the business.

A noncompetitive restricted entry environment would seem most vulnerable to instability because of disputes between customer and collector. Abuse by the collector would be hard to police, while effective customer choice among collectors would be absent. A contract system would be easier to police and would allow for some systematic long-run choice of collectors on an areawide basis. A free entry competition, or a limited entry competition between private and nonprofit agencies would offer individual customer choice but only the latter would offer the additional potential for effective public supervision.

Chapter IV

FINANCING AND DECISIONMAKING

In the previous section we concluded that an intersectoral competitive framework would best provide an efficient and stable refuse collection service. Additional questions remain as to what level of services ought to be produced and how these services ought to be distributed. More to the point, what are the financial and public decision-making arrangements that will lead to the best patterns of service provision? The important criteria are general efficiency in the allocation of economic resources, and fairness or equity in the distribution of services and cost burdens.

SELECTION OF QUALITY AND SERVICE LEVELS

Quality can be judged from two different perspectives: the <u>individual</u> user is concerned with the frequency of service, the location of a pickup, the noise made by collectors, the care with which collectors avoid spillage or damage on his property, and so on; the <u>community</u> as a whole is concerned with the adequacy of the service in maintaining desired levels of overall sanitation and avoiding environmental disturbance, i.e., limiting the refuse accumulations, noise, spillage, and damage which affect others in addition to the immediate customer. From both the individual and community perspectives, quality includes both the <u>level</u> of services (frequency, pickup location, etc.) and the health, safety, and environmental <u>standards</u> that are heeded in providing the chosen level of services. Both of these aspects of quality will normally cost money to increase and effort to enforce.

How good should refuse collection services be, or more to the point, how should this question be decided in a given locality? As with the two perspectives on quality, both individual and collective decision-making mechanisms are required. Communities must prescribe minimum standards and levels of service to satisfy collective judgments on health, safety, and environmental problems. Above that guideline, individual discretion on service levels and standards may be indulged.

Accommodating individual quality preferences in an organizational
framework is no serious problem. The basic requirement is that the
collection agency should be able to determine the costs of requested
additional service components, and should have the incentive to provide
them upon request, for the proper charge.[44]

In view of previous observations, collection by a bureau is clearly
inadequate on these counts, while a directly competitive system is
best. Regulatory or contract systems exhibit some inertia on this
matter. Under regulation, service variations and charges would have to
be approved by the regulatory body; under a contract arrangement,
options would have to be written into the specifications.

Arrangements which properly recognize community quality
judgments will take into account the nature of the "external effects"
that give rise to collective preferences about refuse collection. An
adequate decision-making structure will recognize the spatial extent
of the external effects, usually neighborhoods, and will also be concerned with the secondary impacts which these same external effects
produce elsewhere because of inter-neighborhood "transfers."

There are two basic kinds of collective quality decisions, those
which should be differentiated by neighborhood and those which
should apply uniformly over a wide area. The dichotomy is based
on the primary and secondary impacts of external effects. The direct
impacts of refuse collection externalities such as the odors, unsight-
liness, and hazards of spilled refuse, health and safety risks from
uncollected refuse, and the noise made by discourteous or indifferent
collectors are fairly self-contained within local nieghborhood areas
defined by natural borders such as main roads or obvious changes in
land use. Refuse collection practices in local areas so defined, would
have only minor direct effects on neighborhoods outside. Residents
within these local areas should be able to make their own collective
judgments about how much it is worth to reduce the external effects,
assuming that these same residents foot the bill. Thus, local areas
should prescribe their own minimum levels of collection frequency
and corresponding minimum charges, and minimum standards on trucks

and containers. Furthermore, they should be integrally involved in the specification and selection processes for enfranchising their own collectors. To the extent, however, that local quality of services has wider impacts, the local standards must be superseded and local financing supplemented on an area-wide basis, as discussed below.

While the direct impacts of external effects may, as we have suggested, be substantially self-contained within local areas, some direct and indirect impacts of collection will be felt more widely. Collection trucks will inevitably cross neighborhoods going to and from disposal sites or garage facilities. Noise or spillage may occur en route.
Such effects require area-wide prescription of minimum truck and container standards. Perhaps more important than these minor spillovers, however, are the inter-area secondary effects. While the immediate health and safety impacts of collection may be locally confined, the fact that people within certain areas of cities live in unsanitary environments has wider ramifications. To the extent that a poorly maintained living environment is broadly detrimental to human development and social stability, the provision of universal adequate sanitation is desirable. Area-wide intervention in support of minimum levels of local collection, prescription of basic standards -- and financial support to achieve them -- are required for general efficiency, if not simply on humanitarian grounds.

It is of some interest to speculate on the nature of area-wide standards, the purpose of which is to achieve minimum levels of sanitation in all neighborhoods. Sanitation is an output that may require various levels of input, such as differing frequencies of collection, depending on the physical conditions of particular neighborhoods. In principle, therefore, an area-wide authority should prescribe the minimum levels of service required in each type of neighborhood to achieve the desired minimum levels of sanitation. Thus, there is a need for some means of measuring output directly and of then correlating it with input. The research done recently in Washington, D.C., in conjunction with that city's "operation clean-sweep" makes a significant step in this direction. In that work, a visual inspection system developed by The Urban Institute,[45] is used to assess the sanitary condition of streets and alleys on an ordinal scale. The output values can be correlated with sanitation department input to determine where collection and street-cleaning forces can be deployed most effectively.

It is clear by now that we are evolving a three-level structure for determining quality in urban refuse collection services. An area-wide, or city, authority would prescribe basic minimum standards on equipment, service frequencies by type of neighborhood, and so on, and establish a policy of financial assistance in support of these standards. Local areas could impose standards above those established on an area-wide basis, and would participate in the design and selection stages of the enfranchisement process. Finally, individual users would have the option to select, and pay for, services above the minimum prescriptions.

In theory, decision-making processes at the three levels would be similar. Area-wide authorities would prescribe minimum standards, as well as a schedule of financial support, so that the marginal benefits from reducing secondary effects and direct inter-area spillovers, would be roughly equated to the marginal costs. Local areas would select minimums above area-wide requirements such that the marginal value of reducing damages due to intra-neighborhood external effects would just exceed the marginal cost. The individual would then select his own service quality at a point above prescribed local minimums where his marginal benefit would just exceed his marginal cost.

While in practice these determinations are difficult to make accurately, the three-level structure is the only one in which the levels of choice closely correspond to the locales -- individual, neighborhood, and area-wide -- in which the different classes of benefits are contained. But, how can this three-level structure be incorporated into the organizational arrangements for collection?

The financing might work as follows: a central, municipal administrative bureau, in coordination with the local legislature, establishes a scale of subsidies, differentiated by the physical and demographic characteristics of neighborhoods, that would permit and

encourage local communities to observe the basic area-wide minimums.
The purpose of the subsidies is to foster an efficient allocation of
service benefits and costs, not simply to redistribute income. Given the
established subsidy scale, local neighborhoods, through their representatives (see below), would have the option of raising local minimum
standards above those set area-wide. In addition, residents would be
permitted to purchase individualized services above local minimums.
The collection firms would bill residential and commercial establishments
directly, with charges based on the subsidized rate structure; they would
then submit to the central bureau, the records of services provided in
order to receive reimbursement for the subsidy.

As suggested above, the proposed subsidies are financed out of
general municipal or county tax revenues. A variant of this system would
replace the general subsidies by subsidies "internal" to solid waste
collection. These subsidies would be generated by imposing charges in
excess of costs for services to certain classes of refuse collection accounts
(commercial or high-income residential) to pay for subsidies to other
classes of accounts (for instance, low-income residential). Regulated
industries often employ internal subsidy practices. For example, airline
passengers on high-density routes subsidize passengers on low-density
routes. In order to implement this practice in refuse collection within a
framework that features direct competition for accounts, an explicit
tax or surcharge would have to be imposed on the more price-inelastic
commercial or high-income residential accounts. Under a contract
system, on the other hand, the rate structure could be designed to
accomplish this cross-subsidization implicitly. Either way, the internal
subsidy system involves "taxing" certain classes of users to subsidize
other classes. Thus, it must be compared with other means of taxation
available to a locality. All methods of taxation involve administrative
costs, implications for the distribution of wealth, as well as distorting
effects on the price signals that influence the way economic resources
are allocated.[46]

The adoption of a system of internal subsidies leads to more
distortion in resource allocation within the solid waste sector than
general subsidies would, because the price of collection to certain users
is raised above cost. On the other hand, an increment in general sales,

income, or property taxes would not specifically distort prices in the
solid waste sector, but would have other more diffuse effects. As for
distributional considerations, general taxation may be more or less
regressive than an internal subsidy system, depending on the source of
general taxes. In the absence of definitive information on the incidence
and allocative effects of the alternative tax mechanisms, effects which
could well turn out to be fairly minimal when considered in the context
of the total system of taxation, perhaps the choice of subsidy
mechanism is best decided on administrative grounds.

Under a contract system, the internal subsidy method would
have the advantage of administrative simplicity, for no additional
taxing mechanism would be necessary, and subsidies could be taken care
of automatically, an advantage over the general subsidy system. Under
direct competition, however, a new taxing mechanism as well as a
new subsidy distribution system would be needed, making this less
attractive administratively than general tax-financed subsidies. Under
a mixed system of direct and contract competition the general
subsidy scheme would seem clearly preferable on administrative
grounds, since the alternative is dual systems of internal subsidies,
one for directly competitive accounts and another for contract
accounts.

Subsidy policy is clearly an area-wide function. But other
policy decisions, such as the setting and enforcement of standards,
and the corresponding administrative function that these require,
involve both area-wide and local participation. In the interests of
economy, it is desirable to minimize duplication of effort at these
two levels. If local area decision-making can be accommodated by
input into the central decision-making process, savings would be
achieved. Yet it is also essential that local representation should not
render the area-wide authority indecisive or become impotent
itself.

The risks of either hamstringing the central functions or
duplicating them on a local level seem high. A system of local
membership on a central authority for example, would mean that
decisions on area-wide standards and distribution of subsidies would
become political tugs of war between the local members. On the

other hand, limiting local participation to public testimony before the central agency would seem ineffective. This apparent dilemma may be resolved by considering in more detail the nature of the area-wide or central authority and the requirements for local area representation. The area-wide authority, representing the public in the city or county as a whole, would logically be a department of the general city or county government. Through its accountability to an executive or legislature, it would be responsible for sanitation on an area-wide basis but would not be especially sensitive to local neighborhoods. If the central agency is to bear responsibility for variations in services at the local level, it must have effective liaison with the local communities. This problem is not unique to sanitation. Other functions, such as police, transportation, housing, and so on, also require a special sensitivity to local circumstances.

In the absence of an effectively decentralized general local government, this problem might be resolved by electing general purpose neighborhood representatives as liaison with the existing city or county administrative agencies. The role of these local representatives would be to sponsor the collective judgments of their communities regarding service levels and standards. In refuse collection, the mission would be to indicate local preferences for services above the area-wide minimums and in the light of centrally determined subsidy policies. Under a contract system, representatives would participate in the design of local contract specifications and in the selection of the successful bidder. Under direct competition, the representative would participate in the process of franchising local collectors. Since these kinds of decisions need not be made very frequently they could well fit within the schedule of a general representative, responsible for several local functions in addition to sanitation.

In the absence of such a system of local representation, a central agency could incorporate local preferences on a more limited basis by using various information gathering devices. Through public hearings, surveys, and referendums, local preferences could be gathered on alternative service standards, rate schedules, and so on. The latter suggests the process used in contracting collection for the garbage disposal districts in Los Angeles County, where the county keeps records of local resident complaints and requests, and surveys the local district before writing contract specifications.

Finally, local input to decision making has important implications for delineating the boundaries of local areas. In particular, (1) local areas should conform to natural boundaries within which external effects are substantially self-contained; (2) areas should correspond to the enfranchisement areas of collectors, whether under contract or in direct competition; (3) areas should be relatively homogeneous socioeconomically to permit local consensus on service preferences; and (4) for administrative convenience and coordinated local representation, areas should correspond to service areas drawn up for other municipal functions (such as the general purpose service areas in Washington, D.C.).

GENERAL RESOURCE ALLOCATION

Quality selection is one aspect of the general consideration -- how much resources should be devoted to refuse collection and solid waste management. This question has important implications for refuse collection organization, especially financing.

Collection and Its Alternatives

While inevitably a significant part of solid waste management, refuse collection has its substitutes. On-site incineration, garbage grinding, and littering or unauthorized dumping – all by-pass the collection stage. On the other hand, collection is precursor to a number of other stages in the solid waste cycle, such as landfill disposal or salvaging, as illustrated by the flow chart of Figure 4. Thus, the cost and performance of collection, as perceived by users of this service, play a critical role in determining how resources are allocated within the solid waste management sector. A collection service that is perceived to be convenient and inexpensive will tend to increase the volume of collection activity vis-à-vis other alternatives, and will increase the usage of disposal options that follow from collection. An expensive or inconvenient collection service will encourage use of substitutes such as home garbage disposals or littering, and the subsequent solid waste processing stages that these imply. One example of the substitutive (and perhaps stimulative) effect of better or cheaper waste collection is the experience of Los Angeles County, where in 1955 a study found that the quantity of collected waste increased with the frequency of pickups.[47] Presumably more frequent service reduced the utilization of other

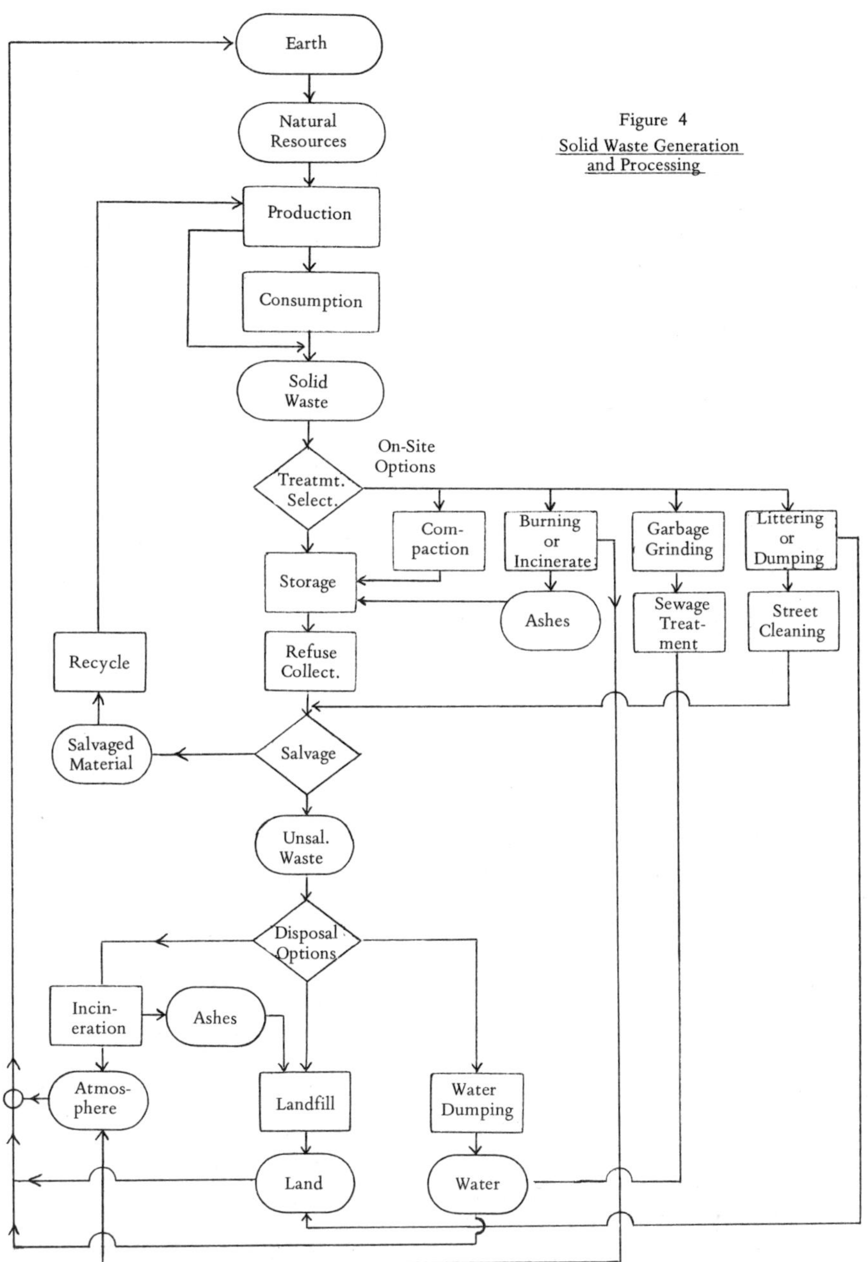

Figure 4
<u>Solid Waste Generation and Processing</u>

options, and perhaps even increased the total volume of refuse produced.
In the same vein, an Oakland report indicates that some individuals
fail to subscribe to collection services because of the cost, and that they
consequently utilize other "free" options such as littering, or depositing
in public litter baskets or in garbage cans belonging to other citizens.[48]
We must conclude that unless the relative costs of options are accurately
reflected to the users proper resource allocation will not be achieved.

Financing -- or more precisely, the question of whether collection
should be paid for out of taxes, or out of service charges that vary
according to usage and cost – is critical in determining how alternative
waste management options are perceived by existing and potential
customers of collection service. (Flat fees on a per household or per
capita basis are like taxes. Service charges, on the other hand, vary with
levels of service usage.) From a general economic point of view, the
rationale for levying cost-based charges for collection (and its substitutes)
is to ensure that economic resources are deployed efficiently among
solid waste management alternatives. The price of collection acts as an
indicator of how much of the service consumers want and how much
collectors can produce.

Without an operative pricing mechanism, decision making at the
level of the individual user would be virtually eliminated. Furthermore,
a system of direct competition for accounts would not even be feasible,
unless the government substituted a pseudo-pricing mechanism by dis-
tributing tax dollars in the form of voucher certificates (in fixed dollar
amounts) to all users of refuse collection services. Under such circumstances, individuals could choose their collector, but their discretion over
service quality would still be very limited unless supplementary payments
were permitted. Under a contract system, on the other hand, vouchers
would serve no purpose, and individual user discretion on services could
only be incorporated through a payment system.

In theory, therefore, rational pricing of collection (and its
alternatives) is clearly desirable. In practice, however, there are a few
complications. While it is quite straightforward to charge for collection
(e.g., by the can), it is not so easy to charge for some of the less desirable
substitutes such as littering, use of neighbor's garbage cans, unauthorized
dumping, accumulating refuse rather than offering it for collection, and

so on. The only way to charge for these activities is to police them vigorously and to impose financial and other penalties which, unfortunately, are by themselves fairly ineffective. Hence, charging for refuse service while some of the less desirable substitutes remain essentially "free" may only encourage use of the latter. On the other hand, collection charges will encourage a proper balance between collection and easily priced options like on-site processing by incineration or garbage grinding and may also improve consumer incentives for conserving economic resources in general, as we will discuss later.

Another objection that is often raised against service charges is the allegedly harsh burden that this imposes on lower income groups. However, it is not entirely clear how much more regressive a rational pricing and subsidy scheme for refuse collection would be than a system that is entirely tax-financed. That depends on the sources of general taxation, since the poor pay property and sales taxes as well as fees and charges. Second, the amount involved in refuse collection service charges, conservatively estimated at $5 per month, is hardly enough to justify foregoing efficiency benefits which if realized might benefit even the poor. But perhaps most important, it is necessary to recognize the problem of poverty as a separate issue, upon which the financing of a service program like refuse collection, involving only $60 per year per customer, will have no measurable impact. Short of an adequate program of income maintenance, a weak palliative measure would be to follow the example of Washington State where additional welfare allowances are granted to cover necessities such as utility bills.

Finally, note that the poverty issue here is separate from the subsidy issue associated with maintaining minimum levels of sanitation. The latter is an efficiency question while the former pertains to distribution on equity grounds. Subsidies of the kind suggested earlier, though they will modify a system of charges for refuse collection, do so in the interests of, rather than at cross-purposes to, improved use of economic resources.

On balance, the arguments for service charges appear convincing. Coupled with subsidized area-wide and neighborhood level requirements for mandatory minimum service levels, charges would present minimal risks of encouraging such practices as littering and dumping. Minimum service requirements, subsidies, policing and fines to control sanitary violations, plus governmental authority to enjoin property of residents who fail to pay their bills, would seem sufficient for minimizing such unwanted behavior.

Level of Resource Use and Waste Generation

Charges for refuse collection help allocate resources to as well as within the waste management sector. The prices associated with disposing of wastes may be reflected in the purchasing behavior of consumers (i.e., how much is bought, in what packaging, of what durability, etc.) and in the ultimate consequences of these decisions on the levels of waste that are generated.

The U. S. generates huge quantities of solid waste at a rate which is increasing at 4 percent per year (along with the GNP). Only half of that increase is attributable to increases in population; the other half is a result of increases in the solid waste generation per capita. Between 1920 and 1965 routinely collected refuse increased from 2.75 to 4.5 pounds per day per capita. Total solid waste in 1965 amounted to eight pounds per day per capita at an annual cost of collection and disposal of more than $3 billion.[49]

In addressing the issue of waste control, we must ask the paradoxical question: how much waste is economically efficient? Waste generation is costly, both in terms of direct collection and disposal expenditures, and of the environmental damage frequently associated with its management, or failure to manage it as well as possible. If the full social costs of waste generation are not reflected in the decisions of consumers and producers then a level of waste will be generated that exceeds what is economically efficient (i.e., the marginal social cost of economic output will exceed the marginal social benefit).[50] This will be true whether excessive generation of wastes is caused by excessive consumption of economic goods, or by excessive waste in the production and packaging of those goods. Hence the organizational arrangements for sanitation, particularly its financing, should facilitate the goal of "economic accountability" in waste generation.

The user charge concept for collection is thus distinctly attractive in helping to limit production and consumption and the consequent generation of waste to economically efficient levels. The charges must be made to reflect not only the costs of collection itself but also the costs of ultimate treatment and disposal. At the same time, collection agencies themselves must be made to account for the full costs of treatment and disposal through an appropriate system of disposal fees. Failure to levy waste management charges commensurate with costs will merely encourage uneconomic waste generation.

EQUITY IN SERVICE PROVISION

In different cities around the country, one observes various policies for the distribution of services and cost burdens among different population groups and neighborhoods, which, on the surface at least, appear to be "unfair." These policies are often directly related to the way refuse collection is organized.

We saw earlier that cities vary considerably in the way they finance collection services. In cities where services are supported by taxation and provided at no charge, an artificial, non-price-related, rationing policy must be implemented to determine who gets what services. The rationing decisions are: (a) what classes of household and commercial establishments are eligible for services, and (b) how shall services be distributed among eligibles.

The answers that cities now provide to these questions lead one to conclude that complete abandonment of the price mechanism is an unfavorable development. First, a fairly arbitrary distinction is often made between commercial and residential accounts in cities (such as Los Angeles, Denver, New York, and Washington, D.C.) that provide some tax-financed collection. Although commercial establishments pay all the appropriate taxes, they are the first to be eliminated from public collection. What is worse, this exclusion of "profit-making" customers is often extended, as in Washington, D.C., and Denver, Colorado, to larger residential dwellings or apartment houses, thereby discriminating against certain classes of taxpaying residents, such as nonhomeowners. Part of the reason for this is that public departments are often incapable of the flexibility required to service the varied needs of commercial and large scale residential accounts. Nevertheless, a clear inequity results from these policies.

Limited evidence from some cities indicates the presence of inequities on a geographic basis, in rationing services among recipients for those classes of accounts that <u>are</u> granted eligibility. For example, in Washington, D. C., researchers found that, although 25 percent of the land area cleaned by the city sanitation department is in the densely populated, low income area east of Anacostia River, that area receives only 15 percent of the services. Visual inspection revealed unsanitary refuse accumulations in this area.[51]

In New York City residential slum areas such as Brownsville in Brooklyn or Hunts Point in the Bronx are overcome with debris while accumulations in Manhattan are kept within tolerable limits. City collection frequencies for these areas are roughly equal.[52] One can argue that neglect of lower income areas is a manifestation of the "squeaky wheel" behavior that government tends to exhibit, especially in the absence of objectively defined criteria for service delivery. In sanitation this means that collection services are concentrated where the politically influential and articulate citizens reside. In New York this is Manhattan, in the District of Columbia it is west of Rock Creek Park.

Another potential inequity arises as a direct result of circumventing the price system in financing collection -- side payments to public collectors may become an additional rationing device. In areas to which collection services are inadequately allocated or where public collection is restricted to a certain set of uniform tasks, (e.g., front of house, once per week pickups) the only way a resident may have to satisfy his special needs is to pay off the municipal collector. An informal price system may rise to fill the vacuum.

Earlier, we touched upon the distribution of service benefits and costs from an efficiency vantage point and found that certain policies of discrimination are sensible. For instance, we concluded, on efficiency grounds, that under an explicit subsidy policy all neighborhoods would utilize collection sufficiently to meet minimum sanitary standards. One effect of such a policy would be some redistribution to poorer, more deteriorated neighborhoods. Finally, we concluded that services might be further differentiated by individual user preferences as long as additions to minimum services were paid for by the recipients.

These efficiency concerns are the appropriate considerations that may result in nonuniform distribution of direct services and financing burdens. Limited evidence indicates that these efficiency guidelines are not widely followed, partly because of faulty organization. A pricing mechanism for financing is required, and this must be coupled with an explicit subsidy policy (effected by a city-wide authority) based on objective evaluation of the sanitary conditions and work force requirements of particular types of neighborhoods. A nonpolitical market-oriented (private or nonprofit) collection agency is also necessary.

We would be remiss in terminating the discussion of equity without mention of the equalization issues presently before the courts. Three recent rulings have focused the equal protection provision (Section 1 of the 14th Amendment to the Constitution) on municipal services. In Hobson vs. Hansen (1966) in the U. S. District Court for the District of Columbia, Judge Skelly Wright ruled that roughly equal expenditure per pupil was required in the provision of public education, regardless of the particular public school that a student attends. In Hawkins vs. Shaw (1971) a Fifth Circuit Court ruled that public services such as lighting, paving, water, and sewers, must be supplied on an equal basis to neighborhoods of both blacks and whites throughout the town of Shaw, Mississippi. Although these two rulings are specifically aimed at racial discrimination, a clearly inappropriate criterion for public service provision, they strongly suggest a wider interpretation of strict equalization of services among citizens and neighborhoods. The third ruling is more explicit on this issue. In August 1971, the California Supreme Court, in an action on existing disparities in revenue per child between rich and poor school districts, struck down the state's financing system for public schools on the grounds that its effect was to provide more money for rich children than for poor. There are similar cases in Illinois, Michigan, Texas, and other states. One case of more direct import to this discussion is the class action suit in Washington, D.C., on behalf of those citizens who reside in the area east of the Anacostia River. That suit singles out trash collection as one service which is alleged to be unfair in its distribution, or more specifically "inadequate and significantly inferior to those provided residents of other parts of the city, particularly the area west of Rock Creek Park."

We can attempt to review the technicalities of the equal protection clause here only superficially. Gershon Ratner, in explaining the possible standards and interpretations by which equal protection cases can be argued, defended, and resolved for municipal services, indicates two "clearly permissible" standards which the courts may find acceptable:[53] (a) the pro rata standard – identical quality and composition of services per resident, and (b) the needs standard – quality, composition, and amount to equally satisfy resident needs. The first of these criteria has been interpreted in terms of equal expenditures per capita or per service recipient. The Hobson Case, for example, resulted in a decision requiring equal expenditure per pupil in public school education. Of course, equalized expenditures are not really the same as equal services, unless the costs of delivering the service to all recipients is the same. In refuse collection, equal expenditures per capita in all areas of a city would result in unequal services. But even a true pro rata standard, involving equal frequencies of collection, does not seem sensible for refuse collection because different customers often have substantially different demands for services.

The second permissible criterion – needs – seems somewhat more sensible. By this standard, services might be adjusted to keep all areas of a city equally free of refuse accumulation. Strictly interpreted, this standard also disallows indulgence of individual and neighborhood preferences with respect to sanitation. If, however, strict equality is replaced by minimum standards of sanitation, objectively measured, for all areas, then an efficient and equitable distribution could be achieved -- which would probably require a greater concentration of services in lower income neighborhoods than these areas currently receive. Again, this result is contingent on the proper organizational structure as we have attempted to outline it here.

Chapter V

CONCLUSION

Our analysis of refuse collection indicates that it is both possible and desirable to harness the forces of competition to provide service in a fair and efficient manner. Much of the difficulty now experienced in large cities may result from failure to recognize this.

Yet we also discover that competition is not synonymous with private industry. Indeed private collection is often provided non-competitively, and indications are that industry and other interests (such as the public utility commissioners) will strive for more regulation, more exclusive franchising, more industry protection, and less competition. This would be an unfortunate development.

Certainly the arrangements under which competition can be used to advantage are not easy to master. Economies of density and scale must be maintained. In commercial, industrial, and heavy residential areas which are dense enough to support several collectors simultaneously, direct competition between a public nonprofit agency and two or more private firms seems highly desirable, but franchises must be carefully assigned in a manner that will neither unduly dilute nor concentrate any one firm's accounts at a given location.

In lighter residential areas where the density of pickups is insufficient to support direct competition, a system of contract competition seems preferable. Such a system also needs "fine tuning." Well designed specifications, performance bonding, an appropriate contract life, bidding staggered over time for contracts in different local areas, a stringent mid-term contract adjustment process, careful guidelines regarding the size and number of contract areas and the number of contracts allowed per firm – all are important elements in achieving satisfactory performance. No doubt a period of experimentation will be required for cities attempting to develop a competitive contract system.

The suggested competitive arrangements will be unsuccessful without proper public control. Local government, although inappropriate as an institution for actually producing the service, has the responsibility to maintain the system in proper working order. This includes setting standards, monitoring compliance on minimum service levels and collector practices, and administering subsidy programs for maintaining desired levels of service in all areas. These are administrative functions best performed by a bureau in the administrative arm of local government. Neighborhood-level input to the administrative process seems essential and could be accomplished by a system of general purpose representation. Definition of local areas, or neighborhoods, should conform to natural boundaries and franchise areas. Intra-neighborhood homogeneity and conformity with boundary lines drawn for administering other public services is also desirable. Finally, individual choice of service specifications, over the minimum city-wide and neighborhood standards, should be permitted. For this and other reasons a system of financing through service charges that reflect the cost and usage of services is necessary. An explicit subsidy policy oriented toward maintaining desired service levels in each type of area, should be coupled with the service charge system.

Where do we go from here? For one reason or another, various cities, counties, and even states will be making policy decisions on solid waste management in the near future. Some of these will be large cities with governmental collection agencies. Perhaps the first step in these places is to convert the governmental collection operation to a public nonprofit corporation and begin to construct the foundations of an operative competitive system. In places where private industry is seeking permanent enfranchisement, or where the regulatory mode of control is expanding, we would hope for reconsideration and for re-direction toward the construction of a competitive framework.

But any major transition involves difficult problems, especially since change inevitably implies transfers of wealth and income. For whatever the economic arrangements, the status quo will have its vested interests. If collection is currently municipal, public sanitation workers and civil servants will risk loss of jobs, and public employee unions will lose power. If collection is currently enfranchised to private collectors in a noncompetitive environment, a transition will subject these firms to capital losses. The nature of the transition is therefore crucial. Threat of an abrupt decline in economic fortunes will certainly diminish prospects for the political acceptance of change. In addition, fundamental considerations of respect for law and government are involved. The present economic arrangements have come about through explicit or tacit approval of (and granting of franchises by) state or local government. If this approval is summarily withdrawn, a loss of faith in the integrity of local government will result.

For these reasons, it is important that any transition be <u>gradual</u> and that it provide for <u>compensation</u> of the victims of change, if possible. It is not within our scope here to suggest guidelines for transition; these will depend, of course, on the local status quo. In general, the implementation of new systems should probably extend over five to ten years on a piecemeal geographic basis (one section of a city at a time). Compensation schemes must address capital losses and lost jobs, and may require cash awards and job placement assistance. Provisions for gradualness and compensation must not only be carefully planned but must also be understood by the public if the transition is to be orderly.

It is important to note that our knowledge of how particular organizational arrangements will work in different local situations is imperfect. As the history of public programs shows, it is often injudicious to implement new concepts on a large scale without first experimenting on a small scale. The implications of this are twofold. First, the need for experimentation re-enforces the desirability of a gradual transition -- begin on a small scale, say one section of a city, and expand as we learn how to perfect the arrangements. Second, planning for the transition should include the design of an <u>evaluation</u> methodology to be applied during the experimental phase. It is important that evaluation be planned in advance, so that principles of scientific experimentation may be incorporated in the transitional design.[54]

"Economies of scale in learning" suggest that the discussion of evaluation should be extended to a national basis. Cities need not duplicate the work of each other in order to determine the merit of particular organization arrangements under different local circumstances. A national system of evaluation, involving testing and demonstration of organizational concepts for a sample of cities representative of various sizes and economic and social characteristics, would appear to be a program concept worthy of federal development and support.

NOTES

1. According to preliminary data from the 1971 survey of solid waste contractors, sponsored by the National Solid Waste Management Association and the U. S. Environmental Protection Agency ("The Private Sector in Solid Waste Management - A Profile of its Resources and Contribution to Collection and Disposal"), the average age of private collection firms is 14.2 years. 58 percent of the firms were incorporated in present form (by merger or original formation) since 1960. Average fleet size of packer and nonpacker vehicles per firm has grown from 3.15 trucks in 1965 to 4.88 trucks in 1970-1971. (This excludes special collection vehicles such as roll-on/roll-off, hoist, or satellite vehicles. Total fleet size including special vehicles averaged 6.15 in 1970-1971). One, two, and three truck firms now constitute 57 percent of the companies, but collect only 11 percent of the refuse by weight.

2. See Anton J. Muhich, Albert J. Klee, and Paul W. Britton, "Preliminary Data Analysis," _1968 National Survey of Community Solid Waste Practices_, U. S. Department of Health, Education and Welfare, Public Health Service, Solid Wastes Program, Cincinnatti, Ohio, 1968.

3. See American Public Works Association, _Refuse Collection Practice_, Public Administration Service, Chicago, Illinois, 1966.

4. This is the category of cities for which census information is easily available.

5. See Lester A. Haug, and Stanley Davidson, "Refuse Collection and Disposal Survey Indicates Changing Trends in 118 Western Cities," _Western City_, April, May 1964, and Winston R. Updegraff and Francis R. Bowerman "Refuse Collection and Disposal in 194 Western Cities," _Western City_, June, July 1958.

6. See Werner Z. Hirsch, "Cost Functions of an Urban Government Service: Refuse Collection," _The Review of Economics and Statistics_, XLVII, February 1965

7. See Ad Hoc Committee on Solid Waste Management of the Division of Engineering Committees on Pollution Abatement and Control, National Research Council, National Academy of Sciences, Policies for Solid Waste Management, for the Bureau of Solid Waste Management, U. S. Department of Health, Education and Welfare, 1970.

8. See Joint Study by the Department of Sanitary Engineering and Health Services Administration, "Comprehensive Plan for the Storage, Collection and Disposal of Solid Waste in the District of Columbia," Washington, D. C., March 1970.

9. See Residential Refuse Collection Proposal, City of Fort Worth, Texas, October, 1969.

10. See John F. McMahon and Herbert R. Gamache, Refuse Collection: Department of Sanitation vs. Private Carting, Office of Administration, Office of the Mayor, The City of New York, November 1970 (confidential).

11. See C. G. Golueke and P. H. McGauhey, Comprehensive Studies of Solid Waste Management, Second Annual Report, University of California for the Bureau of Solid Waste Management, Public Health Service, U. S. Department of Health, Education and Welfare, 1970. A solid waste management manpower study currently in process for the Office of Solid Waste Management Programs/U.S. Environmental Protection Agency, performed by Applied Management Sciences, indicates that the private sector is more capital intensive than the public sector in its collection operations, even when correction is made for differences in commercial/residential mix.

12. See McMahon and Gamache, op. cit.

13. Residential Refuse Collection Proposal, op. cit.

14. For a discussion of this point see Anthony Downs, Inside Bureaucracy, Little, Brown, and Co., Boston, 1967.

15. Labor unions also serve an important role in defining the degree of management discretion in personnel decisions under either private or civil service systems. Unions are discussed further in the next section.

16. See Harry H. Wellington and Ralph K. Winter, Jr., <u>The Unions and the Cities</u>, The Brookings Institution, Washington, D. C., 1971.

17. Membership in the American Federation of State, County, and Municipal Employees increased from 182,500 in 1960 to 442,749 in 1970, to 525,000 in 1972. Based on a census taken by AFSCME in 1968, roughly 4 percent of the membership are public sanitation workers. According to a Teamster's spokesman about 16,000 public sanitation workers were organized by that union in 1969. In general, it is estimated that 15 percent of private sanitation workers and over 50 percent of public sanitationmen are unionized.

18. See David T. Stanley and Carole L. Cooper, <u>Managing Local Government Under Union Pressure</u>, The Brookings Institution, Washington, D. C. 1972.

19. See John K. Galbraith, <u>American Capitalism</u>: <u>The Concept of Countervailing Power</u>, Houghton Mifflin Co., Boston, 1956.

20. See Wellington and Winter, <u>op. cit</u>. The term "demand elasticity" is used in a very general sense in this paper. Basically, we are referring to changes in demand with respect to cost increases faced by consumers. The cost increases may be manifested in terms of price increase, tax increases, or quality deterioration, depending on institutional context. Our point is that the lack of close substitutes for some public services means that output levels demanded, through the market or the political process, will not appreciably decline as costs increase.

21. See Stanley and Cooper, <u>op. cit.</u>

22. See Wellington and Winter, <u>op. cit.</u>

23. This is not to imply that the sole purpose of local trade associations is political lobbying or that associations are always strong enough to mount powerful efforts for entry restriction. Association functions may be confined to information dissemination, public relations, or industry representation on occasional public issues such as changes in dumping fees.

24. See Frederic M. Scherer, <u>Industrial Market Structure and Economic Performance</u>, Rand McNally and Co., Chicago, 1971.

25. See Harry M. Trebing, "Toward an Incentive System of Regulation," <u>Public Utilities Fortnightly</u>, July 1963.

26. See William Iulo, <u>Electric Utilities - Costs and Performance, A Study of Inter-Utility Differences in the Unit Electric Costs of Privately Owned Electric Utilities</u>, Pullman, 1961. Also, see Joe L. Steele, <u>The Use of Econometric Models by Federal Regulatory Agencies,</u> D. C. Heath and Company, Lexington, Massachusetts, 1971, for a review of the use of econometric models by the Federal Power Commission in the regulatory process.

27. See Harry M. Trebing, <u>op. cit.</u>

28. See Robert A. Colonna, "Public Utility Concept to be Tested in Feasibility Study," <u>Waste Age</u>, May-June 1971.

29. For example, in New York City commercial collection, the regulated maximum price of $4.50 per cubic yard is not always charged.

30. See Roger G. Noll, <u>Reforming Regulation: An Evaluation of the Ash Council Proposals</u>, The Brookings Institution, Washington, D. C., 1971.

31. <u>Ibid.</u>

32. In the City of Minneapolis part of residential collection is performed by the City and part is contracted out by the City to an association of private firms.

33. See Anthony Downs, <u>op. cit.</u>

34. See Marcus M. Truitt, Jon C. Liebman, and Cornelius W. Kruse, "Mathematical Modeling of Solid Waste Collection Policies," Johns Hopkins University for the Bureau of Solid Waste Management, Public Health Service, Department of Health, Education and Welfare, 1970.

Also, see American Public Work Association, <u>Refuse Collection Practices</u>, <u>op. cit.</u>

35. See <u>An Analysis of Refuse Collection and Sanitary Landfill
Disposal</u>, Technical Bulletin No. 8, Series 37, Sanitary Engineering
Research Project, University of California, 1952.

36. $$C_{INT} = \left(\text{interest cost/truck-year} \right) \bullet \left(\text{truck-years/ton} \right)$$

$$= I\tfrac{i}{2} \left(1 + \frac{1}{\text{truck-life}} \right) \bullet \left(\text{truck-years/ton} \right)$$

$$= I\tfrac{i}{2} \left(1 + \frac{m}{M} \right) \left(\text{tons/mile} \right) \bullet \left(\text{miles/ton} \right) \left(\text{truck-years/ton} \right)$$

$$= I\tfrac{i}{2} \left(1 + \frac{m}{M} \right) \left(\text{miles/ton} \right) \frac{\text{truck-years}}{\text{mile}}$$

$$= I\tfrac{i}{2} \left(1 + \frac{m}{M} \right) \left(\frac{1}{d} + h \right) \frac{1}{m}$$

37. See Frank R. Dair, "Time/Crew Size/Costs," <u>Refuse Removal
Journal</u>, August 1967.

38. An analysis of costs of private carting firms in commercial collection
in New York City (see "Private Cartmen and the Department of
Sanitation," a Report by the Environmental Protection Administration and the Department of Sanitation) found the average cost of
containerized collection about one-third the average cost of compac-
tion service. Use of containerization in residential collection also
affords economies, at the expense of some inconvenience resulting
from neighboring households having to share containers. Scottsdale,
Arizona reportedly achieved savings on the order of 45 percent in
residential collection by moving to a system of containerized
residential service. See, <u>The Struggle to Bring Technology to the
Cities</u>, The Urban Institute, Washington, D. C. 1971.

39. The recent analysis of private carting firms by New York City's
Environmental Protection Administration produced cost data by
firm size for a small 10 firm sample (although the analysis was not

specifically focused on the economies of scale question). Casual inspection of this data indicates wide variation in the costs of one truck firms, from \$58.73 per ton to \$22.47 per ton. Other figures are \$21.50 for a three truck firm, \$26.38 for a six truck firm, and \$28.80 for compactor service by a "large" firm. Unfortunately, these data are inconclusive on the economies of scale issue because variations in the sample firms' service characteristics and accounting practices preclude simple comparison; at the same time the sample is too small and the data too incomplete to permit statistical analysis.

40. "The Private Sector in Solid Waste Management - A Profile of Its Resources and Contribution to Collections and Disposal," preliminary data from 1971 National Solid Wastes Management Association Survey.

41. These curves assume fixed values of density (tons/mile) and account size (tons/service). For purposes of this discussion, the effects of density and scale are separated out. Any effort to construct a precise cost function would have to treat these as jointly varying effects.

42. For a discussion of this point, see Albert O. Hirschman, <u>Exit, Voice, and Loyalty,</u> Harvard University Press, Cambridge, Massachusetts, 1970.

43. For a record of work stoppages by public sanitationmen see Wellington and Winter, <u>op. cit.</u>

44. The situation is actually a little more complex. Providing the capability of delivering differentiated services may in itself be costly, aside from the marginal costs of providing additional units of service. Thus, the decision on degree of flexibility must be made collectively by local communities at least under arrangements not featuring direct competition for accounts. The "economic" level of service flexibility will evolve automatically under direct competition.

45. See Louis Blair and Alfred Schwartz, <u>Improving the Measurement of the Effectiveness of D. C. Solid Waste Collection Activities,</u> Urban Institute Working Paper, Washington, D. C., August 1971.

46. For a discussion of this issue see Richard A. Posner, "Taxation by Regulation," The Brookings Institution, Report 226, Washington, D. C. 1972.

47. See "A Report to the Directors of the County Sanitation Districts," Los Angeles County, California, September 1955.

48. See M. Mealey, "Garbage Cleanup, A Staggering Task," Oakland Tribune, Oakland, California, October 1965.

49. See National Academy of Sciences, National Research Council, Waste Management and Control, Publication 1400, Washington, D. C., 1966.

50. For an expanded discussion of this kind of analysis, see Allen V. Kneese and Blair T. Bower, Managing Water Quality: Economics, Technology, Institutions, Resources for the Future, Inc., Washington, D. C., 1968.

51. See Louis Blair and Alfred Schwartz, op. cit., and Leon Dash, "Trash and the City," The Washington Post, Washington, D. C. September 20, 1971.

52. See James M. Markham, "Residents, Not City, Are Called Keys to Cleaner Streets," The New York Times, October 18, 1971 and Stephen Isaacs, "Filth City: New York Wallows," The Washington Post, Washington, D. C., September 6, 1971.

53. See Gershon M. Ratner, "Inter-Neighborhood Denials of Equal Protection in the Provision of Municipal Services," Harvard Civil Rights-Civil Liberties Law Review, Fall 1968.

54. See Thomas K. Glennon, Jr., "Using Experiments for Social Research and Planning," Monthly Labor Review, February 1972.